Clinical Nutrition Case Studies

Fourth Edition

by Wayne Billon
Western Carolina University

THOMSON

WADSWORTH

Australia • Brazil • Canada • Mexico • Singapore • Spain • United Kingdom • United States

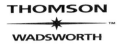

THOMSON
WADSWORTH

Clinical Nutrition Case Studies
Fourth Edition
Wayne Billon

Publisher/Executive Editor: Peter Marshall
Development Editor: Elizabeth Howe
Assistant Editor: Elesha Feldman
Editorial Assistant: Lauren Vogelbaum
Technology Project Manager: Travis Metz
Marketing Manager: Jennifer Somerville
Marketing Assistant: Michelle Colella

Cover Images: Blueberries © Photodisc/Getty Images; Strawberries © Digital Vision/Getty Images; Soy beans © Photodisc/Getty Images

Production Project Manager: Andy Marinkovich
Creative Director: Rob Hugel
Art Director: Lee Friedman
Print Buyer: Lisa Claudeanos
Permissions Editor: Kiely Sisk
Cover Designer: Robin Terra, Terra Studio
Printer: Thomson/West

Thomson Higher Education
10 Davis Drive
Belmont, CA 94002-3098
USA

Library of Congress Control Number: 2005927017

Printed in the United States of America

1 2 3 4 5 6 7   08 07 06 05

ISBN 0-534-51612-2

For more information about our products, contact us at:
Thomson Learning Academic Resource Center
1-800-423-0563

For permission to use material from this text or product, submit a request online at
http://www.thomsonrights.com.
Any additional questions about permissions can be submitted by email to **thomsonrights@thomson.com.**

TABLE OF CONTENTS

PREFACE

About fifteen years ago, I was sitting in my office making out a case study to use as a test for my clinical nutrition class when a young salesman from West Publishing walked in and asked if there was anything by way of nutritional textbooks I needed. I replied, "A case study book." I explained that I had used case studies in my classes for years and would like to see a book of case studies. His reply was simple: "Why don't you write one?" At first I chuckled, but as the days passed and I considered the idea, I decided it was a possibility. Now, the fourth edition is in print. The intent has not changed, to prepare students in clinical dietetics for clinical practice.

I believe this edition has been greatly improved. Abbreviations, medications, laboratory values, and formulas have been added or updated. Many changes have taken place in diabetes, cardiovascular disease, weight reduction, blood pressure, and more. The cases have been updated to reflect the new standards and guidelines. New cases have been added along with some new "brief" cases. A lot of SOAP notes and tube feeding drills have also been added per suggestions from reviewers.

One complaint from some of the reviewers was that the cases were too long. Actually, in this edition they are longer, but they are now divided into parts in such a way that the students can complete a part of a case and still accomplish an objective. I encourage the instructors to be creative with the questions. I use this book in my classes but I do not have the students answer all the questions. *I have intended this book to be used a guide and not a Bible of nutrition. It is at the discretion of the instructor to add to or delete from the case studies to meet the needs of their students. This book is not intended to be a main text but a supplement to a textbook.* Most cases cover more than one topic in an attempt to include a greater variety of situations. I hope that the studies will stimulate thought that *will generate additional questions.*

Appendix D has been combined with Appendix A and much of D has been omitted. There are so many suggestions on how to determine stress factors that, since this is not a primary text, I decided to let the instructor teach the students how they think caloric and protein needs should be determined as directed in their primary text. If, by writing this book, I can impart some knowledge or understanding that will help someone become a better person and be able to more efficiently help someone else, I will be fulfilled. To the person studying this book, I hope you will enjoy learning about nutrition as much as I enjoy teaching nutrition.

Wayne E. Billon, PhD, RD, LDN
Health Sciences Department
Western Carolina University

ACKNOWLEDGEMENTS

Producing this book was no easy task. The fourth edition took much more effort than either of the previous editions. I received assistance and encouragement from many individuals, including my students, who added comments as they completed case study assignments. These comments, along with those of several reviewers and consultants, gave insight into the development of the fourth edition. To all of these I give my most sincere thanks.

I particularly want to thank my loving wife, Cathy, for her encouragement, understanding, and typing skills; and my daughter Ashley who was understanding when I could not spend time with her because of the book. This edition was as hard on them as it was on me. Peter Marshall of West/Wadsworth Publishing has been extremely helpful and especially Elesha Feldman who has been a tremendous help in the coordination of the editing, reviewing, and publishing, but also with her insight and encouragement.

Many of the improvements in the fourth edition are the result of ideas I received from allied health professionals that reviewed cases or gave advice. They include:

Cynthia York-Camden MS, RD, LDN , clinical dietitian, Heartland Regional Medical Center, Marion, Illinois, preceptor for dietetic internship program at Southern Illinois University at Carbondale, consultant dietitian, and webmaster at http://www.rdlink.com/. Cynthia reviewed Cases #23 and 25.

Ralph Kahler, MD, Infectious Diseases, Hattiesburg Clinic, Hattiesburg, MS. Provided answers to technical medical questions and advice on medications.

Angele D. Miller MS RD LD, Renal Dietitian, Hattiesburg Clinic Dialysis Unit, Hattiesburg, MS. Angele, a former graduate student of mine, reviewed Case #33.

Julian Robinson, RPh, Pharmacist in Hattiesburg, MS for help with current medications.

Phillip Rogers, MD, nephrologists, Hattiesburg Clinic, Hattiesburg, MS. Provided answers to technical medical questions, advice on medications, and gave ideas about the brief case studies..

Beth T. Silvers, RD, CDE, MS, BC-ADM, LDN, part time WIC Nutritionist in Cleveland County, NC and part time for Silvers Consulting, Inc in Belmont, NC. Beth, a former undergraduate of mine, reviewed case #24.

Erica Stark, MHS, RD, LDN, CDE, BC-ADM. Diabetes Nutrition Specialist, Cherokee Diabetes Program, Cherokee, NC. Erica reviewed cases #23 and 25.

Dan Southern, MS, CLSp(H)NCA Professor and Director of Clinical Lab Sciences, Department of Health Sciences, Western Carolina University. Dan helped with advice on many of the laboratory values.

David C. Trigg, M.D. Director of the Emergency Medical Care Program, Health Sciences Department, Western Carolina University. David provided answers to technical medical questions and advice on medications.

Karen White, MS, RD, Visiting Assistant Professor, Western Carolina University. Karen helped with the metabolic syndrome brief case.

There are also a number of professors that reviewed the third edition and gave recommendations for this fourth edition that were most helpful. For this I am most grateful and would like to extend a special thank you to the following reviewers:

Judith Ashley
University of Nevada, Reno

Joelle E. Romanchik-Cerpovicz, Ph.D., RD
Georgia Southern University

Joseph C. Bonilla
University of the Incarnate Word

Previous edition reviewers: Susan Appelbaum, St. Louis Community College – Florissant Valley; Erin Bettinger, SUNY College of Technology and Agriculture; Dorothy Chen-Maynard, California State University – San Bernardino; Barbara Cosper, Western Carolina University; Judy Gaare, New York Institute of Technology; Janet W. Gloeckner, James Madison University; Jeffrey Harris, West Chester University; Betsy Holli, Rosary College; Mary Hubbard, Grossmont College; Sara Long, Southern Illinois University at Carbondale; and Mardell Wilson, Illinois State University.

INDEX TO OTHER NUTRITION TEXTBOOKS

Key: *CNCS* - Billon's *Clinical Nutrition Case Studies* 4e
           UNCN - Rolfes/Pinna/Whitney's *Understanding Normal and Clinical Nutrition* 7e
           NDT   - Cataldo/DeBruyne/Whitney's *Nutrition and Diet Therapy* 6e
           FCAN - Grodner/Long/DeYoung's *Foundations and Clinical Applications of Nutrition* 3e
           BNDT - Williams's *Basic Nutrition and Diet Therapy* 11e
           ENDT - Williams's *Essentials of Nutrition and Diet Therapy* 8e
           KFNDT- Mahan/Escott-Stump's *Krause's Food, Nutrition, and Diet Therapy* 11e

CNCS case #	*UNCN* chapter	*NDT* chapter	*FCAN* chapter	*BNDT* chapter	*ENDT* chapter	*KFNDT* chapter
1	6	4	6			
2	8	10, 16	9, 10	16	15	17, 18, 21
3	8, 17, 20	10, 16, 20	9, 10	16	15	17, 18, 21, 23
4	9	7				25
5	19	15				19
6, 7, 8, 9	8, 9, 16	7	9	15	6	24
10	16, 23	18	17	18	18	29
11	8, 9, 16, 23	18	17	18	18	29
12, 13	15, 20	12, 20	11	10	12	9, 23
14	23, 20	18, 20	17	18	18	29
15, 35, 37	24, 20, 21	19, 20, 21	17	18	18	30, 23
16	18	17				16
17	18, 25, 20	23, 20		18	18	31, 23
18, 19	27, 20	25, 20	20	19	19	35, 23
20	20, 22, 25, 27	20	15		19	38, 23
21-27, 38	8, 9, 26, 20	20, 24	19	20	20	33, 23
28	20	20	15	20	25	42, 43, 23
29	25, 20	23, 20	18	18	18	31, 23
30 - 32	20, 21, 29	28, 20, 21	22	23	24	40, 23
33, 34, 36	28, 20	26, 20	21	21	21	39, 23
39	18	17				
40	19, 28	15	16			19

TABLE OF CASE STUDIES AT A GLANCE

A quick look at content of cases:

CS	Vits/Mins/Herbs	Special Concerns	SOAP	Tube Feeding
1	Organic vs synthetic	Vegetarian, anemia	No	No
2	Vit C, Echinacea, astragalus	Anorexia, anemia, assessment form, dialogue	No	No
3	I.V. Vits & minerals	Dehydration, anemia, elderly, updated meds, chart note to read	Yes	Yes x 2
4	None	Anorexia, bulimia, dialogue	Yes	No
5	None	Anemia, elderly, updated meds	Yes	No
6	None	Ethnic (Italian), obesity	No	No
7	Multivit/mineral	Obesity, bariatric surgery	No	No
8	None	Obesity, very low kcals	No	No
9	Chart note to read	Ethnic (Mexican), obesity, labs updated, I.V. glucose	No	No
10	None	Elderly, updated meds	No	No
11	None	Elderly, updated meds	No	No
12	None	Peds, updated meds	Yes	Yes
13	None	Peds, updated meds	No	No
14	None	Two parts, diet & surgery, anemia, peptic ulcer	Yes	Yes
15	None	Two parts, diet & surgery, diverticulosis, dialogue, ethnic (German)	Yes	Yes x 2
16	Fe	**New!** Nutritional genomics, Fe abuse	Yes	No
17	None	Cystic fibrosis	No	Yes
18	Folic acid, B_6, B_{12}, E, garlic, CoEQ	Three parts, updated meds	Yes x 2	
19	None	Two parts, MI and CHF, updated meds, ethnic (Japanese)	Yes x 2	Yes x 2
20	Vits	**New!** Three parts, cholecystectomy, open heart surgery, COPD, up-to-date meds, blood gases, home health	Yes	Yes x 2
21	No	Hypoglycemia	No	No
22	No	Type 1 DM	Yes	No
23	No	Two parts, Type 2 DM and metabolic syndrome, several meds, advanced, ethnic (Native American)	Yes x 3	No

C S	Vits/Mins/Herbs	Special Concerns	SOAP	Tube Feeding
24	No	Type 2 DM, ethnic (Cuban)	Yes	Yes
25	Folic acid	Gestational DM	Yes	No
26	No	**New!** Metabolic syndrome	Yes	no
27	No	**New!** Low-carbohydrate diet	Yes	No
28	No	Two parts, closed head injury and home health	Y x 2	Y x 3
29	No	Two parts, Pancreatitis/hepatitis/cirrhosis	Yes x 2	Yes
30	No	Two parts, esophageal cancer/TPN, dialogue	Yes x 2	Yes
31	No	**New!** Colon cancer, latest meds, dialogue	Yes	Yes
32	No	AIDS	Yes	Yes
33	No	Peritoneal dialysis, updated meds	No	No
34	No	Three parts, HTN/hemodialysis/kidney transplant, updated meds, dialogue	Yes	Yes
35	No	Two parts, Crohn's/TPN, ethnic (Jewish)	Yes x 2	Yes
36	No	**New!** OTC drug abuse	Yes	No
37	No	**New!** College student with Crohn's, latest meds	No	Yes
38	No	**New!** Metabolic syndrome	No	No
39	No	**New!** Non-diabetic peripheral neuropathy	No	No
40	St. John's wort	**New!** Diet-drug interaction	No	No

CASE STUDY #1
VEGETARIANISM

INTRODUCTION

The purpose of each of the case studies is to gradually introduce the student to one or more of the following processes: reading and understanding a patient's chart, interviewing a patient, interpreting pertinent data, and assimilating that data into an appropriate nutritional care plan. The first study is a warm-up that includes a small number of abbreviations and lab values. The cases will become more difficult as the book progresses. This study is about a person who is a true vegan and is concerned about environmental issues. Review information about vegetarian diets, possible deficiencies, and complications. The reference list at the end of each case study is a good place to begin looking for information about the case. Most answers should appear in a basic or an advanced clinical nutrition textbook. It would be wise to make copies of the appendices to refer to as you prepare for and read the case study.
****

SKILLS NEEDED

ABBREVIATIONS:
Knowledge of the following abbreviations is required in order to understand this case. You should learn these abbreviations before you begin to read the study. (See Appendix C.)
BUN, Ca, CBC, Cl, Cr, glu, hct, hgb, IBW, lymph, MCH, MCHC, MCV, Mg, Na, P, RBC, ser alb, WBC, and YOWF.

LABORATORY VALUES:
An ability to interpret the nutritional significance of the following laboratory values will be needed for this case study: BUN, Ca, Cl, Cr, glu, hct, hgb, K, lymph, MCH, MCHC, MCV, Mg, Na, P, RBC, ser alb, and WBC (Appendix B).

FORMULAS:
The formulas used in this case study are for ideal body weight and percent ideal body weight. The formulas can be found in Appendix A, Tables 7 and 8.
****

SR is a 23 YOWF college student who is very concerned about the pollution of the environment. She believes mankind should do everything possible to preserve nature and protect wildlife. SR is very health conscious and advocates that everyone should be a vegetarian. She is a vegan and has been for two and one-half years. She is 5'2" and weighs 98 lbs. Her diet includes tofu, alfalfa sprouts, and legumes of various types. Instead of cow's milk, she drinks soy milk. SR does not take a vitamin or mineral supplement on a regular basis because she believes they are not necessary and her needs can be met from her diet. However, when stressed out, she takes a vitamin and mineral supplement, but it has to be "all-natural and organic." SR has not felt stressed in a long time, so she has not been taking her vitamin and mineral tablets. She takes no other nutritional supplement, does not smoke or consume alcoholic beverages, and does not eat bleached flours. Most of the bread SR eats is home-made with only "all-natural" ingredients. A microwave is never used. She takes in a variety of fruits and vegetables and eats a grain with every meal that has legumes.

SR has been feeling progressively weaker over the last year. She is not very active and gets little exercise. In spite of her health consciousness, she is a very sedentary person. Her appearance is very pale, her hair lacks luster, she has pale gums, and her nail beds take several seconds to return to their normal pink color when depressed. If she uses the stairs to get to her office, the climb up three flights causes her to exhibit shortness of breath. SR made a visit to her physician to obtain a checkup. He completed some routine labs and found the following:

CBC

TEST	RESULT	REFERENCE UNITS Conventional	SI	TEST	RESULT	REFERENCE UNITS Conventional	SI
Hgb	10 g/dl	12-16 g/dl	120-160 g/L	WBC	5.2 10^3/µl	4.5-10.5 x 10^3/cells/mm^3	4.5-10.5 x10^9/L
Hct	30 %	36-48%		% Lymph	23%	25 – 40% of total WBC	1500-4000 cells/mm^3
RBC	4.2x10^6/µ	3.6-5.0x10^6/L	3.6-5.0 x10^{12}/L	MCH	23 pg/cell	26-34 pg/cell	0.40-.53 fmol/cell
MCV	72 µm^3	82-98µm^3	82-98 fL	MCHC	33 g/dl	32-36 g/dl	320-360 g/L

BASIC METABOLIC PACKAGE

TEST	RESULT	REFERENCE UNITS Conventional	SI	TEST	RESULT	REFERENCE UNITS Conventional	SI
Glu	80 mg/dl	70-110 mg/dl	3.8-6.1 mmol/L	Na	138 mEq/L	136-145 mEq/L	136-145 mmol/L
BUN	5 mg/dl	6-20 mg/dl	2.1-7.1 mmol/L	K	3.8 mEq/L	3.5-5.2 mEq/L	3.5-5.2 mmol/L
Cr	0.3 mg/dl	0.6-1.1 mg/dl	53-97 µmol/L	Cl	101 mEq/L	96-106 mEq/L	96-106 mmol/L
Ca	8.8 mg/dl	8.8-10.0 mg/dl	2.20-2.60 mmol/L	Mg	1.8 mEq/L	1.8 - 2.6 mEq/L	136-145 mmol/L
Ser alb	3.1 g/dl	3.5-4.8 g/dl	39-50 g/dl	P	2.5mg/dl	2.7-4.5 mg/dl	4.7-6.0 kPa

****

QUESTIONS:

1. Define the following terms:

   Vegan:

   Ovo-vegetarian:

   Lacto-vegetarian:

   Pesco-vegetarian:

   Pollo-vegetarian:

   Natural vitamins:

   Organic vitamins:

   Synthetic vitamins:

2. Determine SR's IBW and the percent of her IBW (Appendix A - 7 & 8).

3. SR likes tofu, alfalfa sprouts, legumes, lentils, chick peas, and soy milk. What are these foods good sources of, if anything?

4. What are the sources of calcium in SR's diet?

5. What are the sources of complete protein in SR's diet?

6. What possible nutritional deficiencies could SR have based on the information given?

7. Do you agree or disagree with SR's theory about vitamin/mineral supplements for vegans? Explain.

8. Does stress increase our need for vitamins and minerals? Explain.

9. Which type of vitamin functions the best in the human body—natural, organic, or synthetic? Explain.

10. Are "all-natural" or organically-grown foods healthier than processed foods?

11. Is irradiation safe? Explain.

12. If you were counseling SR about her diet and she insisted on remaining a vegan, what recommendations would you give her to improve her nutritional intake? What animal products might she include in her diet that the consumption of which would actually help preserve the animals from which the products are derived?

13. Besides those that are in SR's diet, name three examples of complementary proteins.

14. The clinical evaluation of SR included paleness, dull hair coat, nail beds that did not return to normal color rapidly after being depressed, and pale gums. What do these clinical signs suggest?

15. What can you tell from the fact that SR has decreased hgb and hct levels?
    a. SR has a microcytic anemia.
    b. SR has a macrocytic anemia.
    c. SR has an anemia of chronic disease.
    d. SR has an anemia.

16. If you include MCV and MCH with hgb and hct, what does it tell you?
    a. SR has a microcytic anemia.
    b. SR has a macrocytic anemia.
    c. SR has an anemia of chronic disease.
    d. SR has an anemia.

17. Briefly explain why you answered the above questions the way you did.

18. Based on the information available on SR's diet, what would you predict to be the cause of anemia?
    a. folate deficiency
    b. B_{12} deficiency
    c. B_6 deficiency
    d. iron deficiency

19. Briefly explain why you answered the above question the way you did.

20. What would be a plausible explanation for BUN, Cr, and ser alb being depressed?

RELATED READING

1. Fischbach, F.T. (2003). A Manual of Laboratory & Diagnostic Tests. 7th Ed. Philadelphia. J.B. Lippincott Company.

2. Food and Nutrition Board, National Research Council, National Academy of Sciences.
   Dietary Reference Intakes for Water, Potassium, Sodium, Chloride, and Sulfate. Panel on Dietary Reference Intakes for Electrolytes and Water, Standing Committee on the Scientific Evaluation of Dietary Reference Intakes (2004).
   Dietary Reference Intakes for Vitamin C, Vitamin E, Selenium, and Carotenoids. Panel on Dietary Antioxidants and Related Compounds, Subcommittees on Upper Reference Levels of Nutrients and Interpretation and Uses of DRIs, Standing Committee on the Scientific Evaluation of Dietary Reference Intakes, Food and Nutrition Board (2000).
   Dietary Reference Intakes for Vitamin A, Vitamin K, Arsenic, Boron, Chromium, Copper, Iodine, Iron, Manganese, Molybdenum, Nickel, Silicon, Vanadium, and Zinc. Panel on Micronutrients, Subcommittees on Upper Reference Levels of Nutrients and of Interpretation and Use of Dietary Reference Intakes, and the Standing Committee on the Scientific Evaluation of Dietary Reference Intakes (2000).
   Dietary Reference Intakes for Thiamin, Riboflavin, Niacin, Vitamin B6, Folate, Vitamin B12, Pantothenic Acid, Biotin, and Choline. A Report of the Standing Committee on the Scientific Evaluation of Dietary Reference Intakes and its Panel on Folate, Other B Vitamins, and Choline and Subcommittee on Upper Reference Levels of Nutrients, Food and Nutrition Board, Institute of Medicine (1998).

3. Position paper of the American Dietetic Association. (1995): Biotechnology and the future of food. *J. Am. Diet. Assoc.* 95:1429.

4. The American Dietetic Association and The Dietitians of Canada Position Statement on Vegetarian diets. Authors: A. R. Mangels, V. Messina, and V. Melina. [On –line] Available http: http://www.eatright.org/Public/NutritionInformation/92_17084.cfm

5. Position paper of the American Dietetic Association: Dietetics professionals can implement practices to conserve natural resources and protect the environment. *J Am Diet Assoc* 2001;101:1221. WEB site: http://www.eatright.org/Public/NutritionInformation/92_adar2_1001.cfm

6. Position paper of the American Dietetic Association: Food and water safety. *J Am Diet Assoc.* 2003;103:1203-1218. WEB site: http://www.eatright.org/Public/GovernmentAffairs/92_adap0297.cfm

7. Position paper of the American Dietetic Association: Food fortification and dietary supplements. *J AM Diet Assoc* 2001;101:115. WEB site: http://www.eatright.org/Public/NutritionInformation/92_8343.cfm

8. *Learning Medical Terminology: A Worktext* by Miriam G., B.A. Austrin, Harvey R. Austrin Publisher: C.V. Mosby; 9th edition (January 15, 1999)

9. Statement of FANSA[1] (1997): What does the public need to know about dietary supplements? *J. Am. Diet. Assoc.* 97:728.

10. Walter, P. (1997). Effects of vegetarian diets on aging and longevity. *Nutrition Reviews*. International Life Sciences Institute, Washington, DC. 55:1, pp. S61-S68.

11. Rolfes, S.R., Pinna, K. and Whitney, E. (2006). *Understanding Normal and Clinical Nutrition*, 7th Ed. West/Wadsworth.

[1] The Food and Nutrition Science Alliance, a partnership of four professional scientific societies: American Dietetic Association, American Society for Clinical Nutrition, American Society for Nutritional Sciences, and the Institute of Food Technologists.

CASE STUDY #2
NUTRITIONAL SCREENING

INTRODUCTION

This study provides the student with the opportunity to screen a patient by means of medical history, nutritional history, biochemical data, anthropometric data, and clinical data. An interview is included but, although it was conducted by a registered dietitian, this does not mean that it was done correctly. The purpose of each of the case studies is to gradually introduce the student to the process of reading and understanding a patient's chart, interpreting pertinent data, and assimilating that data into an appropriate nutritional care plan. This case study introduces the student to hospital procedures, particularly nutritional screening. Abbreviations, medical terms, and lab values are more important in this case study than they were in the previous study.
****

SKILLS NEEDED

ABBREVIATIONS:

Knowledge of the following abbreviations is required in order to understand this case. You should learn these abbreviations before you begin to read the study (see Appendix C).

AIDS, ASAP, BMI, BUN, Ca, CBC, CHF, Cl, cm, CO_2, C/O, Cr, CVA, dl, Dx, FH, GI, glu, hct, hgb, HIV^+, HTN, IBW, ICU, K, L, lymph, MAC, MAMC, MCH, MCHC, MCV, mEq, Mg, MH, m^3, mm, Na, NH, NH_3, N/V, P, pg, RBC, Rm, SBR, ser alb, SH, TF, LC, TPN, TSF, UBW, and YOWF.

LABORATORY VALUES:

You will need to be able to interpret the nutritional significance of the following laboratory values for this case study: BUN, Ca, Cl, CO_2, Cr, Glucose, hct, hgb, K, Lymphocytes, MCH, MCHC, MCV, Mg, Na, NH_3, P, RBC, ser alb, and WBC (Appendix B).

FORMULAS:

The formulas used in this case study include ideal body weight using the Hamwi formula, percent ideal body weight, percent usual body weight, mid-arm muscle circumference, total lymphocyte count, basal energy expenditure using the Harris-Benedict equation, total energy expenditure using an appropriate activity factor, and effects of fever on energy needs (Appendix A).
****

MK is a 21 YOWF college student who has been bothered by a cold for most of the semester. She has several colds a year but they usually do not last as long as this one. She had the usual symptoms: a sore throat, blocked sinuses, and a hacking cough with moderate quantities of slightly yellowish sputum. Two days ago her cough was considerably worse. The amount of sputum increased and was purulent. MK also had a temperature of 99.8° and C/O of pain in the left side of her chest on breathing. Her respirations were shallow. She felt weak and ached all over. She felt so bad that she did not feel like eating anything. Yesterday she was getting ready to take a final exam when she collapsed in her room. Her roommate and some friends brought her to the campus infirmary. The MD listened to her breath sounds and diagnosed pneumonia with exhaustion. She was admitted to a local hospital. Her admission orders included SBR, appropriate antibiotics, respiratory treatments, and a regular diet.

Normally, dietitians do not visit patients with an order for a regular diet unless they are requested to do so. However, this hospital has an excellent nutritional screening process that requires a diet technician to review admission criteria, height, weight, and admission lab values. All of the above information goes into the hospital computer on admission. The technician accomplishes the screening by simply pulling up the new admissions for the previous day on the computer and reviewing for the four parameters previously mentioned. This can be done while sitting in the dietary offices. The techs have a form to fill out as they review the computerized chart. The form will vary from hospital to hospital, but there will be a thread of commonality in all screening forms. If the form requires extensive information, not all of the information required may be obtainable from the computer. There are times when the tech will have to visit the patient to obtain additional information. The day after admission, MK was screened using the computer and a brief interview by the diet tech. The following information was obtained:

MK's MH was unremarkable except for frequent colds. Her weight history was very significant. She claimed that her UBW was 115 lbs and that she had lost 17 lbs over the last three months. She attributed this weight loss to a very strenuous semester. The computer indicated her height and weight to be:

➢ **Height 5'4"**

➢ **Weight 98 lbs**

In order to complete the screening form, the tech had to complete some calculations. Answer the following questions and compare your answers to those found in the following screening form.

QUESTIONS:
1. Determine MK's IBW (Appendix A, Table 7).

2. Calculate the percent of her IBW, and the percent of her UBW. Please show work for all calculations completed in this report (Appendix A, Table 8).

3. Calculate MK's BMI and explain what the results mean (Appendix A, Tables 10 & 11).

Fasting blood was drawn the morning after admission and the results were as follows:

BASIC METABOLIC PACKAGE

TEST	RESULT	REFERENCE UNITS Conventional	SI	TEST	RESULT	REFERENCE UNITS Conventional	SI
Glu	75 mg/dl	70-110 mg/dl	3.8-6.1 mmol/L	Na	136 mEq/L	136-145 mEq/L	136-145 mmol/L
BUN	7 mg/dl	6-20 mg/dl	2.1-7.1 mmol/L	K	3.0 mEq/L	3.5-5.2 mEq/L	3.5-5.2 mmol/L
Cr	0.8 mg/dl	0.6-1.1 mg/dl	53-97 μmol/L	Cl	101 mEq/L	96-106 mEq/L	96-106 mmol/L
Ca	8.9 mg/dl	8.8-10.0 mg/dl	2.20-2.60 mmol/L	Mg	1.9 mEq/L	1.8 - 2.6 mEq/L	136-145 mmol/L
Ser alb	3.1 g/dl	3.5-4.8 g/dl	39-50 g/dl	P	2.8mg/dl	2.7-4.5 mg/dl	4.7-6.0 kPa

CBC

TEST	RESULT	REFERENCE UNITS Conventional	SI	TEST	RESULT	REFERENCE UNITS Conventional	SI
Hgb	11 g/dl	12-16 g/dl	120-160 g/L	WBC	14 x 10^3/μl	4.5-10.5 x 10^3/cells/mm^3	4.5-10.5 x10^9/L
Hct	33 %	36-48%		% Lymph	9%	25 – 40% of total WBC	1500-4000 cells/mm^3
RBC	4.1x10^6/μ	3.6-5.0x10^6/L	3.6-5.0 x10^{12}/L	MCH	27 pg/cell	26-34 pg/cell	0.40-.53 fmol/cell
MCV	80 μm^3	82-98μm^3	82-98 fL	MCHC	33 g/dl	32-36 g/dl	320-360 g/L

4. Calculate her TLC (Appendix A, Table A - 13).

5. MK's elevated WBC indicates:
   a. anemia of chronic disease.
   b. dehydration.
   c. infection.
   d. protein malnutrition.

6. What can you tell from the fact that MK has decreased hgb and hct levels?
   a. MK has a microcytic anemia.
   b. MK has a macrocytic anemia.
   c. MK has an anemia of chronic disease.
   d. MK has an anemia.

7. If you include MCV and MCH with hgb and hct, what does it tell you?
   a. MK has a microcytic anemia.
   b. MK has a macrocytic anemia.
   c. MK has an anemia of chronic disease.
   d. MK has an anemia.

8. Briefly explain why you answered the above questions the way you did.

MK's screening indicated a high nutritional risk. The diet tech brought the results to the dietitian who went to see MK to obtain a nutritional history and to do a complete nutritional assessment. Since MK's first day in the hospital was not typical, the dietitian asked MK to describe her intake and activity on a typical day. The dietitian also obtained a food frequency, and a family, medical, and social history. MK's MH was as previously mentioned. Her FH was unremarkable. Her SH was another story. She came from a well-to-do family that expected a lot from her. MK was active in many organizations on campus, including a sorority, cheerleaders, student government, and others. She was an honor student and a perfectionist. She claimed to drink socially because it was the "in thing" to do. MK denied the use of drugs. She admitted to smoking when alone but not in public. Her classes were the hardest yet and she held an office in three major organizations. She strongly denied anorexia nervosa or bulimia, but admitted that she watched her weight very closely. Between cheerleader practice, aerobics, swimming, and intramurals, her exercise was classified as heavy. She also admitted to taking laxatives "rather often" for constipation but would not admit to an amount or frequency.

The dietitian's interview of MK's "typical day recall" went like this:

RD: MK, I want you to take me through a typical day at school, when you are feeling well. When you get up in the morning, what is the first thing you have to eat or drink?

MK: I don't eat breakfast on a usual day. I do not have time. I usually have some coffee later in the morning. I need coffee to keep me going.

RD: What do you put in your coffee?

MK: Nothing. I never use sugar or cream . . . fattening.

RD: How much coffee do you have in a typical day?

MK: About six or seven cups, mostly at night to help me stay awake to study.

RD: Is this decaffeinated or regular coffee?

MK: Regular! I drink it for the caffeine.

RD: Well, after your morning coffee, what is the next thing you have to eat or drink?

MK: Sometimes I'll pick up a pack of peanut butter or cheese crackers with the coffee if I have time. Otherwise, it will be lunch before I'll eat.

RD: And what is a typical lunch like?

MK: Oh, a hamburger or hot dog with some fries and a diet soda. Sometimes it's a pack of crackers again with a diet soda, depending on how much time I have.

RD: Do you put mayonnaise on your hamburger?

COUNTY HOSPITAL
NUTRITION SERVICES
NUTRITION SCREENING

Name MK   **MD** Dr. JK   **Rm #** 1102

Admission Date 3/21/05   **Dx** Pneumonia with exhaustion   **Age** 21

Diet Order Regular diet   **Ht** 5'4"   **Wt** 98 lbs   **UBW** 115 lbs   **IBW**

BMI   **Criteria for Nutritional Risk:**

	MILD RISK		MODERATE RISK		SEVERE RISK
	Undefined weight loss of 5 to 10 lbs in 6 mos		Undefined weight loss of 10 to 15 lbs in 6 mos	X	Undefined weight loss of <15 lbs in 6 mos
	> 20% over IBW		Morbid obesity		> 20,% over IBW
	BMI = 19 or BMI =25 to 30		BMI = 17 – 18 or BMI =30 to 35	X	BMI < 17or BMI > 35
	Mild N/V, diarrhea		Prolonged N/V, diarrhea		Malabsorption
X	Decreased appetite		Very poor appetite		TPN or TF dependency
	Chewing or swallowing problems, other mild nutritional problems		Mild decubitus or other open wounds		Severe decubiti or other wounds that are not healing
	HTN		Renal disease		Severe pancreatic disease
	Atherosclerosis, elevated lipid profile		Early stages of cancer and/or chemotherapy and/or radiation therapy/HIV+		Advanced cancer with cachexia AIDS
	Recent minor surgery/hospitalization		Recent major surgery/hospitalization		GI surgery or major surgery
X	Anemia		Diabetes in poor control	?	Malnutrition
	Ulcer		GI diseases or GI bleeding, ileus, etc.		ICU patient, burns
	Confined or nursing home patient		CHF		Sepsis
?	Simple dehydration		CVA		Multiple trauma
X	Albumin 3.2 – 3.4 mg/dl		Albumin 2.8 – 3.1 mg/dl		Albumin <2.8 mg/dl
X	TLC1200 – 1500 cells/mm^3		TLC 900 – 1200 cells/mm^3		TLC < 900 cells/mm^3
	Mild depression		Moderate depression		Severe depression
X	Other: mild temp/cold		Other:		Other:

High Risk   = 1 or more severe risk factors or 3 or more moderate risk factors or 6 or more mild risk factors

Moderate Risk   = 2 or more moderate risk factors or 4-5 mild risk factors

Low Risk   = < 4 mild risk factors

High Risk   = RD to see patient ASAP, do complete assessment, chart, re-evaluate in 3-5 days.

Moderate Risk   = RD to see patient in within 3 days, assessment and chart as necessary, re-evaluate in 3-5 days.

Low risk   = Basic nutrition services, diet tech to re-evaluate within 7-10 days.

MK: No, mustard . . . less calories.

RD: Do you ever eat in the cafeteria on campus?

MK: Are you kidding? My daddy buys me a meal ticket every semester, but I only eat there in the evenings . . . sometimes. The lines are too long, and I don't like their food . . . too much fat in it . . . and the "mystery meat," ugh!

RD: OK, I understand. When do you eat again?

MK: Well, I have cheerleader practice at 5 P.M. and usually grab a diet soda and a candy bar before practice. I don't like eating sweets, but I have found that if I don't, I will not make it through practice. Besides, I have one of those good candy bars, you know, with nuts in it for energy.

RD: These diet sodas you are drinking, what kind are they? Do they contain caffeine?

MK: Yep! The highest in caffeine I can find.

RD: Do you eat after practice?

MK: Yea. By the time I get cleaned up, it is time for the cafeteria to close and the lines are not too long. I usually have a salad.

RD: Describe the salad for me.

MK: Well, you know, whatever they have, lettuce, tomatoes, celery, stuff like that.

RD: Do you put anything on your salad?

MK: You mean like dressing? Yeah, usually low-fat Thousand Island.

RD: And do you have anything to drink with this salad?

MK: Yeah, I have coffee. I usually have a meeting to go to after eating, and then I have to study. I have a 3.5 GPA you know.

RD: Do you have anything to eat or drink before you go to bed?

MK: Like I told you, I drink coffee while I'm studying to help me stay awake. Sometimes I snack on some cookies or something.

RD: You did not mention milk. Do you ever drink milk?

MK: Sometimes, if I ever eat breakfast, I use some on my cereal.

RD: What about cheese or ice cream?

MK: I like cheese. I eat it when I'm at home, but I don't have a place to keep it here. I eat ice cream occasionally. It's too fattening. Sometimes I get some low-fat frozen yogurt.

RD: You did not mention fruit. Do you ever eat fruit?

MK: I like fruit, but I don't buy it here; I do at home. If I eat breakfast, I drink orange juice.

RD: What about vegetables? Other than the salad and the potatoes, you did not mention vegetables.

MK: I don't like vegetables. I eat some carrots or green beans at home. I only like them the way my mother fixes them.

RD: Are there any supplements, like vitamins, minerals, or herbs, that you take?

MK: I usually take 1 gram of vitamin C, echinacea, and astragalus every day during flu season, but I didn't take'em this year.

The dietitian finished her interview and obtained some anthropometric measurements, the results of which were as follows: **TSF 18 mm** **MAC 25.7 cm**

While the dietitian was talking to MK, she noticed her hair was very dull and stringy for a cheerleader. She was very thin and appeared weak and malnourished. She was pale and, upon examination, her nail beds were pale and slow to return to their normal color when pressed. Her skin was dry and appeared to be "itchy." MK scratched her arms several times while the dietitian was there.
****

QUESTIONS CONTINUED:

9. Calculate MK's daily energy requirements using the Harris-Benedict equation and an activity factor (Appendix A, Table 17).

10. At the onset of MK's sickness, she had a temperature of 99.8°. How many kcals would this require above her hospitalized BEE (Appendix A, Table 18)?

11. Convert 99.8° F to °C (Appendix A, Table 4).

12. Calculate MK's mid-arm muscle circumference (Appendix A, Table 12). What percentile is MK in for TSF, MAC, and MAMC and what do these mean?

13. Analyze MK's nutritional intake and name the possible vitamin and mineral deficiencies that could exist.

14. Explain how MK's lifestyle and/or diet may have affected the lab values you mentioned above.

15. After the interview was over and the anthropometric measurements were taken, the RD made some observations concerning MK's hair, general appearance, color, nail beds, and skin. What are these observations called? What does each indicate?

16. The RD asked some questions at the end of her interview in an attempt to obtain the intake of certain specific nutrients. Which specific nutrients should any registered dietitian be concerned about regardless of the disease state of the client being interviewed?

17. As a health care professional, you will counsel patients like MK. You will not be expected to be their psychologist, but you will be expected to be sensitive to their needs and be able to offer some alternatives to their lifestyle. Unless MK makes some changes, she is not going to have time to eat and will never be able to correct her nutritional deficiencies. What are some suggestions you could give MK about the stressful situations that are causing stress in MK's life, including mental, physical, and social stress?

18. There are a few techniques the RD used in the interview that were wrong. See if you can find the errors and indicate how you would correct them. List at least three good points about this interview.

19. MK strongly denied anorexia nervosa and bulimia, but there were several indications in her interview that suggested either anorexia or bulimia. List these indications.

20. Caffeine was high in MK's intake. What are the possible effects of caffeine on the human body?

21. Would the laxatives have an effect on any of the lab values? If so, which ones and what would the effects likely be?

22. What are the claims for taking vitamin C, echinacea, and astragalus during the flu season? Discuss the peer reviewed research and he non-peer reviewed articles about these supplements.

23. Briefly outline how you would counsel MK on her diet. Include in your outline behavior modification tips and the following topics:
    a) The nutrients she is lacking and how she could increase those nutrients through diet.
    b) The substances she has an excess of and how she could avoid those substances.
    c) How she can incorporate these principles into her lifestyle.
    d) How you would try to convince MK of the importance of these changes.

RELATED READINGS

1. Arrowsmith, H. (2000). A critical evaluation of the use of nutrition screening tools by nurses. *Br J Nurs*. Jan 12;8(22):1483-90.

2. Corish, C.A., Flood, P., & Kennedy, N.P. (2004). Comparison of nutritional risk screening tools in patients on admission to hospital. *J Hum Nutr Diet*. Apr;17(2):133-9.

3. Davis, C., Kaptein, S., Kaplan, A.S., Olmsted, M.P., & Woodside, D.B. (1998). Obsessionality in anorexia nervosa: the moderating influence of exercise. *Psychosom. Med*. 60(2):192-197.

4. Elmore, M.F., Wagner, D.R., Knoll, D.M., Eizember, L., Oswalt, M.A., Glowinski, E.A., & Rapp, P.A. (1994). Developing an effective adult nutrition screening tool for a community hospital. *J. Am. Diet. Assoc*. 94(10):1113-1118.

5. Grindel, C.G. & Costello, M.C. (1996). Nutrition screening: an essential assessment parameter. *Medsurg. Nurs*. 5(3):145-154.

6. Kerekes, J. & Thornton, O. (1996). Incorporating nutritional risk screening with case management initiatives. *Nutr. Clin. Pract*. 11(3):95-97.

7. Kovacevich, D.S., Boney, A.R., Braunschweig, C.L., Perez, A, & Stevens, M. (1997). Nutrition risk classification: a reproducible and valid tool for nurses. *Nutr. Clin. Pract*. 12(1):20-25.

8   Lee, R.D., Nieman, D.C., & Nieman, D. (2002). *Nutritional Assessment*. 3rd Ed. McGraw-Hill.

9. Position paper of the American Dietetic Association. (2001). Nutrition intervention in the treatment of anorexia nervosa, bulimia nervosa, and eating disorder not otherwise specified (EDNOS). *J Am. Diet Assoc*; 101:810. http://www.eatright.org/Public/NutritionInformation/92_adap0701.cfm

10. Position paper of the American Dietetic Association. (2002). Weight management *J Am Diet Assoc*. 2002;102:1145-1155.

11. Pryor, T., & Wiederman, M.W. (1998). Personality features and expressed concerns of adolescents with eating disorders. *Adolescence*. 33(130):291-300.

12. Stratton, R.J., Hackston, A., Longmore, D., Dixon, R., Price, S., Stroud, M., King, C., & Elia, M. (2004). Malnutrition in hospital outpatients and inpatients: prevalence, concurrent validity and ease of use of the malnutrition universal screening tool ('MUST') for adults. *Br J Nutr*. Nov;92(5):799-808.

13. Sullivan, P.F., Bulik, C.M., Carter,F.A., Gendall, K.A., & Joyce, P.R. (1996). The signifance of a prior history of anorexia in bulimia nervosa. *Int. J. Eat. Disord*. 20(3):253-261.

14. Rolfes, S.R., Pinna, K. & Whitney, E. (2006). *Understanding Normal and Clinical Nutrition*, 7th Ed. West/Wadsworth.

15. Wills-Brandon, C. (1989). *Eat Like a Lady. Guide for Overcoming Bulimia*. Deerfield Beach, Flordia. Health Communications, Inc.

CASE STUDY #3
NUTRITIONAL ASSESSMENT

INTRODUCTION

This study is concerned with nutritional assessment, general problems facing the elderly, anemia, dehydration, and normal laboratory values. It is also a good introduction to the use of some medications.

****

SKILLS NEEDED

ABBREVIATIONS:

Knowledge of the following abbreviations is required in order to understand this case. You should learn these abbreviations before you begin to read the study (Appendix C).

ALP, ALT, amp, ASA, AST, BR, BUN, Ca, CC, cc, Cl, CPK, Cr, D_5NS, DBIL, DBW, d, dl, Dx, ER, ETOH, FF, fmol, Fx, g, GI, glu, HA, hct, hgb, H&H, Hx, IBW, IM, I.V., K, L, lymph, MCH, MCHC, MCV, mEq, Mg, mg, MH, mm^3, MNT, MOM, M.T.E.,MVI, Na, nmol, N/V, P, pg, po, pt, R, RBC, RDA, ,ser alb, TBIL, t.i.d., TLC, TP, UBW, U/L, WBC, YO, YOM, YOWM, 3d, μm^3, μmol, ♂, @, ↓,↑, and ø.

LABORATORY VALUES:

You will need to be able to interpret the nutritional significance of the following laboratory values for this case study: ALP, ALT, amylase, AST, BUN, Ca, Cl, CPK, Cr, DBIL,glu, hct, hgb, K, Lymph, MCH, MCHC, MCV, Mg, Na, P, RBC, Ser alb, serum amylase, TBIL, total protein, and WBC (Appendix B).

FORMULAS:

The formulas used in this case study include ideal body weight using the Hamwi formula, percent ideal body weight, total lymphocyte count, basal energy expenditure using the Harris-Benedict equation, and an appropriate stress factor (Appendix A).

MEDICATIONS:

Become familiar with the following medications before reading this case study. Note the diet-drug interactions, dosages and method of administration, gastrointestinal tract reactions, etc.
1. Milk of Magnesia; 2. Haldol (haloperidol); 3. Norpace (disopyramide phosphate); 4. Pepcid (famotidine); 5. Mobic (meloxicam); 6. Ambien (Zolpidem tartrate); 7. Di-Gel Liquid; 8. Aspirin (acetylsalicylic acid).

****

Mr. D is a 73 YOWM who has lived with his son for the past five years. He ambulates well but his mental powers are slipping. He has a hard time remembering from one day to the next. His son noticed his father's condition deteriorating significantly over the last six months. Because of his condition and the family's inability to provide proper attention at home, he should have been in a nursing home, but he refused to go. His son knows it is best for his father but he does not have the heart to admit him.

Mr. D had not been eating well. He had been losing weight and growing weaker. He said he just did not feel like eating. Nothing tasted the same. He had dentures but refused to wear them. He claimed they were too loose and would fall out if he tried to eat with them. His daughter-in-law does the cooking, but she does not always have the time to fix soft foods especially for him. She tried feeding him pureed food, but he absolutely refused to eat "baby food." His eyesight and hearing have also been failing. He was being treated for many disorders, none of which were serious, but he was taking several medications. This created another problem in light of his failing memory. He either forgot to take his medicine, or he took too much. His medications included: haloperidol (Haldol); disopyramide phosphate (Norpace); Milk of Magnesia; famotidine (Pepcid); meloxicam (Mobic), Di-Gel Liquid; Zolpidem tartrate (Ambien), and aspirin for frequent headaches. One day his son and daughter-in-law returned home from work and found him on the floor, unable to get up. He was in pain and was not able to move his left leg. His son called for an ambulance and he was brought to the hospital. His Dxs were:

➢ Fx left femur
➢ Cachexia
➢ Dehydration
➢ R/O malignancy

His lab values on admission were as follows:

BASIC METABOLIC PACKAGE							
TEST	RESULT	REFERENCE UNITS Conventional	SI	TEST	RESULT	REFERENCE UNITS Conventional	SI
Glu	186 mg/dl	70-110 mg/dl	3.8-6.1 mmol/L	Na	140 mEq/L	136-145 mEq/L	136-145 mmol/L
BUN	40 mg/dl	6-20 mg/dl	2.1-7.1 mmol/L	K	4.2 mEq/L	3.5-5.2 mEq/L	3.5-5.2 mmol/L
Cr	1.3 mg/dl	0.9-1.3 mg/dl	80-115 µmol/L	Cl	106 mEq/L	96-106 mEq/L	96-106 mmol/L
Ca	8.9 mg/dl	8.8-10.0 mg/dl	2.20-2.60 mmol/L	Mg	1.6 mEq/L	1.8 - 2.6 mEq/L	136-145 mmol/L
Ser alb	3.2 g/dl	3.5-4.8 g/dl	39-50 g/dl	P	3.0mg/dl	2.7-4.5 mg/dl	4.7-6.0 kPa

LIVER FUNCTION							
TEST	RESULT	REFERENCE UNITS Conventional	SI	TEST	RESULT	REFERENCE UNITS Conventional	SI
AST	18 U/L	14-20 U/L	0.23-0.33 µkat/L	TBIL	1.6 mg/dl	0.3-1.0 mg/dl	5.0-17.0 µmol/L
ALT	18 U/L	10-40 U/L	0.17-0.68 µkat/L	DBIL	0.1 mg/dl	0-0.2 mg/dl	0-3.4 µmol/L
ALP	63 U/L	25-100 U/L	17-142 U/L	CPK	325 U/L	38–174 IU/L	0.63-2.90 µkat/L
TP	5.8 g/dl	6.5-8.3 g/dl	65-83 g/dl	Amylase	62 U/L	25–125 U/L	0.4-2.1 µkat/L

CBC							
TEST	RESULT	REFERENCE UNITS Conventional	SI	TEST	RESULT	REFERENCE UNITS Conventional	SI
Hgb	12.8 g/dl	14 - 17.4 g/dl	140-174 g/L	WBC	4.3 10^3/µl	4.5-10.5 x 10^3/cells/ mm^3	4.5-10.5 x 10^9/L
Hct	38%	42 – 52%		% Lymph	18%	25 – 40% of total WBC	1500-4000 cells/mm³
RBC	4.3x10^6/µ	3.6-5.0x10^6/L	3.6-5.0x10^{12}/L	MCH	26 pg/cell	26-34 pg/cell	0.40-.53 fmol/cell
MCV	78.8 µm³	82-98µm³	82-98 fL	MCHC	29 g/dl	32-36 g/dl	320-360 g/L

Normally, weighing a patient with a broken leg would not be attempted, but Mr. D was so thin, a bed weight was obtained after stabilization of the Fx. Mr. D weighed 133 lbs and was 6'0" tall. His son was embarrassed by the Dx and his father's weight. He said: "I knew my father was losing weight. I did not realize he lost this much." Mr. D weighed 165 lbs a year ago.

Mr. D's Medical Nutrition Therapy (MNT) included:

➢ High protein mechanical soft (edentulous) diet with snacks
➢ Force fluids
➢ Have dietitian see pt.
➢ Thiamin, 50 mg IM each hip every day x 3d
➢ Magnesium sulfate, 1 g right hip every day x 3d
➢ Folic acid 1 mg po every day
➢ D_5W @ 75 cc/h
➢ 1 amp of MVI-12 (vials 1 and 2) and M.T.E.- 5 (see Appendix D) in one I.V. bottle every day

Lab values several days later after I.V. hydration:

BASIC METABOLIC PACKAGE							
TEST	RESULT	REFERENCE UNITS Conventional	SI	TEST	RESULT	REFERENCE UNITS Conventional	SI
Glu	127 mg/dl	70-110 mg/dl	3.8-6.1 mmol/L	Na	135 mEq/L	136-145 mEq/L	136-145 mmol/L
BUN	16 mg/dl	6-20 mg/dl	2.1-7.1 mmol/L	K	4.4 mEq/L	3.5-5.2 mEq/L	3.5-5.2 mmol/L
Cr	0.9 mg/dl	0.9-1.3 mg/dl	80-115 µmol/L	Cl	104 mEq/L	96-106 mEq/L	96-106 mmol/L
Ca	7.9 mg/dl	8.8-10.0 mg/dl	2.20-2.60 mmol/L	Mg	2.2 mEq/L	1.8 - 2.6 mEq/L	136-145 mmol/L
Ser alb	2.4 g/dl	3.5-4.8 g/dl	39-50 g/dl	P	3.7mg/dl	2.7-4.5 mg/dl	4.7-6.0 kPa

LIVER FUNCTION							
TEST	RESULT	REFERENCE UNITS Conventional	SI	TEST	RESULT	REFERENCE UNITS Conventional	SI
AST	17 U/L	14-20 U/L	0.23-0.33 µkat/L	TBIL	0.9 mg/dl	0.3-1.0 mg/dl	5.0-17.0 µmol/L
ALT	20 U/L	10-40 U/L	0.17-0.68 µkat/L	DBIL	0.1 mg/dl	0-0.2 mg/dl	0-3.4 µmol/L
ALP	222 U/L	25-100 U/L	17-142 U/L	CPK	150 U/L	38–174 IU/L	0.63-2.90 µkat/L
TP	5.8 g/dl	6.5-8.3 g/dl	65-83 g/dl	Amylase	56 U/L	25–125 U/L	0.4-2.1 µkat/L

CBC							
TEST	**RESULT**	**REFERENCE UNITS** Conventional	SI	**TEST**	**RESULT**	**REFERENCE UNITS** Conventional	SI
Hgb	10.6 g/dl	14 - 17.4 g/dl	140-174 g/L	WBC	4.7 10^3/µl	4.5-10.5 x 10^3/cells/mm^3	4.5-10.5 x 10^9/L
Hct	35.3%	42 – 52%		% Lymph	19%	25 – 40% of total WBC	1500-4000 cells/mm^3
RBC	4.4x10^6/µ	3.6-5.0x10^6/L	3.6-5.0x10^{12}/L	MCH	24 pg/cell	26-34 pg/cell	0.40-.53 fmol/cell
MCV	79.0 µm^3	82-98µm^3	82-98 fL	MCHC	30 g/dl	32-36 g/dl	320-360 g/L

The RD went to Mr. D's nursing station and read his chart. In so doing, she was able to verify the physician's orders and his synopsis of the patient. After reading the chart, the RD visited Mr. D but, because of his mental status, did not try to interview him. She interviewed his son to obtain his father's likes and dislikes. Anthropometric measurements were not obtained since it had already been determined that Mr. D was a nutritional risk. His anticipated hospital stay was not long. The son was now planning to place his father in a nursing home so follow-up was not likely. After visiting the patient and collecting as much information as she could, the RD left a chart note to document her visit. In her chart note, she indicated her observations and stated that she, or her diet tech, would visit the patient on a daily basis during the noon meal to evaluate meal acceptance. She also indicated that she would initiate a calorie count to determine daily energy and protein intakes. She did not recommend further tests, as for anergy, since malnutrition had already been established and was being treated.

Chart notes are often difficult to read because they are written in haste. What follows are examples of a physician's and a dietitian's progress note. The legibility of the notes is good when compared to many in real life. The patient's chart will also contain a Doctor's Order sheet on which he will record his orders. This sheet is not included here but the physician repeats his orders in his progress note. This is the procedure that many physicians often follow. Locate each of the orders mentioned above and note how they are written. Attempt to read the following notes as practice for the real world. There is always more than one way to write a chart note. The dietitian's note should describe the patient's problem (or problems) from a medical, physical, social, and nutritional point of view. The information box below describes how to accomplish this. See if the chart note complies with the information box. As you read the notes, think about what changes you would make, if any, to make the note more readable or informative. The RD used a widely accepted style called a SOAP note:

Information Box 3 - 1

Subjective: In the first part of the note, subjective information is recorded. This is any information obtained verbally from the patient or anyone associated with the patient, such as a family member or visitor who knows the patient. Examples of the information in this section include:
- Nutritional history, food likes and dislikes, current intake, appetite.
- Usual body weight.
- Usual activity, type of work, exercise.
- Socioeconomic status, cultural habits, pertinent information about family.
- Physical impairments, dentures.

Objective: The second section records the objective information. This includes all information that can be measured or documented in some way:
- All anthropometric information, as height, weight, and skinfolds.
- Ideal body weight.
- Recorded information in the chart, as diet order, age, diagnosis.
- Pertinent results of diagnostic tests, laboratory results.
- Documented nutritionally important results of surgical procedures.
- Nutritionally related medications and those that may have diet/drug interactions.
- Results of calorie counts, computerized diet analysis.

Assessment: The third section includes the RD's assessment based on the information obtained in **S** and **O**:
- Evaluation of nutritional status based on history, appetite, intake.
- Evaluation based on anthropometrics, usual body weight.
- Interpretation of lab values, diagnostic tests, and medications as they pertain to nutritional deficiencies or requirements.
- Estimation of nutrient deficiencies and requirements based on above information.
- Assessment of appropriateness of diet order to meet the patient's needs.
- Assessment of the patient's comprehension, ability, and enthusiasm about following diet.
- Estimation of the patient's level of compliance.

Plan: The last section is the plan and relates what the RD is going to do about the assessment:
- Goals for nutritional therapy.
- Recommendation for changes in diet order and/or additional supplements, or approval of the current regimen, as appropriate.
- Plans for follow-up, future visits, encouragement at mealtime.
- Suggestions for additional tests necessary for a more complete assessment, if appropriate.
- Suggestions for referrals to a social worker, physical therapist, etc., as appropriate.
- Description of nutritional education given, to be given, or requested to be given, as appropriate.

PROGRESS NOTES

8/1/98

CC: This malnourished cachexic 73 YOW ♂ admitted via ER c̄ fx ® femur, malnutrition & dementia. Pt found @ home on floor conscious but in pain & unable to move ® leg. X-ray confirms ® femur fx. Severely malnourished. Labs pending — suspect they will confirm dehydration.

MH: Hx of GI distress - gastric ulcers, constipation. Frequent HA resulting in ASA abuse. Arthritis. Pt retired, & eyesight & hearing. ↓ ETOH abuse / tobacco abuse.

Rx: BR, FF to hydrate, ↑ prot ↑ mech soft diet c̄ nourishments t.i.d. Rx NS @ 75 cc/h c̄ ↑ amp MVI ↑ MTE - 4 q d. Thiamin 50 mg ↑ M ea hip q d x 3 d, Mg SO₄ ↑ q ® hip q d x 3d, folate ↑ mg p o q d. R/O malignancy / Alzheimer's. R.D. to see pt.

                              _S____ M.D.

8/1/98
1530

Nutrition: S: Pt's son states: "My father has been depressed and has not been eating well. He has lost wt. gradually over the past yr." Food preferences were obtained from the son.

O: 73 YO ♂ Ht. 6' Wt 133 UBW 165 RBW 178 ± 10%. Labs: ↑ glu 181 mg/dl, ↑ BUN 40 mg/dl, ↓ CPK 325 U/L; ↑ Hct ↑. Diet order: High protein mechanical soft diet c̄ nourishments. Dxr: Malnutrition, fx ® femur, dementia, dehydration.

A: 92# wt loss in past year. 75% of RBW & 81% UBW. Pt dehydrated — when rehydrated, expect to see labs change & provide more indications of malnutrition. Agree c̄ nutritional plan.

P: Will send diet as ordered c̄ ↑ kcal ↑ prot nourishments t.i.d. Will visit pt. c̄ diet tech during meal time to evaluate intake and will start a calorie count x 3 days to determine ↑ cal ↑ prot. intake. Will reevaluate p̄ 3 days of kcal. counts & pt. has been hydrated.

                             _____ R.D.

QUESTIONS:
1. Briefly define the following terms:

    Cachexia:

    Edentulous:

    Anergy:

    Anorexia:

    Alzheimer's Disease:

2. Determine Mr. D's IBW and his percent of IBW. Please show work for all calculations (Appendix A, Tables 7 and 8).

3. Calculate Mr. D's BMI and interpret the results (Appendix A, Tables 10 and 11).

4. List the lab values affected by hydration and explain why.

5. Calculate Mr. D's TLC (Appendix A, Table 13).

6. List each lab value that suggests a nutritional deficiency. Identify the nutritional deficiency in each case and explain how the circumstances in Mr. D's history contributed to each deficiency.

7. Taking multiple medications is a problem that is common with the elderly. Not only does this create possible diet-drug interactions, but it is expensive. Considering many elderly live on fixed incomes, they may be left with insufficient funds for the food they need. Find out if there are any programs in your area that provide assistance for these problems and discuss.

8. Diet-drug interactions are important in any nutritional assessment. The medications a person has to take and the effects these medications have on nutrient availability must be considered and planned for. Therefore, it is necessary to be familiar with the more common medications. Look up each of the following drugs mentioned in the case study and identify their action. Using the table below, identify those that could have the following complications.

DRUG	ACTION	N/V	CONSTIPATION	DIARRHEA	ANOREXIA
Haldol					
Norpace					
MOM					
Pepcid					
Mobic					
Ambien					
Di-Gel					
Aspirin					

9. Identify the medications that are sources of nutrients and indicate the nutrients.

10. Which medications could cause gastric bleeding? Briefly explain how.

11. What are possible causes of Mr. D's lack of taste?

12. Do you agree or disagree with the RD's decision not to take anthropometric measurements or recommend anergy determinations? Discuss why or why not.

13. When hospitalized, Mr. D was given 50 mg of thiamin IM every day x 3d. What is the current RDA for thiamin for a 73 YOM? How could such a dose be justified, especially since he is to receive one amp of MVI-12 every day?

14. Look up and record the RDAs for folic acid and Mg for a 73 YOM. Discuss how you could justify such a dose of folic acid and Mg. Mr. D is also receiving M.T.E.- 5 (see Appendix D).

15. Compare the RDAs for a 51 YO, a 73 YO, and a 90 YO. Considering the results of these comparisons, what do you think about the sufficiency of the RDAs?

16. Calculate Mr. D's basal energy expenditure using the Harris-Benedict equation. Determine a stress factor to multiply this by and determine total energy needs (Appendix A, Table 17).

17. Considering Mr. D's mental and physical condition, his nutritional deficiencies, his medications, and his calculated energy needs, plan a 3-day sample menu for Mr. D that would meet his needs. (Turn in on a separate sheet of paper.)

18. Discuss how you might influence Mr. D to eat.

19. Comment on the dietitian's chart note. Was it adequate? Were the components in the right place? Did it need additional information?

ADDITIONAL OPTIONAL QUESTIONS:
Tube Feeding Drill:

20. Using a table below, compare several of the enteral nutritional supplements that provide about 1 kcal/ml and can be taken orally or with a feeding tube (there is room for seven comparisons).

21. Using a table below, compare several of the enteral nutritional supplements that provide 1.5 kcals/ml and that can be taken orally or with a tube.

Product	Producer	Form	Cal/ ml	Non-pro cal/g N	g/L			Na mg	K mg	mOsm /kg water	Vol to meet RDA in ml	g of fiber /L	Free H$_2$O /L in ml
					Pro	CHO	Fat						

Product	Producer	Form	Cal/ ml	Non-pro cal/g N	g/L			Na mg	K mg	mOsm /kg water	Vol to meet RDA in ml	g of fiber /L	Free H$_2$O /L in ml
					Pro	CHO	Fat						

RELATED READINGS

1. Delacorte, R.R., Moriguti, J.C., Matos, F.D., Pfrimer, K., Marchinil, J.S., & Ferriolli, E. (2004). Mini-nutritional assessment score and the risk for undernutrition in free-living older persons. *J Nutr Health Aging*. 8(6):531-4

2. Fischbach, F.T. (2003). *A Manual of Laboratory & Diagnostic Tests*. 7th Ed. Philadelphia. J.B. Lippincott Company.

3. Food and Nutrition Board, National Research Council, National Academy of Sciences. *Dietary Reference Intakes for Water, Potassium, Sodium, Chloride, and Sulfate*. Panel on Dietary Reference Intakes for Electrolytes and Water, Standing Committee on the Scientific Evaluation of Dietary Reference Intakes (2004).
   Dietary Reference Intakes for Vitamin C, Vitamin E, Selenium, and Carotenoids. Panel on Dietary Antioxidants and Related Compounds, Subcommittees on Upper Reference Levels of Nutrients and Interpretation and Uses of DRIs, Standing Committee on the Scientific Evaluation of Dietary Reference Intakes, Food and Nutrition Board (2000).
   Dietary Reference Intakes for Vitamin A, Vitamin K, Arsenic, Boron, Chromium, Copper, Iodine, Iron, Manganese, Molybdenum, Nickel, Silicon, Vanadium, and Zinc. Panel on Micronutrients, Subcommittees on Upper Reference Levels of Nutrients and of Interpretation and Use of Dietary Reference Intakes, and the Standing Committee on the Scientific Evaluation of Dietary Reference Intakes (2000).
   Dietary Reference Intakes for Thiamin, Riboflavin, Niacin, Vitamin B_6, Folate, Vitamin B_{12}, Pantothenic Acid, Biotin, and Choline. A Report of the Standing Committee on the Scientific Evaluation of Dietary Reference Intakes and its Panel on Folate, Other B Vitamins, and Choline and Subcommittee on Upper Reference Levels of Nutrients, Food and Nutrition Board, Institute of Medicine (1998).

4. Lee, R.D., Nieman, D.C., & Nieman, D. (2002). *Nutritional Assessment*. 3rd Ed. McGraw-Hill.

5. Kovacevich, D.S., Boney, A.R., Braunchweig, C.L., Perez, A., & Stevens, M. (1997). Nutritional risk classification: a reproducible and valid tool for nurses. *Nutr. Clin. Pract.* 12(1):20-25.

6. McLaren, S. & Green, S. (1998). Nutritional screening and assessment. *Prof. Nurse.* 13(6S):S9-S15.

7. Pepersack, T., Rotsaert, P., Benoit, F., Willems, D., Fuss, M., Bourdoux, P., & Duchateau, J. (2001). Prevalence of zinc deficiency and its clinical relevance among hospitalized elderly. *Arch Gerontol Geriatr.* Nov;33(3):243-53.

8. Prendergast, A. & Fulton, F.L. (1997) *Medical terminology: A Text/Workbook.* 4th Ed. Redwood City, California. Addison-Wesley Nursing.

9. Pronsky, Z.M., Redfern, C.M., Crowe, J. & Epstein, S. (2003) *Food Medication Interactions*, 13th Ed Phoenix, Arizona. Food-Medications Interactions, Publishers and Distributors.

10. Rolfes, S.R., Pinna, K. & Whitney, E. (2006). *Understanding Normal and Clinical Nutrition*, 7th Ed. West/Wadsworth.

11. Schlenker, E.D. (1997). *Nutrition in Aging.* St. Louis, Missouri. Mosby-Year Book, Inc.

12. Stratton, R.J., Hackston, A., Longmore, D., Dixon, R., Price, S., Stroud, M., King, C., & Elia, M. (2004). Malnutrition in hospital outpatients and inpatients: prevalence, concurrent validity and ease of use of the malnutrition universal screening tool ('MUST') for adults. *Br J Nutr.* Nov;92(5):799-808.

13. Weddle, D.O., & Kuczmarski, F. (2000). Nutrition, aging and the continuum of care *J Am Diet Assoc. 100:580-595.*

14. Zulkowski, K. & Coon, P.J. (2004). Comparison of nutritional risk between urban and rural elderly. *Ostomy Wound Manage.* May; 50(5):46-8, 50, 52.

CASE STUDY #4
ANOREXIA NERVOSA-BULIMIA NERVOSA

INTRODUCTION

The occurrence of anorexia nervosa is increasing in our society. In the past, the actual incidence of this disorder was not widely known since it has been a disease kept in a "closet." Because of this, the number of cases of anorexia nervosa may be higher than previously realized. The consequences of this eating disorder can be devastating. It is important for health care professionals to understand what anorexia nervosa is, how to recognize it, and what can be done for someone who is suffers from this disorder.

****

SKILLS NEEDED

ABBREVIATIONS:

Knowledge of the following abbreviations is required in order to understand this case. You should learn these abbreviations before you begin to read the study: BMI, BMR, IBW, and YOWF (Appendix C).

FORMULAS:

The formulas used in this case study include ideal body weight, percent ideal body weight (Appendix A, Tables 7 - 10), and basal metabolic rate using the Harris-Benedict equation (Appendix A, Table 17).

MEDICATIONS:

Become familiar with the following medications before reading the case study. Note the diet-drug interactions, dosages, methods of administration, gastrointestinal tract reactions, etc.
1. Emetics; 2. Diuretics; 3. Laxatives.
****

SP is a 19 YOWF in her second year of college. She is the only child of an upper-middle-class family. She lives at home with her parents, both of whom have flourishing careers and expect her to be highly successful. With all the good intentions in the world, her parents decided to help her reach success by placing tight restraints on her and pressuring her to be the best in everything she attempts. SP has very few opportunities to make decisions for herself. She does not see this as a sign of her parents' love but, rather, views it as the placement of unreasonable restrictions designed to hinder her social life. SP feels she has to perform to receive love and encouragement, instead of receiving love and encouragement to help her perform. Her parents want her to be a successful doctor but SP wants to be a special education teacher.

SP's parents expect her to be active in as many prestigious campus organizations as she can and still maintain an "A" average. Because of this emphasis on excellence, SP has set very high goals for herself, but her grades in school have been poor because she does not like what she is studying. She cannot put her heart into her studies. In the past, when she failed to reach a goal, she would blame herself and become very depressed. Now she is blaming her parents. At least this is the theory her psychologist has proposed to explain her refusal to eat. He believes she is rebelling against her parents' dominance.

During her freshman year, SP took a health course and learned about anorexia nervosa. After taking the course, SP started talking about how she needed to lose a few pounds and went on a diet. She was 5'2" with a medium frame and weighed 120 lbs. She wanted to go on a diet "the right way," so she obtained a book from a newsstand on basic nutrition and calorie content and began counting calories. She learned that fat provides more calories than carbohydrate or protein, so she tried to eliminate fat from her diet entirely. SP discovered that sugar provides "empty calories," so she tried to eliminate sugar. Some friends of hers were on low-carbohydrate diets and convinced her that carbohydrate causes you to gain weight, so she tried to avoid carbohydrates also. Her nutrition and calorie counter book said that white flour was harmful, so she eliminated white flour. She also read that a diet high in meat, particularly red meat, was also high in fat and could cause cancer, so she eliminated red meat. That did not leave much for SP to eat.

Her nutrition and calorie counter book also emphasized the importance of exercise for weight loss and a healthy body. She started an exercise program that was very vigorous. She attended aerobics classes three times a week, rode her bicycle almost everywhere she went, and played tennis on a regular basis. In addition, she was very active at school.

SP did not think she was losing weight fast enough so she reduced her calories even more. She avoided eating with her parents as much as possible to keep them from seeing her starve herself. If she did eat with them, she would eat a normal amount and then go force herself to throw-up. When she was down to 105 lbs, her mother noticed a difference and asked her about the weight loss. SP told her she was on a diet. Her mother told her to stop dieting immediately; she had lost enough weight. In rebellion against her parents, this encouraged SP to stay on the diet longer. When she reached 100 lbs, she was on a plateau and could not lose additional weight. Her friends were continually telling her how thin she looked. This reinforced her desire to lose weight and gave her a feeling of accomplishment. Her mother nagged her constantly. The more people talked to her about her diet, the more determined she was to lose more weight. She was convinced that she needed to lose a few more pounds. SP continued to decrease her intake and increased her exercise. She began to become tired very easily, could not concentrate, and amenorrhea and headaches were a problem. Her grades were getting worse and SP started spending most of her time alone.

One day SP collapsed at school after standing up rapidly. She had to be brought home. Her mother was furious. She took her to a physician who examined SP and said she had orthostatic hypotension and bradycardia. A clinical examination revealed lanugo, and SP admitted having amenorrhea. Her weight was 90 lbs. The doctor easily made a diagnosis of anorexia nervosa. SP denied it and her mother agreed with her at first, refusing to believe her daughter was starving herself. The physician recommended a psychologist and a registered dietitian. Both SP and her mother refused to see them. SP insisted that nothing was wrong with her. Her mother insisted that she was going to handle her daughter her way.

The situation continued until SP became so weak she had to drop out of school. At this point her father demanded she return to the doctor and follow his recommendations. SP started receiving counseling from the psychologist and registered dietitian. She weighed 85 lbs.
****

QUESTIONS:

1. Determine SP's IBW and percent IBW (Appendix A, Tables 7 and 8). Show all work.

2. After her first visit to the physician, SP weighed 90 lbs. Her weight before her diet was 120 lbs. What was her percent loss of weight (Appendix A, Table 8)?

3. SP's weight after her last visit was 85 lbs. Recalculate her percent loss of weight.

4. Calculate SP's BMI and comment on its interpretation (Appendix A, Tables 10 and 11).

5. Define the following terms:

    Emetics:

    Diuretics:

    Orthostatic hypotension:

    Bradycardia:

    Amenorrhea:

    Lanugo:

6. Discuss anorexia nervosa relative to the following points:
    ➢ What social class(es) of people usually has/have anorexia nervosa?

    ➢ What physical, social, mental, or psychological characteristics do individuals with anorexia nervosa frequently have?

    ➢ What are the theories about the possible causes of anorexia nervosa?

7. SP went on a low-carbohydrate diet. How much carbohydrate is "low"?
   a. 100 grams
   b. 150 grams
   c. 200 grams
   d. 250 grams

8. What is a high-carbohydrate diet?
   a. 100 grams
   b. 150 grams
   c. 200 grams
   d. 250 grams

9. Would the answers you gave in the above two questions be the same in every case, for every individual? Explain.

10. What are the physiological effects of a low-carbohydrate diet?

11. Future evaluation for SP should include diagnostic assessment for (circle all that apply):
    a. protein and calorie malnutrition.
    b. microcytic anemia.
    c. macrocytic anemia.
    d. dehydration.
    e. percent body fat.
    f. weight.

12. List the above assessments in order of the most important to the least important to know. Give the time frame as to when they might be completed.

13. What goals for nutritional therapy would you use to improve the assessment parameters listed in question 11?

14. SP's problem is a very complex one and requires counseling from several different members of the health care team. As a member of that team, you must be careful to reinforce, and not contradict, the information SP is receiving from the other team members. Discuss what you think your boundaries are and how the team effort should be coordinated.

15. List the symptoms of anorexia nervosa SP demonstrated. List all additional possible symptoms that SP could have demonstrated.

16. When SP's friends and family told her how thin she looked, it encouraged her. This is typical for many anorexics. What approach should be used to discourage rather than encourage a person with anorexia?

****

When SP went to see the RD, her mother insisted on going with her. The first interview included the following:

RD: SP, when did you first start on your diet?

SP: Well . . .

Mom: She started a long time ago. Those kids she hangs around with, they talked her into it.

RD: Yes ma'am. When you first started on your diet, how did you see yourself?

SP: I . . .

Mom She has a very healthy perception of herself; always did. She just wanted to lose a few pounds and then got sick and lost a lot, that's all.

RD: Yes ma'am. SP, I want you to tell me everything you have to eat or drink in a typical day from the time you get up in the morning to the time you go to bed at night, everything.

Mom: Now tell the lady what you eat honey, don't leave out anything. She is just trying to help . . . .

This interview is not intended for comic relief. Such behavior is not uncommon and has to be dealt with. During the interview, the RD obtained some valuable information though much of the time was wasted. The obvious conclusion was the dominance of SP's mother.
****

<u>QUESTIONS CONTINUED</u>:

17. How would you handle SP's mother in the above situation?

18. If blood was drawn and analyzed, what results would you expect to find? Explain your expectations.

Refeeding someone after a period of starvation should be done with caution. A starved person should not start eating large meals. Generally, the longer the starvation period, the slower the refeeding. Each case is different and should be evaluated on its own circumstances. SP has been dieting for about a year, the last several months being a starvation diet. She lost from 120 to 85 lbs. The psychologist, RD, and physician worked as a team with SP's father and convinced him that SP needed to have more of a voice in her life. In turn, he convinced his wife. They agreed to allow SP more freedom. They gave her their blessing to change her major to special education. This greatly changed the home atmosphere and gave the psychologist and RD a chance to work with SP. By now she had created a tremendous fear of being fat and did not want to gain her weight back. They were able to show her that her dieting hurt her social life more than it hurt her parents. They also helped her to dream of being the teacher and role model she wanted to be for children. She slowly started to eat more but gained several pounds very fast. She was afraid she would continue to gain weight at that rate and would get fat. The RD explained the occurrence of rapid weight gain to her and calmed her fears. SP continued to gain weight. As she did, she began to feel stronger. Still fearing to gain too much, she restarted her vigorous exercise routine. She remembered how much she enjoyed eating and began to overeat, using the excessive exercise as an excuse. She enjoyed what she was doing but felt guilty for overeating. She gained 30 lbs back and was now 115 lbs. SP was released from the care of her physician and counselors.

She started to binge and purge often. She was in a real dilemma. She wanted to eat but did not want to gain weight. She was willing to purge to keep her weight down but she found that gross. She did not like sticking her finger down her throat. One day a friend introduced her to ipecac syrup, an over-the-counter drug that would make her throw-up. SP began using this drug with laxatives and diuretics to keep her weight down while overeating.
****

<u>QUESTIONS CONTINUED</u>:

19. Assume that SP will submit to ending her starvation diet. Calculate SP's BMR using the Harris-Benedict equation. What activity factor would you initially use? On a separate sheet of paper, outline a refeeding plan for SP and include in your plan: the number of kcals you would start with per day, the rate at which you would advance, and your final kcals per day.

20. If you feed too much too fast, what problems would you expect SP to have?

21. Explain why there would be a rapid weight gain right after going off a starvation diet.

22. Would you counsel SP any differently then the team did in this case?

23. List the characteristics and complications of bulimia.

24. Describe the action, nutritional complications, and any adverse reactions of ipecac syrup.

25. What are the principles behind using laxatives and diuretics in this case?

26. If SP took ipecac syrup, laxatives, and diuretics on a daily basis, predict the probable complications. What lab values would most likely be affected? Be specific and explain.

SP thought she could binge and lose the food she ate with the over-the-counter drugs and no one would know. Her binging increased. Some days she would throw up once, twice, or ten times. A typical binge could include a large bag of chocolate chip cookies, a liter of soda, two peanut butter sandwiches, a large bag of potato chips, almost a half-gallon of ice cream, and several candy bars. She might throw up four or five times during this binge. Sometimes she would spend $30.00 to $40.00 a day for binge food. SP went to her dentist for a check up. Upon examining her, he noted perimolysis. When he asked her if she had been vomiting a lot, she denied it.

****

QUESTIONS CONTINUED:

27. Describe the nutritional approach you would use to counsel SP now that she is bulimic. Would your nutritional goals change? Explain.

28. What is perimolysis? Explain its relationship with bulimia.

29. Using any of the given information, compose a SOAP note about SP.

S:
O:
A:
P:

RELATED READINGS

1. Davis, C., Kaptein, S., Kaplan, A.S., Olmsted, M.P., & Woodside, D.B. (1998). Obsessionality in anorexia nervosa: the moderating influence of exercise. *Psychosom.* Med. 60(2):192-197.

2. Kordella, T. (2003). To "Low-Carb" Or Not To "Low-Carb". Diabetes Forecast, December. http://www.diabetes.org/diabetes-forecast/dec2003/research.jsp

3. Le Grange, D. Binford, , & Loeb, K.L. (2005). Manualized family-based treatment for anorexia nervosa: a case series. *J Am Acad Child Adolesc Psychiatry.* Jan;44(1):41-6.

4. Maine M. (2004). Altering women's relationships with food: A relational, developmental approach. *J Clin Psychol.* Dec 21;57(11):1301-1310.

5. Makino, M., Tsuboi, K., & Dennerstein, L. (2004). Prevalence of eating disorders: a comparison of Western and non-Western countries. *MedGenMed.* Sep 27;6(3):49.

6. Mayo Clin Health Lett. 2004 Low-carb diets. Answers to your questions Nov;22(11):4-5.

7. NIDDK. Weight-loss and Nutrition Myths. Myth: *Fad diets work for permanent weight loss.* Myth: High-protein/low-carbohydrate diets are a healthy way to lose weight. Myth: *Starches are fattening and should be limited when trying to lose weight.* Myth: *Eating red meat is bad for your health and makes it harder to lose weight.* NIH Publication No. 04-4561, March 2004. http://win.niddk.nih.gov/publications/myths.htm

8. NIH. Binge eating disorders: http://win.niddk.nih.gov/publications/binge.htm. Very low calorie diets: http://win.niddk.nih.gov/publications/low_calorie.htm

9. Pearce, J.M. (2004). Richard Morton: Orgins of Anorexia nervosa. *Eur. Neurol.* Nov 10;52(4):191-192.

10. Perkins, P.S., Klump, K.L., Iacono, W.G., McGue, M. (2004). Personality traits in women with anorexia nervosa: Evidence for a treatment-seeking bias? *Int J Eat Disord.* Dec 22;37(1):32-37.

11. Position paper of the American Dietetic Association. (2001). Nutrition intervention in the treatment of anorexia nervosa, bulimia nervosa, and eating disorder not otherwise specified (EDNOS). *J Am Diet Assoc*; 101:810. http://www.eatright.org/Public/NutritionInformation/92_adap0701.cfm

12. Position paper of the American Dietetic Association. (2002). Weight management *J Am Diet Assoc.* 2002;102:1145-1155.

13. Powers, P.S. & Santana, C. (2004) Available pharmacological treatments for anorexia nervosa. *Expert Opin Pharmacother.* Nov;5(11):2287-92.

14. Pryor, T., & Wiederman, M.W. (1998). Personality features and expressed concerns of adolescents with eating disorders. *Adolescence.* 33(130):291-300.

15. Siegel, M., Brisman, J. & Weinshel, M. (1989). *Surviving an Eating Disorder.* New York: Harper & Row.

16. Sullivan, P.F., Bulik, C.M., Carter, F.A., Gendall, K.A., & Joyce, P.R. (1996). The significance of a prior history of anorexia in bulimia nervosa. *Int. J. Eat. Disord.* 20(3):253-261.

17. Tong, J., Miao, S.J., Wang, J., Zhang, J.J., Wu, H.M., Li, T., & Hsu, L.K. (2004). Five cases of male eating disorders in Central China. *Int J Eat Disord.* Dec 22;37(1):72-75.

18. Rolfes, S.R., Pinna, K. and Whitney, E. (2006). *Understanding Normal and Clinical Nutrition*, 7th Ed. West/Wadsworth.

19. Weaver K, Wuest J, & Ciliska D. (2005). Understanding Women's Journey of Recovering From Anorexia Nervosa. *Qual Health Res.* Feb;15(2):188-206.

20. Williamson, D.A., Gleaves, D.H., Stewart, T.M. (2004). Categorical versus dimensional models of eating disorders: An examination of the evidence. *Int J Eat Disord.* Dec 22;37(1):1-10.

21. Wills-Brandon, C. (1989). *Eat Like a Lady. Guide for Overcoming Bulimia.* Deerfield Beach, Florida. Health Communications, Inc.

CASE STUDY #5
POLYPHARMACY

INTRODUCTION
This case study describes a typical situation that occurs often, particularly with the elderly. It involves several complications that by themselves are not serious, but together lead to disaster. Several medications are included in this study and the Nutritional Screening Initiative is introduced.
****

SKILLS NEEDED

ABBREVIATIONS:
Knowledge of the following abbreviations is required in order to understand this case. You should learn these abbreviations before you begin to read the study. Many of the simpler abbreviations that have been used in previous case studies will not be listed here (Appendix C).
ALT, ALP, AST, b.i.d, BMI, BUN, Ca, Chol, Cl, C/O, CPK, Cr, DBIL, D/C, Dx, glu, hct, hgb, hs, IBW, K, MCH, MCHC, MCV, mEq/L, Mg, mm^3, Na, P, po, prn, PVC, q6h, RBC, ser alb, t.i.d., TBIL, TP, UBW, UTI, WBC, YOWF, μm^3, and 1/4NS.

FORMULAS:
The formulas used in this case study are: reference body weight and percent reference body weight (Appendix A, Tables 7 and 8).

LABORATORY VALUES:
You will need to be able to interpret the nutritional significance of the following laboratory values for this case study: ALT, ALP, AST, BUN, Ca, chol, Cl, CPK, Cr, DBIL, Glucose, hct, hgb, K, Lymphocytes, MCH, MCHC, MCV, Mg, Na, P, RBC, ser alb, TBIL, TP, and WBC (Appendix B).

MEDICATIONS:
Become familiar with the following medications before reading this case study. Note the diet-drug interactions, dosages and method of administration, gastrointestinal tract reactions, etc.1. Mobic (meloxicam); 2. FML Liquifilom Ophthalmic; 3. Maxitrol Ointment; 4. Diovan (valsartan); 5. Lasix (furosemide); 6. Norpace (disopyramide phosphate); 7. Ambien (zolpidem tartrate); 8. Ativan (lorazepam); 9. Bactrim DS (trimethoprim and sulfamethoxazole); 10. Tagamet (cimetidine); 11. Ventolin (albuterol).
****

Mrs. SJ is a 75 YOWF who has been a widow for 15 years. Until recently, she had been active in various groups such as the "Quilters" and the "Crafters." Arthritis in her hands and arms started making it increasingly difficult for her to sew or make crafts. Arthritis in her knees and hips also made it difficult for her to move freely. She has to walk with a cane. Her Family Practice physician sent her to a rheumatologist. She has been taking 7.5 mg of Mobic (meloxicam) po once daily for a number of years. Mrs. SJ smoked a pack of cigarettes a day for 40 years before being forced to quit by her physician and family. A severe cough, difficulty breathing, and the diagnosis of chronic pulmonary emphysema also helped to convince her to quit. She has been taking Ventolin for three years for this condition.

Mrs. SJ has also been having problems with her eyes. Not only does she have to get her glasses changed more frequently, but her eyes have been very watery and burn a lot. Her doctor has not determined if she has an allergy or if she has an infection. She has not yet responded to treatment. Her ophthalmologist prescribed FML Liquifilm Ophthalmic for allergies and Maxitrol Ointment for infection. Ophthalmology visits are expensive and are not covered by her health insurance. Mrs. SJ has been underweight all her life even though she had a ravenous appetite until recently. She is a 5'5" small-framed woman and weighs 100 lbs. In her prime, the most she ever weighed was 111 lbs with very little variation from year to year. This is the least she has weighed since high school. Since about age 60, she has been having a problem with hypertension and has been taking Diovan (valsartan), 160 once every day, po. She had a small but noticeable amount of edema in her feet and C/O the rings on her fingers being too tight. Her doctor prescribed Lasix (furosemide) 20 mg every other day prn. Mrs. SJ started having arrhythmias with frequent PVCs around age 65 and had to see a cardiologist. He prescribed Norpace (disopyramide phosphate), 150 mg,q6h, po. Mrs. SJ became depressed about a year ago. Several factors brought this about. The death of her older sister was a shock to her. Mrs. SJ was the fourth of five children but now is the oldest alive. She still has a younger brother who lives 200 miles away. She has two children but they both moved to another state. After her sister died, two of her closest friends in her craft club passed away within three months of each other. They were both younger than she is and used to be her means of transportation since they both had cars and could drive well. She fears that she is now the next to die and that thought scares her. All the deaths took place during the winter when Mrs. SJ has the most trouble with her arthritis. The past winter was particularly bad with a lot of snow. Mrs. SJ was stuck indoors for weeks at a time. She lives in an efficiency apartment in a complex inhabited by elderly tenants.

The depression has aggravated her arrhythmias. Her heart rate is usually good but, when the arrhythmias occur, Mrs. SJ becomes very weak and dizzy. At these times she does not want to go anywhere for fear of having an attack. The more fearful she becomes, the more the arrhythmias occur. This makes her even more fearful. It also increases her blood pressure, which adds to the stress. Mrs. SJ has still another problem, gastritis. After years of complaining about a burning sensation in her stomach, she consulted a gastroenterologists. A mild case of gastritis was diagnosed. Most of the time this did not bother her but, with the added stress, the burning sensation returned. The gastroenterologists prescribed cimetidine which Mrs. SJ has been taking for years.

This downward spiral has been going on for several months and affects her sleep. She did not tell her Family Practice physician everything, but she told her about not sleeping. Since her rest is important, her Family Practice physician gave her 10 mg of Ambien (zolpidem tartrate) at hs for sleep and Ativan (lorazepam), 1 mg t.i.d. for anxiety. Neither of these seemed to work fast enough for her so she doubled the doses. The additional stress also caused her to have anorexia which resulted in weight loss and weakness. All of this lowered her immune system and she ended up with a bladder infection. For this her physician gave her Bactrim DS (trimethoprim and sulfamethoxazole), 1 DS tablet q12h and told her to force fluids.

Mrs. SJ felt too weak and sick to go to the corner grocery to buy food and too sick to prepare it. She stayed inside and ate cereal and milk until she ran out of milk. She ate soft foods like rice with a little margarine and hot tca. After several days of this, she became too weak to get out of bed. When she did not show up in the recreation room for Friday night BINGO, something she never missed, some of the tenants went to check on her. She was found in bed very confused and disoriented and could not even sit up. They called 911 and had her sent to the hospital. Mrs. SJ was admitted with a Dx of UTI, dehydration, anemia, and depression. Her admission lab values were as follows:

BASIC METABOLIC PACKAGE							
TEST	RESULT	REFERENCE UNITS Conventional SI		TEST	RESULT	REFERENCE UNITS Conventional SI	
Glu	165mg/dl	70-110 mg/dl	3.8-6.1 mmol/L	Na	149 mEq/L	136-145 mEq/L	136-145 mmol/L
BUN	14 mg/dl	6-20 mg/dl	2.1-7.1 mmol/L	K	5.1 mEq/L	3.5-5.2 mEq/L	3.5-5.2 mmol/L
Cr	0.8 mg/dl	0.6-1.1 mg/dl	53-97 µmol/L	Cl	102 mEq/L	96-106 mEq/L	96-106 mmol/L
Ca	8.2 mg/dl	8.8-10.0 mg/dl	2.20-2.60 mmol/L	Mg	1.8 mEq/L	1.8 - 2.6 mEq/L	136-145 mmol/L
Ser alb	3.6 g/dl	3.5-4.8 g/dl	39-50 g/dl	P	2.5mg/dl	2.7-4.5 mg/dl	4.7-6.0 kPa

CBC							
TEST	**RESULT**	**REFERENCE UNITS** Conventional SI		**TEST**	**RESULT**	**REFERENCE UNITS** Conventional SI	
Hgb	17 g/dl	12-16 g/dl	120-160 g/L	WBC	14 10^3/µl	4.5-10.5 x 10^3/cells/mm^3	4.5-10.5 x10^9/L
Hct	48 %	36-48%		% Lymph	13%	25 – 40% of total WBC	1500-4000 cells/mm^3
RBC	$4.2x10^6$/µ	$3.6-5.0x10^6$/L	3.6-5.0 $x10^{12}$/L	MCH	26 pg/cell	26-34 pg/cell	0.40-.53 fmol/cell
MCV	78 µm^3	82-98µm^3	82-98 fL	MCHC	32 g/dl	32-36 g/dl	320-360 g/L

LIVER FUNCTION							
TEST	**RESULT**	**REFERENCE UNITS** Conventional SI		**TEST**	**RESULT**	**REFERENCE UNITS** Conventional SI	
AST	81 U/L	10-36 U/L	0.17-0.60 µkat/L	TBIL	0.6 mg/dl	0.3-1.0 mg/dl	5.0-17.0 µmol/L
ALT	20 U/L	7-35 U/L	7-56 U/L	DBIL	0.1 mg/dl	0-0.2 mg/dl	0-3.4 µmol/L
ALP	82 U/L	25-100 U/L	17-142 U/L	CPK	52 IU/L	26–140 U/L	0.42-2.38 µkat/L
TP	5.8 g/dl	6.5-8.3 g/dl	65-83 g/dl	Amylase	68/L	25–125 U/L	0.4-2.1 µkat/L

****

QUESTIONS:

1. Define:

    Rheumatologist:

    Ophthalmologist:

    Cardiologist:

    Arrhythmias:

2. Mrs. SJ is taking a lot of medications. This is typical for the elderly and is cause for concern, particularly when they are seeing more than one physician and not telling each physician what the others are prescribing. Research each medication Mrs. SJ is taking and list the possible nutritional complications for each.

MEDICATION	ACTION	NUTRITIONAL COMPLICATION
Mobic (meloxicam)		
Diovan (valsartan)		
Lasix (furosemide)		
Norpace (disopyramide phosphate)		
Ambien (zolpidem tartrate)		
Ativan (lorazepam)		
Bactrim DS (trimethoprim and sulfamethoxazole)		

3. Each of these medications is given to correct a problem but each could possibly cause a side effect that may negate the effects of another medication or increase the intensity of another symptom. Example: Mobic is a nonsteroidal anti-inflammatory for mild to moderate pain caused by osteoarthritis or rheumatiod arthritis. Possible side effects include peptic ulcer, anxiety, palpitations, dysrhythmias, and insomnia. List the possible side effects that could occur with the following medications.

MEDICATION	INTERACTION WITH OTHER MEDS
Mobic (meloxicam)	
Diovan (valsartan)	
Lasix (furosemide)	
Norpace (disopyramide phosphate)	
Ambien (zolpidem tartrate)	
Ativan (lorazepam)	
Bactrim DS (trimethoprim and sulfamethoxazole)	

4. Discuss Mrs. SJ's symptoms in light of her medications. Do you think some of her problems could have been caused by drug interactions? Explain.

5. Considering her diseases and medications, describe an adequate home diet for Mrs. SJ. Interject in your discussion nutrients that she needs to include and substances she should avoid or ingest sparingly.

****

When Mrs. SJ's physician saw all of the drugs she was taking from four different doctors, she told her that one of her problems was "polypharmacy." She D/C'd all of her at-home medications and started I.V. antibiotics with 1/4NS and an antihypertensive medication. All other medications were given on a prn basis. Within a couple of days, Mrs. SJ's infection was under control and she was awake and alert. The dietitian visited her to do an assessment using Level I of the Nutrition Screening Initiative and obtained the following information:

BODY WEIGHT HISTORY

Ht 5'5"   Wt 100 lbs   Wt 1 yr ago 111 lbs   **Wt 6 mos ago 111 lbs**

The following statements on the Level I Screening Initiative were all answered positively by Mrs. SJ.

EATING HABITS
- ✓ **Usually eats alone**
- ✓ **Has poor appetite**
- ✓ **Eats vegetables two or fewer times daily**
- ✓ **Eats milk products once or not at all daily**
- ✓ **Eats fruit or drinks fruit juice once or not at all daily**
- ✓ **Eats breads, cereals, pasta, rice, or other grains five or fewer times daily**
- ✓ **Has difficulty chewing or swallowing**

LIVING ENVIRONMENT
- ✓ **Lives alone**
- ✓ **Is housebound**

FUNCTIONAL STATUS: Usually or always needs assistance with
- ✓ **Walking or moving about**
- ✓ **Traveling (outside the home)**
- ✓ **Preparing food**
- ✓ **Shopping for food or other necessities**

****

QUESTIONS CONTINUED:

6. Obtain a guideline for the Nutrition Screening Initiative (available from: ADA, see http://www.eatright.org/Public/SearchResults.cfm). Using this guide, identify the agencies that should be contacted for each of the problems in the outline above. With the Nutrition Screening Initiative as a guide, discuss possible solutions to the problems mentioned above.

7. Consider other problems Mrs. SJ had, such as, money for all the medications and physicians and all the causes for depression, etc. Discuss how these problems have to be addressed if Mrs. SJ is to improve. List the possible solutions.

8. What did the physician mean by "polypharmacy"?

9. What is Mrs. SJ's IBW and percent of IBW (Appendix A, Tables 7 and 8)? Please show all work.

10. What is her UBW and percent UBW (Appendix A, Table 8)?

11. What is Mrs. SJ's BMI (Appendix A, Tables 10 and 11)? Would her age affect her BMI?

After a few more days, Mrs. SJ's labs were repeated and the following obtained:

BASIC METABOLIC PACKAGE							
TEST	**RESULT**	**REFERENCE UNITS** Conventional SI		**TEST**	**RESULT**	**REFERENCE UNITS** Conventional SI	
Glu	95 mg/dl	70-110 mg/dl	3.8-6.1 mmol/L	Na	140 mEq/L	136-145 mEq/L	136-145 mmol/L
BUN	6 mg/dl	6-20 mg/dl	2.1-7.1 mmol/L	K	3.8 mEq/L	3.5-5.2 mEq/L	3.5-5.2 mmol/L
Cr	0.6 mg/dl	0.6-1.1 mg/dl	53-97 µmol/L	Cl	100 mEq/L	96-106 mEq/L	96-106 mmol/L
Ca	8.7 mg/dl	8.8-10.0 mg/dl	2.20-2.60 mmol/L	Mg	1.9 mEq/L	1.8 - 2.6 mEq/L	136-145 mmol/L
Ser alb	3.1 g/dl	3.5-4.8 g/dl	39-50 g/dl	P	2.3mg/dl	2.7-4.5 mg/dl	4.7-6.0 kPa

LIVER FUNCTION							
TEST	**RESULT**	**REFERENCE UNITS** Conventional SI		**TEST**	**RESULT**	**REFERENCE UNITS** Conventional SI	
AST	45 U/L	10-36 U/L	0.17-0.60 µkat/L	TBIL	0.5 mg/dl	0.3-1.0 mg/dl	5.0-17.0 µmol/L
ALT	55 U/L	7-35 U/L	7-56 U/L	DBIL	0.1 mg/dl	0-0.2 mg/dl	0-3.4 µmol/L
ALP	77 U/L	25-100 U/L	17-142 U/L	CPK	97 IU/L	26–140 U/L	0.42-2.38 µkat/L
TP	5.9 g/dl	6.5-8.3 g/dl	65-83 g/dl	Amylase	80/L	25–125 U/L	0.4-2.1 µkat/L

CBC							
TEST	RESULT	REFERENCE UNITS Conventional	SI	TEST	RESULT	REFERENCE UNITS Conventional	SI
Hgb	11 g/dl	12-16 g/dl	120-160 g/L	WBC	6.5 10^3/μl	4.5-10.5 x 10^3/cells/mm^3	4.5-10.5 x10^9/L
Hct	33 %	36-48%		% Lymph	24%	25 – 40% of total WBC	1500-4000 cells/mm^3
RBC	4.3x10^6/μ	3.6-5.0x10^6/L	3.6-5.0 x10^{12}/L	MCH	26 pg/cell	26-34 pg/cell	0.40-.53 fmol/cell
MCV	77 μm^3	82-98μm^3	82-98 fL	MCHC	33 g/dl	32-36 g/dl	320-360 g/L

****

QUESTIONS CONTINUED:

12. Using the first set of lab values, list the parameters that are abnormal and give the possible explanations.

13. Do the same for the second set of lab values.

14. What can you tell from the fact that SR has decreased hgb and hct levels?
    a. Mrs SJ has a microcytic anemia.
    b. Mrs SJ has a macrocytic anemia.
    c. Mrs SJ has an anemia of chronic disease.
    d. Mrs SJ has an anemia.

15. If you include MCV and MCH with hgb and hct, what does it tell you?
    a. Mrs SJ has a microcytic anemia.
    b. Mrs SJ has a macrocytic anemia.
    c. Mrs SJ has an anemia of chronic disease.
    d. Mrs SJ has an anemia.

16. Briefly explain why you answered the above questions the way you did.

17. Mrs SJ's Ca was low in both sets of lab values probably because:
    a. her calcium intake was poor.
    b. she was dehydrated.
    c. she has osteoporosis.
    d. her serum albumin was low.

18. Briefly explain why you answered the above question as you did.

19. In the second set of lab values, glu, BUN, Cr, ser alb, hgb, and hct all dropped. This probably means that Mrs SJ was:
    a. bleeding.
    b. eating poorly in the hospital.
    c. dehydrated when the first labs were drawn.
    d. over hydrated when the second set of labs was drawn.

20. What caused lymphocytes, WBC, AST, and ALT to change between the two sets of labs?

21. What could be concluded from the low Cr level in the second set of lab values? (☺ *Hint: Consider Mrs. SJ's weight and muscle status.*)

22. Explain how Mrs. SJ's lifestyle and diet could have contributed to some of the results in the first set of lab values.

23. Considering Mrs. SJ's anthropometrics, medical history, and nutritional history, on a separate sheet of paper, outline a patient care plan for her. Be sure to include a teaching plan.

24. As if you were the dietitian assessing Mrs. SJ, write an appropriate SOAP note based on the information stated above.

    S:

    O:

    A:

    P:

EPILOGUE

In an attempt to make the cases more interesting, it would be noteworthy to leave some final remarks about some of the cases that are based on real occurrences. This case was embellished slightly to enable the student to learn, but most of it is factual information about my mother.

RELATED READING

1. Agostini, J.V., Han, L., & Tinetti, M.E. (2004). The relationship between number of medications and weight loss or impaired balance in older adults. *J Am Geriatr Soc*. 2004 Oct;52(10):1719-23.

2. Atkin, P.A., Stringer, R.S., Duffy, J.B., Elion, C., Ferraris, C.S. Misrachi, S.R., & Shenfield, G.M. (1998). The influence of information provided by patients on the accuracy of medication records. *Med. J. Aust.* 169(2):85-88.

3. Barone, L., Milosavljevic, M., & Gazibarich, B. (2003). Assessing the older person: is the MNA a more appropriate nutritional assessment tool than the SGA? *J Nutr Health Aging.* ;7:433-437.

4. Beers, MH, Munekata, M, & Storrie, M. (1990). The accuracy of medication histories in the hospital medical records of elderly persons. *J. Am. Geriatr. Soc.* 38(11):1183-1187.

5. Chumlea, W.M. & Sun, S.S. (2004). The availability of body composition reference data for the elderly. *J Nutr Health Aging*;8:76-78.

6. Delacorte, R.R., Moriguti, J.C., Matos, F.D., Pfrimer, K., Marchinil, J.S., & Ferriolli, E. (2004). Mini-nutritional assessment score and the risk for undernutrition in free-living older persons. *J Nutr Health Aging.* 8(6):531-4

7. Fischbach, F.T. (2003). *A Manual of Laboratory & Diagnostic Tests.* 7th Ed. Philadelphia. J.B. Lippincott Company.

8. Lamy, P.P. (1987). Age-associated pharmacodynamic changes. *Methods Find Exp Clin Pharmacol.* 9(3):153-159.

9. Lee, R.D., Nieman, D.C., & Nieman, D. (2002). *Nutritional Assessment*. 3rd Ed. McGraw-Hill.

10. Nutrition Screening Initiative. (1991). A project of the American Academy of Family Physicians, the American Dietetic Association, and the National Council on Aging, funded in part by Ross Laboratories. http://www.eatright.org/Public/SearchResults.cfm

11. Weddle, D.O., & Kuczmarski, F. (2000). Nutrition, aging and the continuum of care *J Am Diet Assoc*. 100:580-595.

12. Prendergast, A. & Fulton, F.L. (1997) *Medical terminology: A Text/Workbook.* 4th Ed. Redwood City, California. Addison-Wesley Nursing.

13. Pronsky, Z.M., Redfern, C.M., Crowe, J. & Epstein, S. (2003) *Food Medication Interactions,* 13th Ed Phoenix, Arizona. Food-Medications Interactions, Publishers and Distributors.

14. Price, D., Cooke, J., Singleton, S., & Feely, M. (1986). Doctors' unawareness of the drugs their patients are taking: a major cause of over prescribing? *Br. Med. J.* 292(6513):99-100.

15. Rolfes, S.R., Pinna, K. & Whitney, E. (2006). *Understanding Normal and Clinical Nutrition,* 7th Ed. West/Wadsworth.

16. Schlenker, E.D. (1997). *Nutrition in Aging.* St. Louis, Missouri. Mosby - Year Book, Inc.

17. Soini, H., Routasalo, P., & Lagström, H. (2004). Characteristics of the Mini-Nutritional Assessment in elderly home-care patients. *Eur J Clin Nutr.*;58:64-70.

18. Spratto, G.R. & Woods, A.L. (2005). *PDR Nurse's Drug Handbook.* Thompson Delmar Learning, NY.

19. Torrible, S.J., & Hogan, D.B. (1997). Medication use and rural seniors. Who really knows what they are taking? *Can. Fam. Phy.* 43:893-898.

20. Troncale, J.A. (1996). The aging process. Physiologic changes and pharmacologic implications. *Postgrad Med.* 99(5):111-114.

CASE STUDY #6
OBESITY TREATED WITH DIET

INTRODUCTION
This is the first of several studies that specifically pertain to the treatment of obesity in adults. Each study involves a different mode of treatment. In this study, dietary modification and exercise, the preferred components of treatment, are employed.

****

SKILLS NEEDED

ABBREVIATIONS:
Knowledge of the following abbreviations is required in order to understand this case. You should learn these abbreviations before you begin to read the study: BMI, Chol, IBW, lbs, Na, YOWM.

FORMULAS:
The formulas used in this case study include ideal body weight and percent ideal body weight (Appendix A, Tables 7 and 8).

****

RB is a 45 YOWM who is married with two children, ages 15 and 18. He is of Italian descent and loves to eat Italian food, although any kind of food will do. He takes pride in his ability to prepare Italian food. RB is a high school mathematics teacher who does not exercise. His love of food and lack of exercise have created a weight problem. For years he has endured much criticism from his family and friends about his health. His family history reveals several areas of concern. His father died of a heart attack and two brothers have had heart attacks. He has a brother and a sister who have high serum cholesterol and are on strict diets. Both of his parents and all of his grandparents had problems with high serum cholesterol. None of this really bothered him until recently. Since his last birthday he has become very concerned about his health and has decided to do something about his weight.

He is 5'10" and weighs 215 lbs. Throughout college he weighed 170 lbs and, according to his wife, "looked good." She wants him to look like that again, so he has decided to lose 45 lbs and get back to his college weight. He has even been talking about starting an exercise program and getting back into his college running condition. Because of his age and his strong family history of cardiovascular disease, his wife convinced him to obtain medical advice first. The family physician found him to be healthy except for his weight. The physician reinforced what the others had been telling him about losing weight and exercising more. He emphasized that he should start slowly and sent him to the clinic RD to discuss his weight problem. The RD interviewed him and obtained the following information:

RB sleeps as late as he can and is usually in a rush in the morning. He occasionally eats breakfast. He drinks a cup of coffee (with sugar) while getting ready for work. He does not eat in the school cafeteria at lunch because he does not like the food. He says it is not real food. The RD discovered that RB does not eat for the sake of eating or boredom; he eats because he enjoys good food. He brings a sandwich from home and drinks a soda. His sandwiches are usually egg salad, chicken salad, deli roast beef, or salami, made with rye, whole wheat, or sometimes French bread. He puts mustard and a little bit of mayonnaise with lettuce and tomato on his sandwiches.

He does not eat again until dinner. He likes to go home and work on his classes before eating. When he sits at the table in the evening, he wants to have the day behind him and nothing left to do but enjoy a good meal and go to bed. He usually helps prepare dinner, or he prepares it himself. This is the meal he lives for. The way RB sees it, he works hard during the day, skips breakfast, eats a light lunch, and does not snack much during the day so he deserves a big meal at night.

RB has never been to Italy but has researched the lifestyle and eating habits there. He has selected those recipes he likes and has combined them with some traditions of this country to come up with his own style of Italian food. The meal has to start with the American traditional tossed salad with about ¼ c of olive oil and vinegar dressing. The Italian tradition of pasta appears at each evening meal. Spaghetti, mostaccioli, fettuccini, or another form of pasta is always included. Tomato sauce, grated cheese, or cheese sauces are essential. Parmesan, Romano, and mozzarella are his favorites. RB and his wife use some chicken and shellfish, but beef and veal are more popular. Lots of Italian seasoning, salt, and olive oil are important. Garlic bread is included in each meal with olive oil and a touch of melted butter. RB insists on real butter for his cooking. He also likes to use real cream in his sauces. Egg batter helps to keep things together. The vegetables are usually eggplant, squash, artichokes, asparagus, or beets. He uses a lot of onions, garlic, bell pepper, celery, and parsley in his cooking. All of this is washed down with several glasses of wine and finished off with pistachio ice cream or an Italian pastry. The serving sizes vary a great deal, depending on the combination of foods served. However, excessive amounts of each food item are the norm rather than the exception. After eating there is some cleaning up to be done before bedtime. Weekend meals are not that much different except that the Sunday meal is usually earlier.
****

QUESTIONS:
1. Determine RB's IBW and percent IBW (Appendix A, Tables 7 and 8). Please show all calculations for this report.

2. Using the Harris-Benedict equation and the appropriate activity factor, calculate his daily energy needs (Appendix A, Table 17).

3. Determine his protein needs.

4. Determine his BMI and interpret the results in relation to health risks (Appendix A, Tables 10 and 11).

5. If RB were to lose one pound per week, he would have to reduce his daily caloric intake by how many kcals?

6. Explain the importance of exercise in RB's weight reduction plan. Include advice you would give RB about the elements of an exercise program, including starting a program, warming-up, duration, intensity, etc.

7. Give some examples of behavior changes you would recommend to RB to promote a healthier lifestyle. This would include nutrition, exercise, daily schedule, etc.

8. Briefly discuss the importance of RB's family medical history.

9. The RD's observation of the reason RB eats is important. Discuss how you would use this information in counseling RB.

10. In column one, list each food in RB's diet that is high in a potentially harmful nutrient. In columns 2 - 6, put a check by the foods that are high in these constituents. In column 7, give an example of a potentially healthier food that can be substituted for the food in column 1.

1)FOOD	2)TOT FAT	3)SAT FAT	4)CHOL	5)Na	6)SUGAR	7)SUBSTITUTE

11. Using the information obtained above, evaluate RB's diet for nutrient deficiencies and/or excesses.

12. RB believes it is all right to skip breakfast, eat light during the day, and eat a big meal at night. Is anything wrong with this kind of thinking? If so, identify the problem and describe the solution.

13. On a separate sheet of paper, plan a day's menu for RB, including kinds of food, amounts, and times eaten.

RELATED READINGS

1. Chisholm, D.J., Samaras, K., Markovic, T., Carey, D., Lapsys, N., & Campbell, L.V. (1998). Obesity: genes, glands or gluttony? *Reprod. Fertil. Dev.* 10(1):49-53.

2. Green, S.M. (1997). Obesity: prevalence, causes, health risks and treatment. *Br. J. Nurs.* 6(20):1181-1185.

3. Goel, M.S., McCarthy, E.P., Phillips, R.S., & Wee, C.C. (2004). Obesity among US immigrant subgroups by duration of residence. *JAMA.* Dec 15;292(23):2860-7.

4. Mancia, G., Volpe, R., Boros, S., Ilardi, M/, & Giannattasio, C. (2004). Cardiovascular risk profile and blood pressure control in Italian hypertensive patients under specialist care. *J Hypertens.* Jan;22(1):51-7.

5. National Heart, Lung, and Blood Institute. (1998). Clinical Guidelines on the Identification, Evaluation, and Treatment of Overweight and Obesity in Adult. National Institutes of Health. Publication 98-4083. http://www.nhlbi.nih.gov/guidelines/obesity/ob_gdlns.htm

6. Position paper of the American Dietetic Association. (2002). Weight management *J Am Diet Assoc.* 2002;102:1145-1155.

7. Rolfes, S.R., Pinna, K. & Whitney, E. (2006). *Understanding Normal and Clinical Nutrition*, 7th Ed. West/Wadsworth.

8. Strumpf, E. (2004). The obesity epidemic in the United States: causes and extent, risks and solutions. *Issue Brief* (Commonw Fund). Nov;(713):1-6.

9. Weight-control Information Network. November, (2001) *Understanding Adult Obesity*. NIH . NIH Publication No. 01-3680, October. http://win.niddk.nih.gov/publications/understanding.htm

10. Weight-control Information Network. March, (2001). *Weight Cycling*. NIH Publication No. NIH Publication No. 01-3901. e-text updated March 2004. http://win.niddk.nih.gov/publications/cycling.htm

11. Weight-control Information Network. May, (2004). *Do you know the health risks of being overweight?* NIH Publication No. 04-4098, e-text posted: November 2004. http//win.niddk.nih.gov/publications/health_risks.htm

12. Weinsier, R.L., Hunter, G.R., Heini, A.F., Goran, M.I., & Sell, S.M. (1998). The etiology of obesity: relative contribution of metabolic factors, diet, and physical activity. *Am. J. Med.* 105(2):145-150.

CASE STUDY #7
OBESITY TREATED WITH SURGERY

INTRODUCTION

This study, like Case Study #6, is also concerned with obesity, but the treatment in this case is centered around surgery rather than diet. Surgery is intended for those who are morbidly obese and cannot obtain weight reduction with diet alone. Most dietitians do not favor this type of treatment for obesity. The old adage, "an ounce of prevention is worth a pound of cure," is the preferred approach. Another way of saying this is to have a "healthy lifestyle" that includes proper diet and exercise to prevent obesity. However, once someone becomes morbidly obese, it is very difficult to lose weight. Exercise may not be a possibility. If the obesity becomes life threatening, some resort to surgery. With the increase in obesity, there has been an increase in this type of surgery. There are many different procedures available. Agreeing or disagreeing with the procedure is not the main point of this case study. If there are those who will have this surgery, then dietitians need to understand the risks, complications, and treatment so that they can provide the patient with the "best" nutritional follow-up.
****

SKILLS NEEDED

ABBREVIATIONS:
Knowledge of the following abbreviations is required in order to understand this case. You should learn these abbreviations before you begin to read the study: c, FH, MH, oz, SH, SOB, T, tsp, and YOWM (Appendix C).

FORMULAS:
The formulas used in this case study include ideal body weight, adjusted body weight (Appendix A, Tables 7 and 9), the Harris-Benedict equation, activity factors, and protein requirements (Appendix A, Table 17).
****

Mr. Y is a 39 YOWM with morbid obesity. He is 6'1" and weighs 320 lbs. He has been overweight all his life, even as a child. He and his doctor have noticed that there is a definite correlation between his increase in age and his increase in weight. He has tried numerous diets without success. He has lost a significant amount of weight with some diets, but they were "so monotonous" he could not stay on them. When he went off a diet, it seemed like he would eat even more, like he was trying to catch up on the food he missed. He is an accountant with a desk job, one at which he can eat all day long without opportunity for exercise. He has never had an exercise program.

His doctor warned him that if he did not do something about his weight, he would not live to see his grandchildren. Mr. Y has been noticing an increased SOB and difficulty accomplishing simple physical tasks. Even though his FH is good concerning heart attacks, strokes, diabetes, cancer, etc., his doctor informed him that he was at a much higher risk for these diseases. He also pointed out that no one in his family was as big as he was. Therefore, Mr. Y decided to take drastic measures to lose weight. He agreed to have gastric partitioning surgery. His doctor explained the risks and benefits of the surgery. He referred him to a surgeon who had a good record with bariatric surgery. He was admitted to the hospital on Monday and was to have surgery on Wednesday. The physician asked the RD to visit him and begin teaching him his new diet. The RD read his chart and made note of his FH, SH, and MH. His lab values were not significant. The RD went into Mr. Y's room to interview him and to determine his usual intake. She obtained the following information:

Mr. Y claimed that he does not eat that much. On a typical day, he gets up at 7 A.M. and eats breakfast with his wife. Usually this consists of:

➢ 2 fried eggs
➢ 1 c grits

➤ 1 glass of orange juice (8 oz)
➤ 2 pieces of toast with 1 pat of margarine and 1 T jelly per slice
➤ 2 c of coffee with 1 tsp of cream and 2 tsp of sugar

Once at work, he snacks on food all day. He always has coffee (the usual cream and sugar) or iced tea (with 2 tsp of sugar per 8 oz) on his desk and "sips" all day. In the morning, glazed doughnuts are usually available. Cheese crackers are one of his favorite snacks, and every now and then, a candy bar appeals to him. Sometimes he brings a big can of roasted peanuts or a bag of candy, like chocolate-covered raisins, and eats "one or two every now and then." By lunch he has worked up an appetite. He and his co-workers usually eat at the sandwich shop across the street. He likes the sloppy roast beef or club special. He must have french fries with the sandwich; the two "sort of just go together." He said he knows that you need fiber in your diet, so a salad is the norm also, with about ¼ c of French dressing. He may have a dessert that consists of homemade pie and/or a scoop of ice cream for calcium.

He follows the same routine in the afternoon as he does in the morning. At suppertime, his wife has a big meal for him. This consists of salad for fiber with ¼ c of salad dressing. He has at least 4 to 5 ounces of meat, as roast with gravy, fried chicken, or fried fish if it's Friday. Sometimes beef steak, ham steak, or fried pork chops are served. Potatoes, rice, or macaroni are always included as the starch ("about 1 cup or so"). She always has a vegetable. Carrots, green beans, and squash are typical. These are usually prepared with salt and butter, fat back, or bacon. Several slices of bread and butter are always served. The drink is tea, sweetened with 2 tsp of sugar per 8 oz. Several glasses per meal is not uncommon. He is still not "big on desserts" but, when his wife fixes something, he eats his share. Mr. Y eats his food very fast, taking little time to chew properly. He enjoys his food so much that he wants to eat it as fast as possible. This is not only true for his evening meal, but for everything he eats. This is a habit he developed as a child.

After supper he is really not that full, so as he sits in front of the TV and relaxes with the newspaper he continues to munch on popcorn (salted, with lots of melted butter), peanuts, cookies, or whatever is in the house. A couple of beers always helps him relax, but he only drinks light beer because it is "less filling." It does not take too long for Mr. Y to become very sleepy. Before he goes to bed, he eats a big bowl of ice cream for calcium.
****

QUESTIONS:
1. Determine Mr. Y's IBW (Appendix A, Table 7). Please show all calculations in this report.

2. Considering the difference between the IBW and the actual body weight, calculate an adjusted body weight (Appendix A, Table 9).

3. Using the adjusted body weight in the Harris-Benedict equation and an activity factor (Appendix A, Table 17), determine Mr. Y's daily energy needs.

4. Calculate Mr. Y's BMI and explain what the results mean (Appendix A, Tables 10 and 11).

5. Determine his daily protein needs.

6. Based on Mr. Y's food record, estimate his energy and protein intake.

7. Assess Mr. Y's diet for possible nutrient deficiencies or excesses.

8. How many calories and how many grams of protein do you recommend for Mr. Y after he as completely healed from surgery?

9. How much food will Mr. Y be able to eat at one sitting after surgery? What are the possible complications if he eats more than the recommended amount?

10. What would be an alternative Ca source?

11. List the foods in Mr. Y's diet that are high in fat or simple sugars and suggest an appropriate substitute.

12. Are there any foods in Mr. Y's diet that contain substances that could bind to or react with essential nutrients and render them unavailable? Identify these foods, the harmful substance they contain, and the nutrient(s) they react with.

13. If we chewed our food very well and ate slowly, could we lose weight? The kind and amount of food we eat is important to our health but how and when we eat is also important. Mr. Y eats very quickly with very little chewing. Discuss the importance of chewing. Include in your discussion the glucostatic theory of hunger and its possible relationship to chewing and the rate at which we eat.

14. Considering the discussion in question 13, why was Mr. Y probably still hungry (when he sat in front of the television) after his evening meal?

15. Mr. Y went to bed after his TV snacks and ice cream, which was not long after supper. How could this contribute to his weight gain?

16. If Mr. Y started an exercise program, should he do aerobic exercise, anaerobic exercise, or both? Explain your answer and give examples of the types of exercises that Mr. Y could do.

17. Describe the ways in which exercise would help Mr. Y lose weight.

18. Define bariatric surgery.

19. Using your textbook or your state or local diet manual, describe the principles of a gastric partitioning diet.

20. There is more than one surgical procedure for gastric partitioning. Most basic clinical texts provide illustrations of the possible procedures. Using such a text (or see the references at the end of this case), sketch at least one surgical procedure and label all anatomical parts related to the surgery.

21. What are the complications of this surgery?

22. If you had to counsel Mr. Y, what are some examples of behavior modifications you would use? Include in your discussion why Mr. Y would have to chew his food extremely well after the surgery.

23. Should Mr. Y take a vitamin and mineral supplement? Why or why not?

24. Do you think Mr. Y could still gain weight after this surgery? If so, explain how.

25. On a separate sheet of paper, plan a day's menu for Mr. Y. Include in your plan the amount of food, the texture, and the time of day that it should be consumed.

RELATED READINGS

1. Chisholm, D.J., Samaras, K., Markovic, T., Carey, D., Lapsys, N., & Campbell, L.V. (1998). Obesity: genes, glands or gluttony? *Reprod. Fertil. Dev.* 10(1):49-53.

2. De Witt Hamer, P.C. & Tuinebreijer, W.E. (1998). Preoperative weight gain in bariatric surgery. *bes. Surg.* 8(3):289-295.

3. Deitel, M. (1998). Commentary: joint pains after various intestinal bypasses and secondary to obesity. *Obes. Surg.* 8(3):265.

4. Fobi, M.A., & Lee, H. (1998). The surgical technique of the Fobi-Pouch operation for obesity (the transected silastic vertical gastric bypass). *Obes. Surg.* 8(3):283-288.

5. Hess, D.S. & Hess, D.W. (1998). Biliopancreatic diversion with a duodenal switch. *Obes. Surg.* 8(3):267-282.

6. Lara, M..D, Kothari. S,,N, & Sugerman, H.J. (2005). Surgical management of obesity: a review of the evidence relating to the health benefits and risks. *Treat Endocrinol.*;4(1):55-64.

7. National Heart, Lung, and Blood Institute. (1998). Clinical Guidelines on the Identification, Evaluation, and Treatment of Overweight and Obesity in Adult. National Institutes of Health. Publication 98-4083. http://www.nhlbi.nih.gov/guidelines/obesity/ob_gdlns.htm

8. Noshiro, H, & Tanaka, M. (2005). Evaluating obesity before surgery. *Ann Surg.* Feb;241(2):383.

9. Position paper of the American Dietetic Association. (2002). Weight management *J Am Diet Assoc.* 2002;102:1145-1155.

10. Rolfes, S.R., Pinna, K. & Whitney, E. (2006). *Understanding Normal and Clinical Nutrition*, 7th Ed. West/Wadsworth.

11. Strumpf, E. (2004). The obesity epidemic in the United States: causes and extent, risks and solutions. *Issue Brief* (Commonw Fund).Nov;(713):1-6.

12. Van Itallie, T.B. (1990). The glucostatic theory 1953- 1988: roots and branches. *Int. J. Obes.* 14 Suppl 3:1-10.

13. Weight-control Information Network. November, (2001) *Understanding Adult Obesity*. NIH . NIH Publication No. 01-3680, October. http://win.niddk.nih.gov/publications/understanding.htm

14. Weight-control Information Network. March, (2001). *Weight Cycling*. NIH Publication No. NIH Publication No. 01-3901. e-text updated March 2004. http://win.niddk.nih.gov/publications/cycling.htm

15. Weight-control Information Network. May, (2004). *Do you know the health risks of being overweight?* NIH Publication No. 04-4098, e-text posted: November 2004. http//win.niddk.nih.gov/publications/health_risks.htm

CASE STUDY #8
OBESITY TREATED WITH VLCD

INTRODUCTION
This is the third study of obesity. The study may seem unusual because the patient is so large, but it is based on an actual case in which the original patient weighed much more than this one. The very-low-calorie weight reduction diet is not favored by nutritionists and MDs, but it is used by some for the treatment of the morbidly obese and it should be understood by health care professionals. Medical terminology is also emphasized in this case study.
****

SKILLS NEEDED
ABBREVIATIONS:
Knowledge of the following abbreviations is required in order to understand this case. You should learn these abbreviations before you begin to read the study, but common abbreviations used several times in previous case studies are not included in this list.
ABGs, BIA, BMI, BMR, C/O, DVT, ER, HCO_3, Hg, LBM, milliIU/L, ng/dl, $PaCO_2$, PaO_2, pg, pH, PT, PVC, qts, SBR, sec, SOB, TSH, T_3, T_4, VLCD, and, 2° (Appendix C).

LABORATORY VALUES:
You will need to be able to interpret the nutritional significance of the following laboratory values for this case study: BUN, Ca, Cl, CO_2, Cr, glucose, hct, hgb, HCO_3, K, lymph, MCH, MCHC, MCV, Mg, Na, P, PaO_2, $PaCO_2$, pH, PT, RBC, ser alb, TSH, T_3, T_4, and WBC (Appendix B).

FORMULAS:
The formulas used in this case study include ideal body weight, percent ideal body weight, adjusted body weight (Appendix A, Tables 7 and 8), and body mass index (Appendix A, Tables 10 and 11).
****

TB is an unemployed, 27 YOWM who used to drive a tractor-trailer rig across country. His boss fired him about two years ago when TB's weight had increased so much that it was impairing his work. During high school, TB was very active as an All-State defensive tackle. He weighed 280 lbs and was 6'3" tall. TB was heavily recruited by several universities and attended college for one year but injured his right knee and was no longer able to play football. He quit college but continued to eat as if he were still playing ball. TB held several odd jobs before he learned how to drive tractor-trailer rigs.

During high school TB ate a huge amount of food but was so active that he had no problem maintaining his weight at 280 lbs. TB's truck driving job was very sedentary and he ate more than he did in high school, mostly out of boredom. He slowly gained weight over the years; he weighed 460 lbs a little over a year ago. He became so large that he could not find a job. His friends made so much fun of him that he avoided them. TB wanted to be active in sports again but was too big to exercise and still had the knee problem. He could not walk more than 50 feet without becoming winded. Unable to fit into most cars, TB was left with nothing to do but sit at home and feel sorry for himself.

His family consisted of his mother, two younger sisters, and a younger brother. They hated to see him sitting around with nothing to do, so, with all the good intentions in the world, they chose to provide him with the one thing he loved—food. His mother and sisters would fix him anything he wanted. Eating became his favorite pass time, his escape from reality. He spent the better part of the day eating, watching TV, and gaining weight. The more weight he gained, the less he moved about, and his self-pity and depression increased. The greater the depression, the more he ate, and the cycle continued.

For the last year TB was severely SOB. He was easily tired and even a small amount of movement caused him to be winded. Recently, he C/O throbbing headaches. His face got flushed and he perspired considerably. He had prolonged drowsiness but did not sleep well at night. Two weeks ago he started with a new symptom; he C/O pain in his left calf and was having such a hard time breathing, his sisters panicked and called 911. The paramedics gave TB some O_2 and brought him to the ER of the county hospital. He was stabilized and weighed in on the freight scales at 552 lbs. The ER physician found TB to be SOB to the point of having cyanotic extremities, particularly the toes. He was experiencing tachycardia with occasional PVCs. His left calf was tender to touch, warm, and seemed to be swollen but it was difficult to examine properly because of his massive size. The ER physician was concerned that TB had a DVT. A venogram was completed and showed filling defects and diverted blood flow, positive for thrombophlebitis. His labs were as follows:

CBC							
TEST	**RESULT**	**REFERENCE UNITS** Conventional	SI	**TEST**	**RESULT**	**REFERENCE UNITS** Conventional	SI
Hgb	17 g/dl	14 - 17.4 g/dl	140-174 g/L	WBC	5.5 10^3/µl	4.5-10.5 x 10^3/cells/ mm^3	4.5-10.5 x 10^9/L
Hct	43%	42 – 52%		% Lymph	29%	25 – 40% of total WBC	1500-4000 cells/mm^3
RBC	4.8x10^6/µ	3.6-5.0x10^6/L	3.6-5.0x10^{12}/L	MCH	24 pg/cell	26-34 pg/cell	0.40-.53 fmol/cell
MCV	90 µm^3	82-98µm^3	82-98 fL	MCHC	36 g/dl	32-36 g/dl	320-360 g/L

BASIC METABOLIC PACKAGE							
TEST	**RESULT**	**REFERENCE UNITS** Conventional	SI	**TEST**	**RESULT**	**REFERENCE UNITS** Conventional	SI
Glu	145 mg/dl	70-110 mg/dl	3.8-6.1 mmol/L	Na	137 mEq/L	136-145 mEq/L	136-145 mmol/L
BUN	13 mg/dl	6-20 mg/dl	2.1-7.1 mmol/L	K	4.8 mEq/L	3.5-5.2 mEq/L	3.5-5.2 mmol/L
Cr	1.2 mg/dl	0.9-1.3 mg/dl	80-115 µmol/L	Cl	106 mEq/L	96-106 mEq/L	96-106 mmol/L
Ca	9.2 mg/dl	8.8-10.0 mg/dl	2.20-2.60 mmol/L	Mg	2.0 mEq/L	1.8 - 2.6 mEq/L	136-145 mmol/L
Ser alb	3.7 g/dl	3.5-4.8 g/dl	39-50 g/dl	P	3.3mg/dl	2.7-4.5 mg/dl	4.7-6.0 kPa

ABGs					
TEST	**RESULT**	**NORM**	**TEST**	**RESULT**	**NORM**
PaO_2	88mm Hg	80-90 mm Hg	$PaCO_2$	58mm Hg	35-45 mm Hg
HCO_3^-	22 mEq/L	24-28 mEq/L	pH	7.31	7.35-7.45

The ER physician diagnosed the patient as follows:
➢ 1. Morbidly obese
➢ 2. Pickwickian syndrome
➢ 3. Mild tachycardia 2° to obesity/Pickwickian syndrome

➤ 4. Mild respiratory acidosis 2° to Pickwickian syndrome
➤ 5. DVT 2° to obesity and immobilization
➤ 6. Polycythemia 2° to Pickwickian syndrome

His treatment included:
- 1. SBR with heat applied to left calf
- 2. Heparin therapy
- 3. Head of bed elevated
- 4. VLCD of 800 kcals

The VLCD is sometimes used with the very obese. Several VLCD plans are available that are sponsored by hospitals, wellness centers, etc. The patients are usually closely monitored by an MD, RD, exercise physiologist, and psychologist. Most plans provide 70 g of protein, 100 g of carbohydrate, and about 800 kcals. The physician in charge of TB's care used a diet like this, allowing him 800 kcals and 100 g of carbohydrate. The usual range is from 600 to 900 kcals. The entire diet is usually in a liquid form for approximately the first three months. Emphasis is placed on maintaining a sodium restriction (2 g of sodium per day), ingesting no more than 300 mg of caffeine per day, consuming at least 2 qts of fluid per day, incorporating an individualized exercise prescription, and attending behavior modification classes. The program also includes a bi-weekly visit with a physician and bi-weekly analyses of blood and urine. This continues for approximately 12 weeks. Solid food is gradually added to the diet, replacing the liquid supplement until about 1000 to 1200 kcals are reached. A registered dietitian teaches weekly nutrition classes and supervises the addition of solid food to the diet. A diet of solid food without supplements is accomplished by the 5th or 6th week after the 12 week fast. A high potency multivitamin and mineral tablet along with 50 mEq K and 800 mg of Ca/d are recommended during the fasting period.
****

QUESTIONS:

1. The events leading up to TB's depression and excessive weight gain are not uncommon. When someone who leads an active lifestyle slows down suddenly, rapid weight gain will occur. List the events that contributed to TB's problem and explain how each of these events contributed.

2. If you had the opportunity to counsel TB about his weight when he weighed 480 lbs, on a separate sheet of paper, describe how you would handle this consultation. There is no single correct answer to this question. The following are some examples of the problems you want to address.
    A. A person of this size is used to consuming huge amounts of food. What could TB do to help keep his mind off of food?
    B. Think about an exercise program for TB. What could he do for exercise?
    C. Determine if there are any support groups for the obese in your area. If so, describe how to involve TB with that support group.

3. Calculate TB's BMI and evaluate the results (Appendix A, Tables 10 and 11).

4. Determine TB's IBW and percent of IBW (Appendix A, Tables 7 and 8). Please show all calculations.

5. There is considerable variation between TB's IBW and actual body weight. Calculate TB's adjusted body weight (Appendix A, Table 9).

6. In this case, do you think that using the adjusted body weight is an accurate way to calculate TB's caloric and protein needs? Explain your answer. If you do not think it is accurate, relate how you would estimate TB's caloric and protein needs.

Information Box 8 - 1

Question 7 is a difficult one. You will not find an answer in any resource that accurately addresses all sides of the issue. Patients of this size are difficult to evaluate. The caloric/protein requirements will depend on a number of factors, including age, level of activity, hormone levels, disease condition, the genetic influences on basal metabolic rate, and body composition. Body composition, or ratio of lean body mass (LBM) to adipose tissue, is an important consideration but is difficult to evaluate with a patient this large. BIA is only accurate when a patient's hydration status is normal. A "normal" hydration status of an obese person that is dieting is also difficult to evaluate. Body composition can be determined by means of skinfold measurements, but the calipers that exist are too small to make this test possible with TB. The patient would be too large to fit into the equipment for underwater weighing. The best answer should come from a dietitian who is experienced in working with the morbidly obese. (**Hint:** *Evaluate the patient the as well as you can based on the information provided and find a RD with experience working with the morbidly obese to obtain an "oral communication" reference.*)

---

7. Calculate TB's protein requirement.

8. Explain the rationale behind the VLCD.

9. Describe the drawbacks and potential hazards of the VLCD. Do the benefits outweigh the disadvantages in this case?

10. Why would caffeine be restricted?

11. Briefly discuss why most weight reduction diets emphasize restricting sodium.

12. What relationship, if any, does potassium have with this diet?

13. Discuss the importance of behavior modification.

14. With a patient of this size, how could the exercise component be implemented?

15. What symptoms can be expected during the first several days of such a fast?

16. When the fast is over, the patient slowly returns to a regular diet. What is the rationale for this?

17. Do you agree with the prescription of a 1000 to 1200 kcal diet for this patient after the fast is over? Discuss your answer. If you do not agree, what kcal level do you recommend?

18. On a separate sheet of paper, plan a 1200 kcal diet for a patient weighing 562 lbs.

19. Review the first table of lab values. Describe the relationship, if any, between the abnormal lab values and TB's nutritional status.

20. Define the following terms:

    Cyanotic:

    Tachycardia:

    Thrombophlebitis:

    Morbid obesity:

    Pickwickian syndrome:

    Respiratory acidosis:

    Polycythemia:

    Decubiti:

21. Would TB be a candidate for gastric surgery to prevent obesity? Explain your answer.

EPILOGUE

This is based on a true case that was modified to make it more believable. This was a patient of mine when I worked with a nutrition support team. The real patient weighed over 800 pounds. Even at that size, his lab values are an accurate portrayal of his real values.

RELATED READINGS

1. Chisholm, D.J., Samaras, K., Markovic, T., Carey, D., Lapsys, N., & Campbell, L.V. (1998). Obesity: genes, glands or gluttony? *Reprod. Fertil. Dev.* 10(1):49-53.

2. Fischbach, F.T. (2003). *A Manual of Laboratory & Diagnostic Tests.* 7th Ed. Philadelphia. J.B. Lippincott Company.

3. Lee, R.D., Nieman, D.C., & Nieman, D. (2002). *Nutritional Assessment.* 3rd Ed. McGraw-Hill.

4. Mayer, J. (1996) Glucostatic mechanism of regulation of food intake. *Obes. Res.* 4(5): 493-496.

5. National Heart, Lung, and Blood Institute. (1998). Clinical Guidelines on the Identification, Evaluation, and Treatment of Overweight and Obesity in Adult. National Institutes of Health. Publication 98-4083. http://www.nhlbi.nih.gov/guidelines/obesity/ob_gdlns.htm

6. Position paper of the American Dietetic Association. (2002). Weight management *J Am Diet Assoc.* 2002;102:1145-1155.

7. Rolfes, S.R., Pinna, K. & Whitney, E. (2006). *Understanding Normal and Clinical Nutrition,* 7th Ed. West/Wadsworth.

8. Strumpf, E. (2004). The obesity epidemic in the United States: causes and extent, risks and solutions. *Issue Brief* (Commonw Fund).Nov;(713):1-6.

9. Weight-control Information Network. November, (2001) *Understanding Adult Obesity.* NIH . NIH Publication No. 01-3680, October. http://win.niddk.nih.gov/publications/understanding.htm

10. Weight-control Information Network. March, (2001). *Weight Cycling.* NIH Publication No. NIH Publication No. 01-3901. e-text updated March 2004. http://win.niddk.nih.gov/publications/cycling.htm

11. Weight-control Information Network. May, (2004). *Do you know the health risks of being overweight?* NIH Publication No. 04-4098, e-text posted: November 2004. http//win.niddk.nih.gov/publications/health_risks.htm

12. Weinsier, R.L., Hunter, G.R., Heini, A.F., Goran, M.I., & Sell, S.M. (1998). The etiology of obesity: relative contribution of metabolic factors, diet, and physical activity. *Am. J. Med.* 105(2):145-150.

CASE STUDY #9
WEIGHT MANAGEMENT WITH CULTURAL CONCERNS

INTRODUCTION

This case study is about a migrant worker from Mexico who is overweight and has additional problems as well. Some cultural practices of Mexico are introduced. A review of the cultural and dietary practices of Mexican-Americans would be beneficial to the understanding of this case.
****

SKILLS NEEDED

ABBREVIATIONS:

Knowledge of the following abbreviations is required in order to understand this case. You should learn these abbreviations before you begin to read the study.

D_5W, ER, Fm^3, GI, I.V., NPO, Trig, and 1/4NS (Appendix C).

LABORATORY VALUES:

You will need to be able to interpret the nutritional significance of the following laboratory values for this case study: BUN, Ca, Cl, Cr, Glucose, hct, hgb, K, Lymphocytes, MCH, MCHC, MCV, Mg, Na, P, RBC, ser alb, and WBC (Appendix B).

FORMULAS:

The formulas used in this case study are ideal body weight and percent ideal body weight (Appendix A, Tables 7 and 8).

MEDICATIONS:

Become familiar with the following medications before reading the case study. Note the diet-drug interactions, dosages and methods of administration, gastrointestinal tract reactions, etc.

1. Phenergan (promethazine hydrochloride); 2. Lomotil (diphenoxylate hydrochloride).
****

Mrs. MG is a 43-year-old Mexican-American who has been living in this country for several years. She and part of her family migrated to Texas from rural Mexico looking for work. Mrs. MG's household includes her husband, five children, and her mother-in-law. Mrs. MG and her husband have been working as migrant farm workers for less than minimum wage. Mrs. MG has been healthy but recently has been experiencing symptoms of gastroenteritis, including bloating, nausea, and diarrhea. She throws-up occasionally but not on a regular basis. She has not been able to eat very much because of her illness. This continued for almost a week before her husband decided to take her to a doctor. By the time she went to the emergency room, she was very weak, dehydrated, confused, and disoriented. Observing her condition and her obvious state of poverty, the ER physician decided to admit her for a couple of days so that she could recover from what he thought was simple dehydration and a stomach virus.

An examination of Mrs. MG revealed the following: Mrs. MG was 5'3" and weighed 165 lbs. She has always been overweight but has slowly been losing weight over the last year. Her labs completed in the ER are posted below with her admission orders.

The dietitian was new to the south Texas area and was not yet familiar with Mexican-American customs. Mrs. MG and her husband spoke very poor English, and the RD did not speak Spanish. She had a very difficult time communicating and could not get Mrs. MG to commit to anything she asked her to do. The RD noticed that Mrs. MG looked at her husband to see his reaction to everything the dietitian said. The RD decided to end the conversation in order to go do some research and obtain the help of an interpreter.

BASIC METABOLIC PACKAGE							
TEST	**RESULT**	**REFERENCE UNITS Conventional**	**SI**	**TEST**	**RESULT**	**REFERENCE UNITS Conventional**	**SI**
Glu	225 mg/dl	70-110 mg/dl	3.8-6.1 mmol/L	Na	151 mEq/L	136-145 mEq/L	136-145 mmol/L
BUN	31mg/dl	6-20 mg/dl	2.1-7.1 mmol/L	K	5.0 mEq/L	3.5-5.2 mEq/L	3.5-5.2 mmol/L
Cr	1.6 mg/dl	0.6-1.1 mg/dl	53-97 µmol/L	Cl	108 mEq/L	96-106 mEq/L	96-106 mmol/L
Ca	9.0 mg/dl	8.8-10.0 mg/dl	2.20-2.60 mmol/L	Mg	2.1 mEq/L	1.8 - 2.6 mEq/L	136-145 mmol/L
Ser alb	4.9 g/dl	3.5-4.8 g/dl	39-50 g/dl	P	4.0mg/dl	2.7-4.5 mg/dl	4.7-6.0 kPa

CBC							
TEST	**RESULT**	**REFERENCE UNITS Conventional**	**SI**	**TEST**	**RESULT**	**REFERENCE UNITS Conventional**	**SI**
Hgb	17 g/dl	12-16 g/dl	120-160 g/L	WBC	8.5 10^3/µl	4.5-10.5 x 10^3/cells/mm^3	4.5-10.5 x10^9/L
Hct	51 %	36-48%		% Lymph	26%	25 – 40% of total WBC	1500-4000 cells/mm^3
RBC	4.5x10^6/µ	3.6-5.0x10^6/L	3.6-5.0 x10^{12}/L	MCH	26 pg/cell	26-34 pg/cell	0.40-.53 fmol/cell
MCV	80 µm^3	82-98µm^3	82-98 fL	MCHC	32 g/dl	32-36 g/dl	320-360 g/L

Doctor's Orders

10/1/98 Admit Mrs. MG to gen med service

I.V. - D5 W 1/2 NS @ 100 cc/h

Phenergan 25mg po q 4h

Lomotil 5mg po qid x 1d then 5mg bid

BRP as able

NPO

RD to see pt.

[illegible]

Through her research on Mexican culture, the RD learned that the family and the extended family are of central importance to an individual's life. Most decisions are made by the male head of the household, who is strongly influenced by his mother. Individual members of the family do not like to make hasty decisions but prefer to talk things over with the family first. This is why the RD could not get Mrs. MG to commit to anything. She also learned that Mrs. MG's culture relies on home remedies first before seeking outside help. When they do seek outside help, it is usually from a folk healer or native healer rather than from a physician.

This explains why Mrs. MG's husband waited so long before he took her to the hospital. Late that afternoon the RD went back to see Mrs. MG with a diet technician who understood the culture and could speak Spanish. Before going to see Mrs. MG again, the RD checked the chart to see if anything new had been entered. She found a new set of lab values that had been completed that afternoon.

BASIC METABOLIC PACKAGE							
TEST	**RESULT**	**REFERENCE UNITS** Conventional	SI	**TEST**	**RESULT**	**REFERENCE UNITS** Conventional	SI
Glu	205 mg/dl	70-110 mg/dl	3.8-6.1 mmol/L	Na	143 mEq/L	136-145 mEq/L	136-145 mmol/L
BUN	17mg/dl	6-20 mg/dl	2.1-7.1 mmol/L	K	3.8 mEq/L	3.5-5.2 mEq/L	3.5-5.2 mmol/L
Cr	1.0 mg/dl	0.6-1.1 mg/dl	53-97 μmol/L	Cl	105 mEq/L	96-106 mEq/L	96-106 mmol/L
Ca	9.2 mg/dl	8.8-10.0 mg/dl	2.20-2.60 mmol/L	Mg	1.9 mEq/L	1.8 - 2.6 mEq/L	136-145 mmol/L
Ser alb	3.9 g/dl	3.5-4.8 g/dl	39-50 g/dl	P	2..8mg/dl	2.7-4.5 mg/dl	4.7-6.0 kPa

CBC							
TEST	**RESULT**	**REFERENCE UNITS** Conventional	SI	**TEST**	**RESULT**	**REFERENCE UNITS** Conventional	SI
Hgb	12 g/dl	12-16 g/dl	120-160 g/L	WBC	7.5 10^3/μl	4.5-10.5 x 10^3/cells/mm^3	4.5-10.5 x10^9/L
Hct	36 %	36-48%		% Lymph	26%	25 – 40% of total WBC	1500-4000 cells/mm^3
RBC	4.4x10^6/μ	3.6-5.0x10^6/L	3.6-5.0 x10^{12}/L	MCH	27 pg/cell	26-34 pg/cell	0.40-.53 fmol/cell
MCV	81 μm^3	82-98μm^3	82-98 fL	MCHC	33 g/dl	32-36 g/dl	320-360 g/L

QUESTIONS:

1. What is Mrs. MG's IBW and percent IBW (Appendix A, Tables 7 and 8)?

2. Calculate Mrs. MG's BMI (Appendix A, Tables 10 and 11).

3. Write out the physician's orders in long-hand and explain abbreviations as appropriate.

4. In the second set of lab values, glu, BUN, Cr, ser alb, hgb, and hct all dropped. This probably means that Mrs MG was:
   a. bleeding.
   b. eating poorly in the hospital.
   c. dehydrated when the first labs were drawn.
   d. over hydrated when the second set of labs was drawn.

5. What can you tell from the fact that Mrs. MG has decreased hgb and hct levels?
   a. Mrs. MG has a microcytic anemia.
   b. Mrs. MG has a macrocytic anemia.
   c. Mrs. MG has an anemia of chronic disease.
   d. Mrs. MG has an anemia.

6. If you include MCV and MCH with hgb and hct, what does it tell you?
   a. Mrs. MG has a microcytic anemia.
   b. Mrs. MG has a macrocytic anemia.
   c. Mrs. MG has an anemia of chronic disease.
   d. Mrs. MG has an anemia.

7. Briefly explain why you answered the above questions the way you did.

Information Box 9 - 1

The number of calories provided by D_5W will contribute to the patient's caloric intake and needs to be accounted for. However, it must be remembered that this intake will never be sufficient to meet anyone's caloric needs. D_5W is equivalent to half-strength Kool-Aid without the added vitamin C. To determine the grams of glucose provided by I.V. infusions, determine the amount of cc infused per day (flow rate X 24 hrs) and multiply by the percent glucose in the solution. In this case it is 5%. To determine the caloric contribution from this, multiply the grams by 3.4. Glucose is normally 4 kcals per gram, but in solution it is in a hydrated state and is 3.4 kcals per gram.[1]

[1] Rombeau, J.L., and Caldwell, M.D. (1993). Clinical Nutrition: PARENTERAL NUTRITION, 2nd Ed. W.B. Saunders Company, Philadelphia pg. 310.

8. Mrs. MG received D$_5$W in 1/4 NS at 100 cc/hr. How many grams of glucose and how many calories would that provide per day?

****

The RD went into Mrs. MG's room with the diet tech and made all of the appropriate introductions. Mrs. MG's husband was there so the RD interviewed both of them with the help of the interpreter. The results were as follows:

Mrs. MG and her family, with the guidance of a local folk healer, thought she had "Empacho." This is something similar to gastroenteritis and is believed to be caused by a blockage in the GI tract. The RD questioned her about symptoms of frequent urination, thirst, and hunger and learned that Mrs. MG experienced all of these in the past few months. The RD also found out that Mrs. MG's father had a disease that caused him to have his foot amputated, but she did not know what it was.

Her diet in this country had not changed much from her native diet in Mexico. Every day she ate some kind of beans, pinto and black beans being her favorites. Tortillas were also part of the everyday diet. She ate fried corn tortillas. Pork was the favorite meat, particularly "chorizos," if it was available. Fried foods were high on her list, and typically lard was used as the fat. Vegetables included tomatoes, onions, squash, garlic, and chili peppers of all kinds. She did not drink very much milk; lactose intolerance seemed to be a problem. Mrs. MG liked cheese and fresh fruit, but both were rarely included in the diet because of the cost. Foods that she has enjoyed since she has been in this country are hamburgers, french fries, potato chips, sodas, and candy.
****

QUESTIONS CONTINUED:

9. Considering Mrs. MG's family medical history, weight history, and most recent set of lab values, what was the RD looking for with her line of questions about frequent urination, thirst, hunger etc.?

10. List the diet principles Mrs. MG should follow and, based on the principles you list, prescribe an appropriate specific diet for Mrs. MG.

11. Based on Mrs. MG's recall, what nutrients are apparently deficient in her diet?

12. List any protein combinations in MG's diet that make complete proteins.

13. Considering her income, education, and cultural practices, on a separate sheet of paper, outline a nutrition care plan you would use for Mrs. MG. Include the teaching techniques you would use.

14. Define empacho and chorizos.

RELATED READINGS:

1. Algert, S.J., Brzezinski, E., & Ellison, T.H. (1998). *Ethnic and Regional Food Practices, A Series: Mexican American Food Practices, Customs, and Holidays.* The American Dietetic Association, Chicago, IL and the American Diabetes Association, Alexandria, VA.

2. Chisholm, D.J., Samaras, K., Markovic, T., Carey, D., Lapsys, N., & Campbell, L.V. (1998). Obesity: genes, glands or gluttony? *Reprod. Fertil. Dev.* 10(1):49-53.

3. Fischbach, F.T. (2003). *A Manual of Laboratory & Diagnostic Tests.* 7th Ed. Philadelphia. J.B. Lippincott Company

4. Green, S.M. (1997). Obesity: prevalence, causes, health risks and treatment. *Br. J. Nurs.* 6(20):1181 1185.

5. Lee, R.D., Nieman, D.C., & Nieman, D. (2002). *Nutritional Assessment*. 3rd Ed. McGraw-Hill

6. National Heart, Lung, and Blood Institute. (1998). Clinical Guidelines on the Identification, Evaluation, and Treatment of Overweight and Obesity in Adult. National Institutes of Health. Publication 98-4083. http://www.nhlbi.nih.gov/guidelines/obesity/ob_gdlns.htm

7. Position paper of the American Dietetic Association. (2002). Weight management *J Am Diet Assoc.* 2002;102:1145-1155.

8. Rolfes, S.R., Pinna, K. & Whitney, E. (2006). *Understanding Normal and Clinical Nutrition*, 7th Ed. West/Wadsworth.

9. Weight-control Information Network. November, (2001) *Understanding Adult Obesity.* NIH . NIH Publication No. 01-3680, October. http://win.niddk.nih.gov/publications/understanding.htm

10. Weight-control Information Network. March, (2001). *Weight Cycling.* NIH Publication No. NIH Publication No. 01-3901. e-text updated March 2004. http://win.niddk.nih.gov/publications/cycling.htm

11. Weight-control Information Network. May, (2004). *Do you know the health risks of being overweight?* NIH Publication No. 04-4098, e-text posted: November 2004. http//win.niddk.nih.gov/publications/health_risks.htm

12. Weinsier, R.L., Hunter, G.R., Heini, A.F., Goran, M.I., & Sell, S.M. (1998). The etiology of obesity: relative contribution of metabolic factors, diet, and physical activity. *Am. J. Med.* 105(2):145-150.

CASE STUDY #10
GASTRITIS IN AN ELDERLY WOMAN

INTRODUCTION
This is part one of a two-part case study involving a typical scenario of aging, weight gain, and the medical complications that accompany this process. It is concerned with weight gain, gastritis, and esophageal reflux, complicated by medications for various other disorders.
****

SKILLS NEEDED
ABBREVIATIONS:
Knowledge of the following abbreviations is required in order to understand this case. You should learn these abbreviations before you begin to read the study.
ac, bid, D/C, EGD, hs, po, prn, qid, UGI, YOWF, and 2xd (Appendix C).

FORMULAS:
The formulas used in this case study include ideal body weight, adjusted body weight, percent ideal body weight, and body mass index (Appendix A, Tables 7 through 10).

MEDICATIONS:
Become familiar with the following medications before reading the case study. Note the diet-drug interactions, dosages and methods of administration, gastrointestinal tract reactions, etc.
1. Lasix (furosemide); 2. Tums (calcium carbonate); 3. Aspirin (acetylsalicylic acid); 4. Mobic (meloxicam); 5. Altace (ramipril); 6. Carafate (sucralfate); 7. Zantac (ranitidine hydrochloride).
****

Mrs. CL is a 79 YOWF with a history of indigestion that goes back many years. For as long as she can remember, she has been taking Tums after most of her meals, particularly the evening meal. Her indigestion worsened over the years and her ingestion of Tums increased proportionately. By the time she was 77, she was taking Tums after every meal and before going to bed at night. The increase was so gradual that Mrs. CL did not realize how many Tums she was taking. She was using a generic brand of calcium carbonate in a very large bottle that she bought in a discount store. This practice had become such an accepted part of her routine that by her 79th birthday it was as natural for her to take a Tums after a meal as it was for her to wipe her mouth with a napkin. Mrs. CL's weight increased with age, while her activity level progressively decreased. At age 79, Mrs. CL was 5'1" and weighed 175 lbs. When she was married 49 years ago, she weighed 110 lbs. Most of her weight gain occurred after age 40, but the most dramatic increase occurred after Mrs. CL retired at age 63. Her weight history can be found in Table 1.

TABLE 1	
AGE	WEIGHT
30	110
40	128
63	148

Mrs. CL was an excellent cook and restaurant manager for ten years prior to her retirement. After her retirement, she helped keep herself busy by cooking for large groups of people at church and civic functions, family gatherings, etc. She developed the habit of tasting everything several times while it was cooking. This turned into almost constant eating while cooking.

As active as Mrs. CL was after retirement, she was not expending nearly as much energy as she did prior to retirement. The lack of exercise, increased eating, and advancing age contributed to the dramatic weight gain. As Mrs. CL aged, her ability to remember and reason diminished. She was on a fixed income, relying on social security, and she lived with her son and daughter-in-law. They did not charge her rent, but she took care of her own medical bills and bought some of the food. She felt like she had to contribute to the household by cooking for the family. They allowed this and enjoyed her cooking most of the time, but they noticed that as she aged, she began to lose her ability to modify recipes and ad lib in the kitchen. She started cooking the same meals very frequently and preparing unbalanced meals, such as rice, potatoes, and peas with bread at the same meal. They prepared a three-week cycle menu for her to follow for variety and balance. Mrs. CL's family did not realize how many Tums she was taking. She never discussed the "burning in her chest" with them. They encouraged her to lose weight on a regular basis without success. Additional factors that affected Mrs. CL's health included arthritis that worsened as she grew older. She took Mobic (meloxicam), 7.5 mg once daily for arthritis. She found that aspirin (acetylsalicylic acid) did her as much good, was cheaper, and could be taken more often. Her aspirin intake also began to increase over the years and by the time she was 79, it was another one of her accepted "natural habits." Mrs. CL also had a problem with hypertension. Her blood pressure was usually about 160/94 without medication and 140/84 with medication. She was taking Altace (ramipril) for her hypertension, 5 mg po every day. She was also taking Lasix (furosemide), 20 mg prn for swelling in her feet.

One evening at supper, Mrs. CL started to panic and indicated to her son and daughter-in-law that she was choking. After her son performed the Heimlich maneuver on her, she coughed up a piece of chicken. The chicken got stuck in her throat and would not go down. She was afraid to eat after that and wanted to go to the doctor. It was at this time that she told her son of the burning she had been experiencing in her chest. She said that it had been getting worse over the past few weeks. He made an appointment for her with the family physician, who sent her to a gastroenterologist. He performed a UGI series and an esophagogastroduodenoscopy (EGD). The results indicated gastritis without ulceration and decreased esophageal motility with reflux esophagitis. He told her to D/C aspirin and Mobic and to see her family physician for replacement drugs. He also prescribed Carafate (sucralfate), 1 g po qid 1 hour ac and hs, and Zantac (ranitidine hydrochloride), 150 mg bid. His prognosis for her gastritis was good, but said that the esophageal reflux would probably give her problems for the rest of her life and she would have to learn to live with it. He told her to follow a soft bland diet.

Mrs. CL went to her family physician and he left her arthritis medication as is and told her not to take it for more than ten days and then wait at least a week before restarting it. He also told her to take it only when she was having continuous severe pain. He did not change the Lasix (furosemide). Mrs. CL followed her physician's orders and took all of the medications until they ran out, which took about one month. She did not get them refilled because she was feeling better and they were too expensive. The Carafate was about $1.00 per tablet. She had Medicare and supplemental insurance, but neither paid for her medications.

****

QUESTIONS:

1. What is Mrs. CL's ideal body weight (Appendix A, Tables 7 and 8)?

2. Calculate her adjusted body weight (Appendix A, Table 9).

3. Calculate her BMI (Appendix A, Tables 10 and 11).

4. Discuss the effects of age and exercise on basal metabolic rate.

5. Discuss the possible reasons for Mrs. CL's gastritis.

6. List the dietary principles to be followed for esophageal reflux.

7. Define:

    UGI series:

    Reflux esophagitis:

    Gastritis without ulceration:

    Esophagogastroduodenoscopy:

8. What is considered to be normal and acceptable blood pressure?

9. Describe the action and side effects of:

   Altace:

   Lasix:

   Carafate:

   Zantac:

10. The physician did not tell Mrs. CL much about her diet. Expound on what he said by writing a nutritional care plan to fit Mrs. CL's nutritional needs and lifestyle.

11. Failing to refill prescriptions because of the cost is typical for elderly who are on fixed incomes. Discuss the limitations that financial restrictions can place on this population and offer some suggestions for techniques that the health care team can use to emphasize the importance of the medications.

12. Some areas have assistance programs for individuals who cannot afford the medications they need. Determine if such a program exists in your area. If so, discuss the characteristics and value of the program. (☺ *Hint: a hospital social worker is a good source of information for this.*)

EPILOGUE

This is another true case that with details very close to what is described here. This case was also based on one of my mother's many unfortunate experiences.

Related Readings

1. Blumberg, J. (1997). Nutritional needs of seniors. *J. Am. Coll. Nutr.* 16(6):517-523.

2. Fischbach, F.T. (2003). *A Manual of Laboratory & Diagnostic Tests.* 7th Ed. Philadelphia. J.B. Lippincott Company.

3. Koskenpato, J., Kairemo, K., Korppi-Tommola, T. & Farkkila, M. (1998). Role of gastric emptying in functional dyspepsia: a scintigraphic study of 94 subjects. *Dig. Dis. Sci.* 43(6):1154-1158.

4. Lovat, L.B. (1996). Age related changes in gut physiology and nutritional status. *Gut.* 38(3):306-309.

5. National Heart, Lung, and Blood Institute. (1998). Clinical Guidelines on the Identification, Evaluation, and Treatment of Overweight and Obesity in Adult. National Institutes of Health. Publication 98-4083. http://www.nhlbi.nih.gov/guidelines/obesity/ob_gdlns.htm

6. Perlman, P.E. & Adams, W. (1989). Physiologic changes as patients get older. *Postgrad Med.* 5(2):213-214.

7. Weddle, D.O., & Kuczmarski, F. (2000). Nutrition, aging and the continuum of care *J Am Diet Assoc.* 100:580-595.

8. Pilotto, A., Franceschi, M., Leandro, G., Novello, R., Di Mario, F., & Valerio G. (2002). Long-term clinical outcome of elderly patients with reflux esophagitis: a six-month to three-year follow-up study. *Am J Ther.* Jul-Aug;9(4):295-300.

9. Pilotto, A. (2004). Aging and upper gastrointestinal disorders. *Best Pract Res Clin Gastroenterol.* 8S:73-81.

10. Prendergast, A. & Fulton, F.L. (1997) *Medical terminology: A Text/Workbook.* 4th Ed. Redwood City, California. Addison-Wesley Nursing.

11. Pronsky, Z.M., Redfern, C.M., Crowe, J. & Epstein, S. (2003) *Food Medication Interactions*, 13th Ed Phoenix, Arizona. Food-Medications Interactions, Publishers and Distributors.

12. Rolfes, S.R., Pinna, K. & Whitney, E. (2006). *Understanding Normal and Clinical Nutrition*, 7th Ed. West/Wadsworth.

13. Saltzman, J.R. & Russell, R.M. (1998). The aging gut. Nutritional issues. *Gastroenterol Clin. North Am.* 27(2):309-324.

14. Schlenker, E.D. (1997). *Nutrition in Aging.* St. Louis, Missouri. Mosby - Year Book, Inc.

CASE STUDY #11
CHEST PAIN IN AN ELDERLY WOMAN

INTRODUCTION

This is part two of a two-part case study involving a typical scenario of aging, weight gain, and the medical complications that accompany this process. It is concerned with gastritis and esophageal reflux, complicated by medications for various other disorders. The patient's symptoms were alleviated in part one, but the patient did not follow up with her medications and now requires additional treatment.

****

SKILLS NEEDED

ABBREVIATIONS:

Knowledge of the following abbreviations is required in order to understand this case. You should learn these abbreviations before you begin to read the study. These are abbreviations not used in the previous case studies: C/O, EKG, mci, and R/O (Appendix C).

FORMULAS:

The formulas used in this case study include ideal body weight, adjusted body weight, Harris-Benedict equation, and activity factors (Appendix A, Tables 7, 9 and 17).

MEDICATIONS:

Become familiar with the following medications before reading the case study. Note the diet-drug interactions, dosages and methods of administration, gastrointestinal tract reactions, etc.
1. Tylenol (acetaminophen); 2. Technesium Cardiolite; 3. Tums (calcium carbonate); 4. Aspirin (acetylsalicylic acid); 5. Mobic (meloxicam; 6. Persantine (dipyridamole); 7. Carafate (sucralfate); 8. Zantac (ranitidine hydrochloride).

****

Mrs. CL followed her bland diet and was careful to chew everything well before swallowing. She also took her medication as prescribed. The swallowing difficulty seemed to go away, and the burning stopped. When the medication ran out, Mrs. CL did not refill her prescription because the medicine was so expensive. She thought that she would wait and see what happened. Several weeks went by and the symptoms did not return. Now and then there would be a little burning and she would take two Tums, but she did not consider it to be unusual. Both physicians, with the help of her son, convinced her not to take any more aspirins. She tried Tylenol (acetaminophen) for her arthritis pain, but it did not help as much so, as time went on, she began taking the Mobic (meloxicam) more frequently. She also began to take some aspirin again. She was told that if she took too much Mobic, since it was stronger than aspirin, it could cause harm to her stomach. She figured that if Mobic was stronger than aspirin, it made sense not to take it as much and take aspirin instead. As time passed, she ended up taking Tums, aspirin, and Mobic as frequently as she had before.

Two years passed since the previous incident and Mrs. CL is now an 81 YOWF with the same history of indigestion (see Case Study #10). She is older, more forgetful, and a little heavier than she was two years ago. Her height is 5'1" and she now weighs 185 lbs. Her son and daughter-in-law have cautioned her about her weight, but there is not much they can do to control her eating during the day when they are working.

Every Friday, her daughter-in-law is off work and is usually at home. One Friday, Mrs. CL came into the kitchen, barely able to walk or breathe. She C/O a severe pain in the center of her chest. Her eyes were dilated, and she appeared to be very frightful. The daughter-in-law, knowing her history, sat her down and calmed her while questioning her. She found out that the pain did not radiate to her shoulder or arm but did go up into her neck. She was not clammy to touch and was not diaphoretic. She did not experience a feeling of heavy pressure pushing in on her chest. Was it a heart attack or gastric reflux? Considering her history, age, weight, hypertension, etc., there was no way to be sure. The daughter-in-law called her husband and the physician. The physician told her to bring Mrs. CL in to see him right away. By the time she arrived at the doctor's office, the pain was gone and she was calm. He did blood work to look at enzymes and did an EKG. All were negative. After she calmed down, she told her son that the pain was similar to the reflux pain she experienced in the past, but more severe. It seemed she had a severe case of reflux esophagitis that went up into her neck.

To R/O a heart problem, the physician decided to test further and scheduled her for a Cardiolite Imaging. This procedure was performed in the Department of Nuclear Cardiology. Mrs. CL reported at 8:00 A.M. and after receiving the appropriate instructions about the risks of the test, signed a consent form. She was then injected I.V. with 8 mci of Technesium Cardiolite. This is a radioactive isotope that enables a gamma camera to record images of the heart. After the injection, there was a minimum waiting period of one hour before she was placed on a special table, and the heart was scanned with a gamma camera for sixteen minutes. The results were recorded in a computer and could be viewed from a computer screen. At that point, the patient is either exercised physically (on a treadmill) or chemically (I.V. injection) and the heart imaged again to determine if there are any differences between resting perfusion and exercise perfusion. Mrs. CL was not able to walk on a treadmill, so she had to be injected I.V. with Persantine (amount depends on patient's weight). This stresses the heart and its effects are equivalent to those of exercise. CL was then injected with 22 mci of Technesium Cardiolite. After a minimum waiting period of thirty minutes, she was again placed on the special table and a gamma camera took images of her heart for sixteen minutes.

The results of this test were also negative, and it was concluded that Mrs. CL experienced severe pain from gastritis and reflux esophagitis. Her physician ordered her to take Carafate (sucralfate), 1 g po qid 1 hour ac and hs as before, but changed Zantac to Axid (nizatidine), 150 mg bid. He told her to continue Mobic (meloxicam) 7.5 mg once daily but not to take it for more than 10 days, and to wait two weeks before resuming the medication. He also told her to avoid aspirin entirely. He gave her a soft bland diet to follow and this time made her an appointment with the clinic dietitian.
****

QUESTIONS:
1. Define:

   Diaphoretic:

   Gastric Reflux:

   Reflux Esophagitis:

   Radioactive Isotope:

   Gamma Imaging:

   Perfusion:

2. Calculate Mrs. CL's BMI (Appendix A, Tables 10 and 11).

3. What is Mrs. CL's ideal body weight (Appendix A, Table 7 and 8)?

4. Calculate Mrs. CL's adjusted body weight (Appendix A, Table 9).

5. With the above information, calculate Mrs. CL's total kcal need using the Harris-Benedict equation and an appropriate activity factor (Appendix A Table 17).

6. List the principles of the diet Mrs. CL should be on.

7. Compare acetylsalicylic acid and acetaminophen as to action and nutritional complications.

8. Explain how the actions of the drugs Mrs. CL was taking could have caused her problems, particularly with her medical history.

9. Describe the action and nutritional implications of Axid.

10. Axid and Carafate both cost about a $1.00 per pill. Add up what this will cost Mrs. CL per day and per month. Mrs. CL is on a fixed income. Discuss what you would do if you had to counsel this patient, knowing that she is going to tell you that she cannot afford the medications.

EPILOGUE

Yet another case based on experiences my mother went through. At this point in her life she was in her 80s, was very overweight, and set in her ways. The fact that I had a PhD in nutrition and was a RD had no effect on her listening to my advice. A high price frequently comes with stubbornness

RELATED REFERENCES

1. Chisholm, D.J., Samaras, K., Markovic, T., Carey, D., Lapsys, N., & Campbell, L.V. (1998). Obesity: genes, glands or gluttony? *Reprod. Fertil. Dev.* 10(1):49-53.

2. Blumberg, J. (1997). Nutritional needs of seniors. *J. Am. Coll. Nutr.* 16(6):517-523.

3. Fischbach, F.T. (1995). *A Manual of Laboratory & Diagnostic Tests.* 5th Ed. Philadelphia. J.B. Lippincott Company.

5. Koskenpato, J., Kairemo, K., Korppi-Tommola, T. & Farkkila, M. (1998). Role of gastric emptying in functional dyspepsia: a scintigraphic study of 94 subjects. *Dig. Dis. Sci.* 43(6):1154-1158.

6. Lee, R.D., Nieman, D.C., & Nieman, D. (2002). *Nutritional Assessment.* 3rd Ed. McGraw-Hill.

7. Lovat, L.B. (1996). Age related changes in gut physiology and nutritional status. *Gut.* 38(3):306-309.

8. National Heart, Lung, and Blood Institute. (1998). Clinical Guidelines on the Identification, Evaluation, and Treatment of Overweight and Obesity in Adult. National Institutes of Health. Publication 98-4083. http://www.nhlbi.nih.gov/guidelines/obesity/ob_gdlns.htm

9. Perlman, P.E. & Adams, W. (1989). Physiologic changes as patients get older. *Postgrad Med.* 85(2):213-214.

10. Position paper of the American Dietetic Association. (2002). Weight management *J Am Diet Assoc.* 2002;102:1145-1155.

11. Prendergast, A. & Fulton, F.L. (1997) *Medical terminology: A Text/Workbook.* 4th Ed. Redwood City, California. Addison-Wesley Nursing.

13. Pronsky, Z.M., Redfern, C.M., Crowe, J. & Epstein, S. (2003) *Food Medication Interactions*, 13th Ed Phoenix, Arizona. Food-Medications Interactions, Publishers and Distributors.

14. Rolfes, S.R., Pinna, K. & Whitney, E. (2006). *Understanding Normal and Clinical Nutrition*, 7th Ed. West/Wadsworth.

15. Saltzman, J.R. & Russell, R.M. (1998). The aging gut. Nutritional issues. *Gastroenterol Clin. North Am.* 27(2):309-324.

16. Schlenker, E.D. (1997). *Nutrition in Aging.* St. Louis, Missouri. Mosby - Year Book, Inc.

CASE STUDY #12
PEDIATRIC GERD

INTRODUCTION
This case study involves a young neonatal/pediatric patient with GERD that required surgery to correct. The study is designed to introduce the student to some facts about gestation, premature births, and pediatric nutrition.
****
SKILLS NEEDED
ABBREVIATIONS:
Knowledge of the following abbreviations is required in order to understand this case. You should learn these abbreviations before you begin to read the study (Appendix C).
GERD, IHDP, oz, PEG, and VLBW.

LABORATORY VALUES:
You will need to be able to interpret the nutritional significance of the following laboratory values for this case study: BUN, Cr, glucose, hgb, Na, K, Cl, and Ser alb (Appendix B).

MEDICATIONS:
Become familiar with the following medications before reading the case study. Note the diet-drug interactions, dosages and methods of administration, gastrointestinal tract reactions, etc.
1. Pepcid (famotidine); 2. Mylanta (simethicone), 3. Reglan (metoclopramide); 4. Ventolin (albuterol), 5. Cefzil (cefprozil).
****

PG is a WM who was admitted to the hospital with recurrent problems resulting from GERD. PG was born prematurely at 30 weeks, weighing 2 lbs 7 oz, and was classified as a VLBW baby. He was 15 inches at birth. Being premature, he was on a ventilator for most of the time he spent in the hospital. After one month, PG was diagnosed with pneumonia. About this time it was noticed that he had difficulty feeding; although nothing therapeutic was done for this, he was watched closely at feeding time. Over the next several months, he continued to have pulmonary problems and was not growing as expected. This was attributed to his condition and the fact that his intake was poor. PG was discharged after three months in the hospital. At six months, PG was taking solid foods better than liquids but it was noted that he was still having problems swallowing. At six and a half months, he was again diagnosed with pneumonia and had to be admitted to the hospital. He was discharged after treatment with no pulmonary problems. PG's mother did not bring him back for regular check-ups as scheduled so his progress could not be routinely measured. At two years and nine months she brought him in with breathing problems. Upon examination, he was again diagnosed with pneumonia and was admitted for a series of tests. Chest X-rays indicated aspiration pneumonia. He also underwent a video fluoroscopy which showed him to be at significant risk for aspiration. During the oral phase of the test, PG had functional control over liquids and had fair propulsion with solids, but a delayed trigger swallow was noted during the pharyngeal phase. It was also noted that PG was well behind normal physical and cognitive development. Upon admission, he weighed 16.5 lbs and his height was 28 inches. PG was diagnosed with pneumonia, GERD, and dehydration. His initial nutritionally relevant lab values were as follows:

TEST	RESULT	NORM	TEST	RESULT	NORM
Glu	95 mg/dl	60-100 mg/dl	Na	140 mEq/L	136-145 mEq/L
BUN	19 mg/dl	5-18 mg/dl	K	4.6 mEq/L	3.4-4.7 mEq/L
Cr	0.5 mg/dl	0.5-1.0 mg/dl	Cl	99 mEq/L	96-106 mEq/L
Ser alb	4.8 g/dl	2.9-5.5 g/dl			

After he was treated for pneumonia, PG underwent surgery to have a Nissan fundoplicatation and a PEG tube placed. PG recovered from surgery without complications and began to receive food via his PEG. Initially, the dietitian recommended that he be fed 3.5 cans of Kindercal (840 ml per day) with Pedialyte as tolerated. This recommendation was not followed but Similac Neocare was used instead, 1180 ml per day. He responded to the feedings without incident. One month after surgery PG was tolerating his feeding well and was showing positive results. He was then offered Similac Neocare po with rice cereal added.

PG's medications included:
Pepcid
Mylanta
Reglan
Ventolin
Cefzil
****

QUESTIONS:
1. Answer the following questions with short answers:
   a. What is the normal range of time in weeks for gestation?

   b. A baby considered to be premature if born before _____ weeks.

   c. What is the average birth weight for babies born in the United States?

   d. What is considered to be a low birth weight baby?

   e. What is considered to be a very low birth weight baby?

2. List the signs that indicate when a baby should be started on solid food.

3. Define the following:
   aspiration pneumonia:

   video fluoroscopy:

   oral phase of swallowing:

   delayed trigger swallow:

   pharyngeal phase of swallowing:

   Pedialyte:

4. What is a Nissan fundoplication and what will it accomplish?

5. Define PEG, describe how it is placed, and give the rationale for its placement in this case.

6. According to the IHDP Growth Percentiles for VLBW Premature Boys (obtainable through Ross Labs; see references 2 and 19), how would you classify PG based on his height and weight for age upon admission for surgery? What should his height and weight be?

7. Knowing that PG is dehydrated, you should be able to predict which lab values would be elevated. List the labs that should be elevated.

8. Cr should be among the labs you listed but it is not elevated. Give a possible explanation for this in PG's case.

9. What is the caloric and protein requirement for a normal baby that is 2 years and 9 months?

10. What would it be for PG immediately after surgery?

11. After recovering from surgery he will not need extra calories for healing but he will need extra calories for catch-up growth. What should his caloric and protein intake be at this time?

12. Give the class of each of the following medications and their action.

Medication	Class	Action
Pepcid		
Mylanta		
Reglan		
Ventolin		
Cefzil		

13. List any nutritional side effects of the following medications:

Medication	Side Effects
Pepcid	
Mylanta	
Reglan	
Ventolin	
Cefzil	

14. What are the potential consequences of giving children Mylanta for an extended period? [*Hint: Check the list of references.*] Is there cause for concern? Explain.

15. In the following table, compare Kindercal with Similac Neocare.

Product	Producer	Form	Cal/ ml	Non-pro cal/g N	g/L			Na mg	K mg	mOsm /kg water	Vol to meet RDA in ml	g of fiber /L	Free H$_2$O /L in ml
					Pro	CHO	Fat						
Kinder-care													
Similac Neocare													

16. Compare the kcals and protein PG would receive from 840 cc of Kindercal and 1180 ml of Neocare Similac.

Information Box 12 - 1
The original **SOAP** note written in a patient's chart should contain all four components, Subjective, Objective, Assessment, and Plan. However, not every **SOAP** note has to contain all four components. After the original note, subsequent notes could contain from one to four of the components. For example, if additional lab values become available that alter the patient's assessment and plan, but no additional subjective information is available, then a second note could be entered into the patient's chart containing only information in the **OAP** sections. If the patient's nutritional therapy changes but nothing else changes, a third note could be entered into the patient's chart with only the **P** section.

17. When PG was two-years and nine months old, his mother brought him to the doctor with breathing problems. He was admitted for a series of tests. No subjective information is given. Using the objective information presented after that admission and your answers to the previous questions, prepare a SOAP note that includes entries in the objective, assessment, and plan sections.

S:
O:
A:
P:

RELATED READINGS

1. Akintorin, S.M., Kamat, M., Pildes, R.S., Kling, P., Andes, S., Hill, J., & Pyati, S. (1997). A prospective randomized trial of feeding methods in very low birth weight infants. *Pediatrics.* 100(4):E4.

2. Casey, P.H., Kraemer, H.C., Bernbaum, J., Yogman, M.W., & Sells, J.C. (1991). Growth status and growth rates of a varied sample of low birth weight, preterm infants: a longitudinal cohort from birth to three years of age. *J. Pediatr.* 119:599-605.

3. Cioffi, U., Rosso, L., & De Simone, M. (1998). Gastroesophageal reflux disease. Pathogenesis, symptoms and complications. *Panminerva Med.* 40(2):132-8.

4. Fischbach, F.T. (2003). *A Manual of Laboratory & Diagnostic Tests.* 7th Ed. Philadelphia. J.B. Lippincott Company.

5. Foldes, J., Balena, R., Ho, A., Parfitt, A.M., & Kleerekoper, M. (1991). Hypophosphatemic rickets with hypocalciuria following long-term treatment with aluminum-containing anatacid. *Bone.* 12(2):67-71.

6. Hamill, P.V.V., Drizd, T.A., Johnson, C.L., Reed, R.B., Roche, A.F., & Moore, W.M. (1979). Physical Growth: National Center for Health Statistics percentilles. *Am. J. Clin. Nutr.* 32:607-29.

7. Henry, S.M. (2004). Discerning differences: gastroesophageal reflux and gastroesophageal reflux disease in infants. *Adv Neonatal Care.* Aug;4(4):235-47.

8. Nevin-Folino, N. (2003). *Pediatric Manual of Clinical Dietetics.* 2nd Ed. Chicago, IL. American Dietetic Association.

9. McCance, K. L. & Huether, S.E. (2002). *Pathophysiology: The Biologic Basis for Disease in Adults and Children.* 3rd Ed. Mosby-Year Book.

10. *Pediatric Nutrition Handbook.* (1998). 4th Ed. American Academy of Pediatrics.

11. Peters, J.H., DeMeester, T.R., Crookes, P., Oberg, S., de Vos Shoop, M., Hagan, J.A., & Bremner, C.G. (1998). The treatment of gastroesophageal reflux disease with laparoscopic Nissen fundoplication: prospective evaluation of 100 patients with Atypical symptoms. *Ann Surg.* 28(1):40-40.

12. Pivnick, E.K., Kerr, N.C., Kaufman, R.A., Jones, D.P., & Chesney, R.W. (1995). Rickets secondary to phosphate depletion. A sequela of antacid use in infancy. *Clin. Pediatr.* 34(2):73-8.

13. Rolfes, S.R., Pinna, K. & Whitney, E. (2006). *Understanding Normal and Clinical Nutrition,* 7th Ed. West/Wadsworth.

14. Prendergast, A. & Fulton, F.L. (1997) *Medical terminology: A Text/Workbook.* 4th Ed. Redwood City, California. Addison-Wesley Nursing.

15. Pronsky, Z.M., Redfern, C.M., Crowe, J. & Epstein, S. (2003) *Food Medication Interactions,* 13th Ed Phoenix, Arizona. Food-Medications Interactions, Publishers and Distributors.

16. Rerksuppaphol, S. and Barnes, G. (2001). Guidelines for evaluation and treatment of gastroesophageal reflux in infants and children: recommendations of the North American Society for Pediatric Gastroenterology and Nutrition. *J Pediatr Gastroenterol Nutr*. 32 Suppl 2:S1-31.

17. Samour, P. Q., Helm, K.K., & Lang, C.E. (2003) *Handbook of Pediatric Nutrition*. 2nd Ed. Jones & Bartlett Publishers

18. Society for Pediatric Gastroenterology, Hepatology and Nutrition. (2003). Treatment of pediatric gastroesophageal reflux disease: current knowledge and future research. Proceedings of a conference sponsored by the Children's Digestive Health and Nutrition Foundation in cooperation with the North American *J Pediatr Gastroenterol Nutr*. Nov-Dec;37 Suppl 1:S1-75.

19. Spratto, G.R. & Woods, A.L. (2005). *PDR Nurse's Drug Handbook*. Thompson Delmar Learning, NY.

20. The Infant Health and development Program: Enhancing the outcomes of low-birth-weight, premature infants. (1990). *JAMA*. 263(22):3035-3042.

21. van der Peet, D.L., Klinkenberk-Knol, E.C., Eijsbouts, Q.A., van den Berg, M., de Brauw, L.M.,& Cuesta, M.A. (1998). Laparoscopic Nissen fundoplication for the treatment of gastroesophageal reflux disease (GERD). Surgery after extensive conservative treatment. *Surg. Endosc*. 12(9):1159-63.

22. Wetscher, G.J., Glaser, K., Wieschemeyer, T., Gadenstatter, M., Klingler, P., Klinger, A., &Hinder, R.A. (1998). Cispride enhances the effect of partial posterior fundoplication onesophageal peristalsis in GERD.

INTRODUCTION

This is the second pediatric case study that is intended to provide an introduction to pediatric terminology, assessment, and nutrition. The physicians in this case were very aggressive in the nutritional treatment of this child.

****

SKILLS NEEDED

ABBREVIATIONS:

Knowledge of the following abbreviations is required in order to understand this case. You should learn these abbreviations before you begin to read the study (Appendix C). BPD, BM, G-tube, IHDP, PEG, PICU, and VLBW.

MEDICATIONS:

Become familiar with the following medications before reading this case study. Note the diet-drug interactions, dosages and methods of administration, gastrointestinal tract reactions, etc.

1. Aldactone (spironolactone); 2. Reglan (metoclopramide); 3. Digoxin (digoxin); 4. Lasix (furosemide); 5. Pepcid (famotidine); 6. Vancocin (vancomycin ydrochloride); 7. Ventolin (albuterol).

****

LV is a 9-month-old BM who was admitted to PICU for ventilator support of BPD. He has had chronic problems with BPD since birth and is oxygen dependent. He has also experienced gastric reflux on occasion and mild hyperkalemia. LV was born premature at 28 weeks gestational age and weighed 1 kg. He was classified as a VLBW baby. He had complications as a result of his prematurity that were primarily respiratory. These included pulmonary emphysema, left tension pneumothorax with chest tube placement, and BPD. He required ventilator support until just prior to discharge and was sent home with oxygen via a nasal cannula.

LV was readmitted at 5 months with additional pulmonary complications. His weight at that time was 3.5 kg and his height was 49.8 cm. His physician was concerned about his weight, so after LV's pulmonary problems cleared up, the physician recommended surgery to have a PEG placed. Other minor surgeries were performed that are common to premature births, i.e. inguinal hernia repair and cryosurgery with laser surgery for premature retinopathy. Similac Neocare was started through the G-tube at a rate of 8.4 Kcal/hr. LV was discharged at 6 months with a social services consult. The concern was that LV's mother had to work and LV has four siblings at home that also need to be provided for.

At 9 months LV has returned for a check-up and weighs 5.2 kg and is 50.1 cms. The G-tube seems to be helping significantly. He is still having some problems with BPD and currently has another pulmonary infection but his reflux and hyperkalemia are resolving and his prognosis has improved. His current feeding is Similac Neocare at the rate of 15.5 ml/hr with 1 tsp of Polycose powder per oz. LV's current medications include:

Aldactone
Pepcid
Ventolin
Reglan
Lasix
Digoxin
Vancomycin

****

QUESTIONS:

1. Define BPD as to the cause, treatment, and prognosis. What is the importance of nutrition in relation to this disorder?

2. Briefly define:
    Pulmonary emphysema:

    Pneumothorax:

    Cryosurgery:

    Polycose:

3. According to the IHDP Growth Percentiles for VLBW Premature Boys (obtainable through Ross labs; see references 3 and 19), how would you classify LV for height and weight for age at 5 months? What should his height and weight be at this age?

4. According to the IHDP Growth Percentiles for VLBW Premature Boys, how would you classify LV for height and weight for age at 9 months? What should his height and weight be at 9 months?

5. At 5 months of age, LV was receiving Similac Neocare at a rate of 8.4 kcals per hour. How many calories and how much protein was this providing? How many calories and how much protein should he be receiving at 5 months?

6. At 9 months of age, LV was receiving Similac Neocare at a rate of 15.5 kcals per hour with 1 tsp of Polycose per oz. How many calories and how much protein was this providing? How many calories and how much protein should he be receiving at 9 months? In your answer show how many mls in an ounce and how much Polycose LV was receiving.

7. How much free water was LV receiving at 5 months? At 9 months? How much should he be receiving at both 5 and 9 months?

8. Give the class of each of the following medications and its action.

Medication	Class	Action
Aldactone		
Pepcid		
Ventolin		
Reglan		
Lasix		
Digoxin		
Vancomycin		

9. List any nutritional side effects of the following medications:

Medication	Side Effects
Aldactone	
Pepcid	
Ventolin	
Reglan	
Lasix	
Digoxin	
Vancomycin	

RELATED READINGS

1. Abrams, S.A. (2001). Chronic pulmonary insufficiency in children and its effects on growth and development. *J Nutr.* 2001 Mar;131(3):938S-941S.

2. Akintorin, S.M., Kamat, M., Pildes, R.S., Kling, P., Andes, S., Hill, J., & Pyati, S. (1997). A prospective randomized trial of feeding methods in very low birth weight infants. *Pediatrics.* 100(4):E4.

3. Casey, P.H., Kraemer, H.C., Bernbaum, J., Yogman, M.W., & `Sells, J.C. (1991). Growth status and growth rates of a varied sample of low birth weight, preterm infants: a longitudinal cohort from birth to three years of age. *J. Pediatr.* 119:599-605.

4. Fischbach, F.T. (2003). *A Manual of Laboratory & Diagnostic Tests.* 7th Ed. Philadelphia. J.B. Lippincott Company.

5. Hjalmarson, O. & Sandberg, K.L. (2005). Lung function at term reflects severity of bronchopulmonary dysplasia. *J Pediatr.* Jan;146(1):86-90.

6. Huysman, W.A., de Ridder, M., de Bruin, N.C., van Helmond, G., Terpstra, N.,Van Goudoever, J.B., & Sauer, P.J. (2003). Growth and body composition in preterm infants with bronchopulmonary dysplasia. *Arch Dis Child Fetal Neonatal Ed.* Jan;88(1):F46-51.

7. Jacob, S.V., Coates, A.L., Lands, L.C., MacNeish, C.F., Riley, S.P., Hornby, L., Outerbridge, E.W., Davis, G.M., & Williams, R.L. (1998). Long-term pulmonary sequelae of severe bronchopulmonary dysplasia. *J. Pediatr.* 133(2):193-200.

8. McCance, K., L. & Huether, S.E. (2002). *Pathophysiology: The Biologic Basis for Disease in Adults and Children.* 4th Ed. Mosby-Year Book.

9. Mueller, D.H. (1998). Timeliness of codifying ABCDE' for BPD. *J. Pediatr.* 133(3):315-6.

10. Nevin-Folino, N. (2003). *Pediatric Manual of Clinical Dietetics.* 2nd Ed. Chicago, IL. American Dietetic Association.

11. Palta, M., Sadek, M., Barnet, J.H., Evans, M., Weinstein, M.R., McGuinness, G., Peters, M.E., Gabbert, D., Fryback, D., & Farrell, P. (1998). Evaluation of criteria for chronic lung disease in surviving very low birth weight infants. Newborn Lung Project. *J. Pediatr.* 132(1):57-63.

12. *Pediatric Nutrition Handbook.* (1998). 4th Ed. American Academy of Pediatrics.

13. Prendergast, A. & Fulton, F.L. (1997) *Medical terminology: A Text/Workbook.* 4th Ed. Redwood City, California. Addison-Wesley Nursing.

14. Pronsky, Z.M., Redfern, C.M., Crowe, J. & Epstein, S. (2003) *Food Medication Interactions*, 13th Ed Phoenix, Arizona. Food-Medications Interactions, Publishers and Distributors.

15. Rolfes, S.R., Pinna, K. & Whitney, E. (2006). *Understanding Normal and Clinical Nutrition*, 7th Ed. West/Wadsworth.

16. Samour, P. Q., Helm, K.K., & Lang, C.E. (2003) *Handbook of Pediatric Nutrition*. 2nr Ed. Jones & Bartlett Publishers.

17. Singer, L., Yamashits, T., Lilien, L., Collin, M., & Baley, J. (1997). A longitudinal study of developmental outcome of infants with bronchopulmonary dysplasis and very low birth weight. *Pediatrics*. 100(6):987-93.

18. Spratto, G.R. & Woods, A.L. (2005). *PDR Nurse's Drug Handbook*. Thompson Delmar Learning, NY.

19. The Infant Health and development Program: Enhancing the outcomes of low-birth-weight, premature infants. (1990). *JAMA*. 263(22):3035-3042.

CASE STUDY #14
PEPTIC ULCER DISEASE RESULTING IN GASTRECTOMY

INTRODUCTION

PART I is a basic study of ulcer disease and involves the treatment of ulcers from two perspectives. Symptoms, treatment, and counseling of the ulcer patient are presented. An emphasis is given to dietary treatment of ulcers. The patient does not take care of herself and in PART II requires surgery. Additional information about PUD is covered with basic information on surgery. Review information for a gastrectomy and the diet for dumping syndrome before completing this study. Treatment of gastric ulcers is so advanced that surgery is not performed as frequently as it was in the past, but there are still many reasons why someone could be required to have a gastrectomy.
****

SKILLS NEEDED

ABBREVIATIONS:
Knowledge of the following abbreviations is required in order to understand this case. You should learn these abbreviations before you begin to read the study. Abbreviations used in most of the previous case studies are not listed here.
ADHD, ASA, BRB, BUT, D_5NS, D_5W, ELISA, ER, exploratory lap, HCl, IgG, LUQ, NH_3, pc, po, post-op, PT, PUD, q6h, RLQ, R/O, and sec (Appendix C).

LABORATORY VALUES:
You will need to be able to interpret the nutritional significance of the following laboratory values for this case study: ALP, ALT, amylase, AST, BUN, Ca, Cl, CO_2, CPK, Cr, DBIL, Glucose, hct, hgb, K, Lymphocytes, MCH, MCHC, MCV, Mg, Na, NH_3, P, RBC, ser alb, TBIL, TP, and WBC (Appendix B).

FORMULAS:
The formulas used in this case study include ideal body weight, percent ideal body weight, the Harris-Benedict equation, and stress factors to determine total caloric needs. The formulas can be found in Appendix A, Tables 7, 8, and 17.

MEDICATIONS:
Become familiar with the following medications before reading the case study. Note the diet-drug interactions, dosages and method of administration, gastrointestinal tract reactions, etc.
1. Carafate (sucralfate); 2. AlternaGel (aluminum hydroxide gel); 3. Nexium (esomeprezole magnesium); 4. Aspirin (acetylsalicylic acid); 5. TUMS (calcium carbonate); 6. Pepcid (famotidine); 7. Amoxil (amoxicillin); 8. Biaxin (clarithromycin).
****

PART I: PEPTIC ULCER DISEASE

GG is a 27 YOWF who was married after one year of college. She has no job skills and has depended on her husband to support her for eight years. Six months ago her husband left her and their 4-year-old son. GG faced the responsibility of supporting herself and her son. She did not receive any financial support from her family and had additional expenses to consider if she were to pursue a divorce settlement, which was necessary to obtain child support for her son. Everyone encouraged her to return to school. Her mother agreed to help by babysitting. GG applied for and received a Guaranteed Student Loan to start school. She obtained a part-time job on campus and returned to school to pursue a degree in accounting.

Adjusting to the new lifestyle was very difficult for GG. Studying was hard for her after such a long time out of school and she had to maintain a good average to keep her loan. The combination of working part-time and trying to be a mother and a father to her son was very demanding. The time demands forced her to eat out frequently and her choices were usually fast foods with a high fat content. Sometimes she did not stop to eat anything. Her home-cooked meals were frequently frozen dinners or fried foods. GG's busy schedule caused her to become fatigued. To overcome this, she started drinking strong, black coffee throughout the day and into the night. GG loved chocolate and usually had chocolate bars during the day for energy. She also started smoking, something she never did before. GG was not sleeping well. To temper this, GG began drinking rum and coke at bedtime.

After her husband left, GG started having severe problems with her son that required psychological intervention. He was diagnosed with ADHD. GG had always been easily upset and often had to take antacids for a burning stomach. She recently started experiencing an increase in the burning and, in the last month, had severe pain in the RLQ. The pain occurred about 30 minutes after eating. It subsided with antacids but returned. She also had a burning sensation in her RLQ after drinking coffee. Stress headaches were not uncommon. Her remedy for this was ASA daily. Recently, GG felt like she really needed a break and convinced her mother to take care of her son for the weekend to give her some time for herself.

That Friday night GG started drinking and had a few too many. During the night she awoke with severe stomach pain that radiated to the right side and up into the chest. GG thought she had indigestion but it was the worse she ever had. She drank some milk because she heard that it would help and she also took some TUMS. The pain subsided after a while and, still somewhat under the influence of alcohol, she went back to sleep. The next morning she again awoke to severe gastric pain. She tried her earlier remedy and it worked for a while but the pain came back. This continued throughout the morning until she decided to go to the urgent care center. After listening to her symptoms, hardships, and intake of caffeine, alcohol, ASA, cigarettes, and high-fat foods, the physician assumed she had gastritis that would clear up with medication and dietary changes. He prescribed the following regimen: Cl liqs x3d; progress to a full liquid diet, then a bland diet. Her medications included: sucralfate (Carafate), 1 tab q6h; aluminum hydroxide gel (AlternaGel), 10 cc po 1h pc and hs; famotidine (Pepcid), 40 mg po hs. He told her to quit drinking alcohol, smoking, and taking aspirin. If the pain did not go away in about a week, she should see her family physician.
****

QUESTIONS:
1. List all the <u>food</u> items that may contribute to GG's condition and explain why.

2. List any additional oral intake that may have contributed to GG's condition and explain why.

3. List the non-oral stimulants (physical or psychological stress) that could contribute to GG's condition and what she could do to change them.

4. List the symptoms of GG's gastritis.

5. Was a bland diet necessary? Explain and list the principles of the diet plan that you think GG should follow.

6. What is the mechanism of action of the following medications GG is receiving: Carafate, AlternaGel, and Pepcid?

7. List the nutrient-drug interactions that are associated with these medications.

■■
GG took the medication as prescribed and refrained from the cigarettes, caffeine, and alcohol as much as possible but, as she started to feel better, she went back to her old ways. One night she went on another binge and drank too much. The next morning she started throwing up BRB and not only had RLQ pain but severe LUQ pain as well. This frightened her so she decided to go to the ER. She was examined and hospitalized to R/O an ulcer. Her chart indicated the following:

➤ Height 5'2"

➤ Weight 98 lbs

➤ Recent loss of weight: 12 lbs in the last six months.
****

QUESTIONS CONTINUED:
8. What are GG's IBW and percent of IBW (Appendix A, Tables 7 and 8)?

9. Estimate her daily energy needs using the Harris-Benedict equation and appropriate stress factor (Appendix A, Table 17).

Lab values on admission:

CBC							
TEST	**RESULT**	**REFERENCE UNITS** Conventional	SI	**TEST**	**RESULT**	**REFERENCE UNITS** Conventional	SI
Hgb	20 g/dl	12-16 g/dl	120-160 g/L	WBC	8.0 10^3/µl	4.5-10.5 x 10^3/cells/mm^3	4.5-10.5 x10^9/L
Hct	60 %	36-48%		% Lymph	23%	25 – 40% of total WBC	1500-4000 cells/mm^3
RBC	3.9x10^6/µ	3.6-5.0x10^6/L	3.6-5.0 x10^{12}/L	MCH	26 pg/cell	26-34 pg/cell	0.40-.53 fmol/cell
MCV	80 µm^3	82-98µm^3	82-98 fL	MCHC	34 g/dl	32-36 g/dl	320-360 g/L

BASIC METABOLIC PACKAGE							
TEST	**RESULT**	**REFERENCE UNITS** Conventional	SI	**TEST**	**RESULT**	**REFERENCE UNITS** Conventional	SI
Glu	160 mg/dl	70-110 mg/dl	3.8-6.1 mmol/L	Na	142 mEq/L	136-145 mEq/L	136-145 mmol/L
BUN	37 mg/dl	6-20 mg/dl	2.1-7.1 mmol/L	K	4.9 mEq/L	3.5-5.2 mEq/L	3.5-5.2 mmol/L
Cr	1.7 mg/dl	0.6-1.1 mg/dl	53-97 µmol/L	Cl	105 mEq/L	96-106 mEq/L	96-106 mmol/L
Ca	8.4 mg/dl	8.8-10.0 mg/dl	2.20-2.60 mmol/L	Mg	1.8 mEq/L	1.8 - 2.6 mEq/L	136-145 mmol/L
Ser alb	4.1 g/dl	3.5-4.8 g/dl	39-50 g/dl	P	2.5mg/dl	2.7-4.5 mg/dl	4.7-6.0 kPa

LIVER FUNCTION							
TEST	**RESULT**	**REFERENCE UNITS** Conventional	SI	**TEST**	**RESULT**	**REFERENCE UNITS** Conventional	SI
AST	32 U/L	10-36 U/L	0.17-0.60 µkat/L	TBIL	0.6 mg/dl	0.3-1.0 mg/dl	5.0-17.0 µmol/L
ALT	20 U/L	7-35 U/L	7-56 U/L	DBIL	0.1 mg/dl	0-0.2 mg/dl	0-3.4 µmol/L
ALP	122 U/L	25-100 U/L	17-142 U/L	CPK	65 IU/L	26–140 U/L	0.42-2.38 µkat/L
TP	5.8 g/dl	6.5-8.3 g/dl	65-83 g/dl	Amylase	350/L	25–125 U/L	0.4-2.1 µkat/L

Her stool was positive for occult blood and an esophagogastroduodenoscopy revealed gastritis superior to the pyloric sphincter with an ulcer on the dorsal wall of the duodenum, just below the pyloric sphincter. During the endoscopy, the physician took a biopsy to R/O *Helicobacter pylori* and carcinoma. Gastric analysis indicated hypersecretion of HCl. An I.V. solution of D_5W was started. Because of the blood in her gut, the physician ordered a backup to the *H. pylori* biopsy with a blood test to detect serum IgG antibody to *H. pylori*. The biopsy for carcinoma was negative but a BUT was positive for *H. pylori*. The ELISA was also positive. As treatment, the physician ordered esomeprezole magnesium 40 mg once daily at hs; amoxicillin 1 g b.i.d.; and clarithromycin 500 mg b.i.d.
****

<u>QUESTIONS CONTINUED:</u>

10. What might be the cause of the LUQ pain along with her usual pain? (*Hint: Consider the enzymes that are elevated.*)

CBC							
TEST	**RESULT**	**REFERENCE UNITS** Conventional	SI	**TEST**	**RESULT**	**REFERENCE UNITS** Conventional	SI
Hgb	10 g/dl	12-16 g/dl	120-160 g/L	WBC	6.5 10^3/μl	4.5-10.5 x 10^3/cells/mm^3	4.5-10.5 x10^9/L
Hct	30 %	36-48%		% Lymph	23%	25 – 40% of total WBC	1500-4000 cells/mm^3
RBC	3.9x10^6/μ	3.6-5.0x10^6/L	3.6-5.0 x10^{12}/L	MCH	25 pg/cell	26-34 pg/cell	0.40-.53 fmol/cell
MCV	77 μm^3	82-98μm^3	82-98 fL	MCHC	33 g/dl	32-36 g/dl	320-360 g/L

Lab values two days after admission:

BASIC METABOLIC PACKAGE							
TEST	**RESULT**	**REFERENCE UNITS** Conventional	SI	**TEST**	**RESULT**	**REFERENCE UNITS** Conventional	SI
Glu	95 mg/dl	70-110 mg/dl	3.8-6.1 mmol/L	Na	141 mEq/L	136-145 mEq/L	136-145 mmol/L
BUN	10 mg/dl	6-20 mg/dl	2.1-7.1 mmol/L	K	3.7 mEq/L	3.5-5.2 mEq/L	3.5-5.2 mmol/L
Cr	0.9 mg/dl	0.6-1.1 mg/dl	53-97 μmol/L	Cl	105 mEq/L	96-106 mEq/L	96-106 mmol/L
Ca	8.5 mg/dl	8.8-10.0 mg/dl	2.20-2.60 mmol/L	Mg	1.9 mEq/L	1.8 - 2.6 mEq/L	136-145 mmol/L
Ser alb	2.4 g/dl	3.5-4.8 g/dl	39-50 g/dl	P	2.5mg/dl	2.7-4.5 mg/dl	4.7-6.0 kPa

LIVER FUNCTION							
TEST	**RESULT**	**REFERENCE UNITS** Conventional	SI	**TEST**	**RESULT**	**REFERENCE UNITS** Conventional	SI
AST	22 U/L	10-36 U/L	0.17-0.60 μkat/L	TBIL	0.6 mg/dl	0.3-1.0 mg/dl	5.0-17.0 μmol/L
ALT	15 U/L	7-35 U/L	7-56 U/L	DBIL	0.1 mg/dl	0-0.2 mg/dl	0-3.4 μmol/L
ALP	108 U/L	25-100 U/L	17-142 U/L	CPK	90 IU/L	26–140 U/L	0.42-2.38 μkat/L
TP	5.9 g/dl	6.5-8.3 g/dl	65-83 g/dl	Amylase	95/L	25–125 U/L	0.4-2.1 μkat/L

11. In the second set of lab values, glu, BUN, Cr, ser alb, Na, K, Cl, hgb, and hct all dropped. This probably means that GG was:
    a. bleeding.
    b. eating poorly in the hospital.
    c. dehydrated when the first labs were drawn.
    d. over hydrated when the second set of labs was drawn.

12. In the second set of lab values, serum amylase, AST, and ALT all dropped. This probably means that:
    a. enzymes were elevated due to alcohol.
    b. her medications caused them to drop.
    c. GG was dehydrated when the first labs were drawn.
    d. GG was over hydrated when the second set of labs was drawn.

13. Refer to the two lab tables again, and note that two days after admission, GG's Alk Phos and CPK remained essentially unchanged. Why?
    a. these enzymes are not affected by alcohol or hydration
    b. her medications caused them to drop
    c. dehydrated when the first labs were drawn
    d. over hydrated when the second set of labs was drawn

Information Box 15 - 1

It is difficult to culture *H. pylori*. The usual detection techniques are either the BUT or the serum antibodies test, but not both. There is evidence to indicate that blood in the stomach could produce a false negative[4] for the BUT, so a backup test would not be completely unreasonable. The two tests were ordered here to help the student to become familiar with the tests. The organism is also difficult to eradicate. The combination of medications that is most effective is still under evaluation but the combinations usually include a H_2-antagonist or a proton pump inhibitor, along with a combination of two antibiotics[1,5]. There is a definite theory behind this approach. *H. pylori* survives in the acidic environment of the stomach by producing urease which deaminates amino acids (hence the reasoning for a BUT). The free amino-group acts as a buffer and raises the pH from 4 to 6. This enables *H. pylori* to survive, but it is unable to reproduce at this pH. Antibiotics are ineffective if the organism is not replicating; thus, single antibiotic therapy does not eradicate the organism. When a H_2-antagonist or a proton pump inhibitor is included with the antibiotics, the pH is raised to between 6 and 8, which allows the organism to replicate. At this point the antibiotics can destroy the organism[9].

---

14. What diagnostic test(s) (not lab values) indicate(s) that GG has an ulcer?

15. Briefly sketch the anatomical position where GG's ulcer can be found.

16. Define:

    H_2 antagonist:

    Proton pump inhibitor:

17. What is the mechanism of action of the following medications GG is receiving: Nexium, amoxicillin, and clarithromycin?

****

PART II GASTRECTOMY

GG's medications were effective and the bleeding stopped. GG was discharged and was instructed to continue taking her medications, Nexium (esomeprezole magnesium), Amoxil (amoxicillin), and Biaxin (clarithromycin), for 14 days with a bland diet. GG followed her diet and took her medications for a while but since she felt so good, she quit taking the medication before she used all of it. She started going to a counselor on campus and her family provided additional help with babysitting. GG made it through the semester. That summer she worked full time and did not try to go to school. She spent more time with her son and that pleased him. The symptoms of ADHD were minimized.

The next fall she started back to school and took a full load. Her classes were hard and it was not long before GG was again too busy to accomplish everything. Her mother got the flu and was not able to baby-sit for her. GG's son went to kindergarten in the morning but needed a babysitter in the afternoon. Kindergarten and a babysitter were additional expenses for GG. Her divorce proceedings began and her husband was trying to fight paying the child support her lawyer was asking. GG started back to her old habits. She did not have time to eat right. She was upset most of the time and started smoking again to help calm herself. Staying up late was necessary and so was the coffee. The burning in her stomach started again. GG was determined not to let it slow her down.

She stopped going to her counselor and felt like she had no one to talk to. Since she was so pressed for time, her son was not getting the quality time with her that he had enjoyed during the summer. The symptoms of ADHD once again became intensely evident. GG was receiving pressure from every side. She was desperately trying to cope but could not perform well under pressure. The burning got worse and more frequent. GG was losing weight and started feeling tired and weak. She was not the type of person to quit so she kept trying. GG needed to unwind. Her drinking restarted and so did the ASA. She noted that her stools were getting darker, but she did not see that as important, so she overlooked it.

One evening, after a very stressful day, GG had several drinks and started vomiting BRB. She called her mother who brought her to the ER where she was diagnosed with PUD. An IV was started with D$_5$NS, and GG received several units of PC. An abdominal tap was done and was positive for red blood cells. GG was rushed to surgery with a perforated ulcer. Her lab values before receiving PC included:

CBC							
TEST	RESULT	REFERENCE UNITS Conventional	SI	TEST	RESULT	REFERENCE UNITS Conventional	SI
Hgb	9 g/dl	12-16 g/dl	120-160 g/L	WBC	11.5 x 10^3/μ	4.5-10.5 x 10^3/cells/mm^3	4.5-10.5 x10^9/L
Hct	27 %	36-48%		% Lymph	17%	25 – 40% of total WBC	1500-4000 cells/mm^3
RBC	3.8x10^6/μ	3.6-5.0x10^6/L	3.6-5.0 x10^{12}/L	MCH	24 pg/cell	26-34 pg/cell	0.40-.53 fmol/cell
MCV	73 μm^3	82-98μm^3	82-98 fL	MCHC	33 g/dl	32-36 g/dl	320-360 g/L

BASIC METABOLIC PACKAGE							
TEST	RESULT	REFERENCE UNITS Conventional	SI	TEST	RESULT	REFERENCE UNITS Conventional	SI
Glu	92 mg/dl	70-110 mg/dl	3.8-6.1 mmol/L	Na	139 mEq/L	136-145 mEq/L	136-145 mmol/L
BUN	26 mg/dl	6-20 mg/dl	2.1-7.1 mmol/L	K	3.6 mEq/L	3.5-5.2 mEq/L	3.5-5.2 mmol/L
Cr	0.9 mg/dl	0.6-1.1 mg/dl	53-97 µmol/L	Cl	101 mEq/L	96-106 mEq/L	96-106 mmol/L
Ca	8.6 mg/dl	8.8-10.0 mg/dl	2.20-2.60 mmol/L	Mg	1.9 mEq/L	1.8 - 2.6 mEq/L	136-145 mmol/L
Ser alb	3.1 g/dl	3.5-4.8 g/dl	39-50 g/dl	P	2.5mg/dl	2.7-4.5 mg/dl	4.7-6.0 kPa

Everyone has a breaking point and the events leading up to GG's reaching hers should be obvious. It is important to spot problem areas so that proper counsel can be provided. If you are not qualified to counsel in a certain area, leave it alone, but be aware of whom you can refer your client to for help.
****

QUESTIONS:

18. GG was not receiving counsel at the time the major bleeding started. If you had the opportunity to counsel GG just before the bleeding, in what areas would you feel competent to counsel her and in what areas would you refer her to someone else? Investigate the agencies in your area that are available to provide assistance to someone like GG.

19. What is the significance of the dark stools?

20. Give the pathophysiology for the cause of the following abnormal values: BUN, NH_3, and WBC.

21. GG was probably dehydrated on admission since she had been drinking. This means that some of her lab values were probably higher/lower (circle one) than indicated.

22. After admission GG received packed cells and IV fluids. How would that affect the next set of lab values?

****

An exploratory lap was done and additional ulceration was found in her stomach just superior to the pyloric sphincter. This was the area that contained gastritis during the previous tests. GG received a partial gastrectomy with a Billroth I and a vagotomy. The ulcer created a small fistula but did not erode a blood vessel. GG was very fortunate; it could have been a lot worse. The post-op period went very well. GG

recovered without complications. She was sent home on a postgastrectomy diet and was placed under the care of a psychiatrist.
****

QUESTIONS CONTINUED:

23. Define the following terms:

    Packed cells:

    Abdominal tap:

    Perforated ulcer:

    Fistula:

    Exploratory Laparotomy:

    Billroth I:

    Vagotomy:

24. Sketch a Billroth I.

25. Compare a Billroth I to a Billroth II as to anatomical changes as well as to dietary changes, if any.

26. Calculate GG's energy and protein needs.

27. List the principles of a postgastrectomy diet and briefly describe the scientific basis for each principle.

28. Is it possible that GG's diet will ever change or do you believe she will be on a postgastrectomy diet for the rest of her life? Explain your answer.

<u>**ADDITIONAL OPTIONAL QUESTIONS**</u>:

Tube Feeding Drill:

29. If GG were to be hospitalized for an extended period of time and required a tube feeding via duodenum or jejunum, what characteristics would be appropriate for the tube feeding you would use?

30. Using the table below, compare several of the enteral nutritional supplements that would be appropriate for GG.

Product	Producer	Form	Cal/ml	Non-pro cal/g N	g/L			Na mg	K mg	mOsm /kg water	Vol to meet RDA in ml	g of fiber /L	Free H$_2$O /L in ml
					Pro	CHO	Fat						

31. Prepare a SOAP note for GG.

S:
O:
A:
P:

RELATED READINGS

1. Ahmed, N. & Sechi, L.A. (2005). Helicobacter pylori and gastroduodenal pathology: New threats of the old friend. *Ann Clin Microbiol Antimicrob.* Jan 5;4(1):1

2. Anda, R.F., Williamson, D.F., Escobedo, L.G., & Remington, P.L. (1990). Smoking and the risk of peptic ulcer disease among women in the United States. *Arch. Intern. Med.* 150(7):1437-41.

3. Basinska, T., Wisniewska, M., & Chmiela, M. (2005). Principle of a New Immunoassay Based on Electrophoretic Mobility of Poly(styrene/alpha-tert-butoxy-omega-vinylbenzyl-polyglycidol) Microspheres: Application for the Determination of Helicobacter pylori IgG in Blood Serum. *Macromol Biosci.* Jan5;5(1):70-77.

4. Chu, K.M., Choi, H.K., Tuen, H.H., Law, S.Y., Branicki, F.J., & Wong, J. (1998). A prospective randomized trial comparing the use of omeprazole-based dual and triple therapy for eradication of Helicobacter pylori. *Am. J. Gastroenterol.* 93(9):1436-1442.

5. Chung, C.S. (1997). Surgery and gastrointestinal bleeding. *Gastrointest. Endosc. Clin. N. Am.* 7(4):687-701.

6. Crabtree, J.E., Shallcross, T.M., Heatley, R.V., & Wyatt, J.I. (1991). Evaluation of a commercial ELISA for serodiagnosis of Helicobacter pylori infection. *J. Clin. Pathol.* 44(4):326-8.

7. Fischbach, F.T. (2003). *A Manual of Laboratory & Diagnostic Tests.* 7th Ed. Philadelphia. J.B. Lippincott Company.

8. Kyzer, S., Binyamini, Y., Melki, Y., Ohana, G., Koren, R., Chaimoff, C., & Wolloch, Y. (1997). Comparative study of the early postoperative course and complications in patients undergoing Billroth I and Billroth II gastrocetomy. *World J. Surg.* 21(7):763-6.

9. Lau, W.Y. & Leow, C.K. (1997). History of perforated duodenal and gastric ulcers. *World J. Surg.* 21(8):890-6.

10. Lee, Y.T., Sung, J.J., Choi, C.L., Chan, F.K., Ng, E.K., Ching, J.Y., Leung, W.K., & Chung, S.C. (1998). Ulcer recurrence after gastric surgery: is Helicobacter pylori the culprit? *Am. J. Gastroenterol.* 93(6):928-31.

11. Leivonen, M., Nordling, S., & Haglund, C. (1998). The course of Helicobacter pylori infection after partial gastrectomy for peptic ulcer disease. *Hepatogastroenterology.* 45(20):587-91.

12. Leung, W.K., Sung, J.J., Siu, K.L., Chan, F.K., Ling, T.K., & Cheng, A.F. (1998). False-negative biopsy urease test in bleeding ulcers caused by the buffering effects of blood. *Am. J. Gastroenterol.* 93(10):1914-8.

13 Levenstein, S., Kaplan, G.A., & Smith, M. (1995). Sociodemographic characteristics, life stressors, and peptic ulcer. A prospective study. *J. Clin. Gastroenterol.* 21(3):185-92.

14. Levenstein, S. & Kaplan, G.A. (1998). Socioeconomic status and ulcer. A prospective study of contributory risk factors. *J. Clin. Gastroenterol.* 26(1):14-7.

15. Prendergast, A. & Fulton, F.L. (1997) *Medical terminology: A Text/Workbook.* 4th Ed. Redwood City, California. Addison-Wesley Nursing.

16. Pronsky, Z.M., Redfern, C.M., Crowe, J. & Epstein, S. (2003) *Food Medication Interactions*, 13th Ed Phoenix, Arizona. Food-Medications Interactions, Publishers and Distributors.

17. Pipkin, G.A., Williamson, R., & Wood, J.R. (1998). Review article: one-week clarithromycin triple therapy regimens for eradication of Helicobacter pylori. *Aliment. Pharmacol. Ther.* 12(9):823-37.

18. Prach, A.T., Malek, M., Tavakoli, M., Hopwood, D., Senior, B.W., & Murray, F.E. (1998). H₂-antagonist maintenance therapy versus Helicobacter pylori eradication in patients with chronic duodenal ulcer disease: a prospective study. *Aliment. Pharmacol. Ther.* 12(9):873-80.

19. Ralphs, D.N. (1981). The dumping syndrome. *Br. J. Clin. Pract.* 35(9):291-3.

20. Rolfes, S.R., Pinna, K. & Whitney, E. (2006). *Understanding Normal and Clinical Nutrition*, 7th Ed. West/Wadsworth.

21. Scott, D., Weeks, D., Melchers, K., & Sachs, G. (1998). The life and death of Helicobacter pylori. *Gut.* Suppl. 1:S56-60.

22. Spratto, G.R. & Woods, A.L. (2005). *PDR Nurse's Drug Handbook.* Thompson Delmar Learning, NY.

23. Svanes, C., Soreide, J.A., Skarstein, A., Fevang, B.T., Bakke, P., Vollset, S.E., Svanes, K., & Sooreide, O. (1997). Smoking and ulcer perforation. *Gut.* 41(2):177-80.

24. Tomita,R., Tanjoh, K. & Fujisaki, S. (2004). Novel operative technique for vagal nerve- and pyloric sphincter-preserving distal gastrectomy reconstructed by interposition of a 5 cm jejunal J pouch with a 3 cm jejunal conduit for early gastric cancer and postoperative quality of life 5 years after operation. *World J Surg.* Aug;28(8):766-74.

25. Vaira, D., Holton, J., Menegatti, M., Landi, F., Ricci, C., Ali, A., Gatta, L., Farinelli, S., Acciardi, C., Massardi, B., & Miglioli, M. (1998). Blood tests in the management of Helicobacter pylori infection. Italian Helicobacter pylori Study Group. *Gut.* Suppl. 1:S39- 46.

26. Vecht, J., Masclee, A.A., & Lamers, C.B. (1997). The dumping syndrome. Current insights into pathophysiology, diagnosis and treatment. *Sacnd. J. Gastroenterol. Suppl.* 223:21-7.

27. Yamashita, Y., Toge, T., & Adrian, T.E. (1997). Gastrointestinal hormone in dumping syndrome and reflux esophagitis after gastric sur

28. Yasunaga, Y., Bonilla-Palacios, J.J., Shinomura, Y., Kanayama, S., Miyazaki, Y., & Matasuzawa, Y. (1997). High prevalence of serum immunoglobulin G antibody to Helicobacter pylori and raised serum gastrin and pepsinogen levels in enlarged fold gastritis. *Can. J. Gastroenterol.* 11(5):433-6.

CASE STUDY#15
DIET AND DIVERTICULOSIS RESULTING IN A COLOSTOMY

INTRODUCTION

This is a two-part study of diverticulosis. In PART I the disease is treated by diet. In PART II the disease progresses and requires surgery. This is a basic study and involves a patient of ethnic background. Review the symptoms, diet, and treatment of diverticulitis prior to completing this study.
****

SKILLS NEEDED

ABBREVIATIONS:

Knowledge of the following abbreviations is required in order to understand this case. You should learn these abbreviations before you begin to read the study. BE, CHD, FH, LLQ, and MI (Appendix C).

FORMULAS:

The formulas used in this case study include ideal body weight and percent ideal body weight. The formulas can be found in Appendix A, Tables 7 and 8.

LABORATORY VALUES:

The normal values for the following parameters will be needed for this case study: BUN, Ca, Cl, CO_2, Cr, glu, hct, hgb, K, % lymph, MCH, MCHC, MCV, Mg, Na, P, RBC, Ser alb, and WBC (Appendix B).

MEDICATIONS:

Become familiar with the following medications before reading the case study. Note the diet-drug interactions, dosages and methods of administration, gastrointestinal tract reactions, etc.
1. Amoxil (amoxicillin); 2. Vasotec (enalapril maleate); 3. Ex-Lax (phenolphthalein).
****

PART I: TREATMENT WITH DIET

Mrs. K is a 68 YOWF who is 5'4" and weighs 170 lbs. She is a German-American widow who lives by herself in central Michigan. She has raised four children, all of whom are well and are living in other cities. Mrs. K has a FH of CHD on her father's side of the family. A brother died of a MI when he was 72, and her father had two MIs before dying of a stroke at 70. Mrs. K's mother died of intestinal cancer when she was 81.

Mrs. K does not smoke. She drinks a glass of wine occasionally. Other than a cold each winter, Mrs. K has been relatively healthy. She had pneumonia five years ago and required hospitalization but she recovered quickly. She has been taking enalapril maleate (Vasotec) for hypertension. Mrs. K has been on a weight reduction diet in the past but without much success. Almost a year ago, Mrs. K was bothered by some abdominal discomfort, particularly in the LLQ, where she had some colicky pains. The discomfort lasted for a couple of days and passed. She noted an increased amount of flatus also. She did not pay any attention to the problem since it ceased to bother her. A few weeks later she experienced a similar discomfort in the LLQ, again with increased flatus. That episode also passed after a couple of days. Mrs. K continued to have attacks on a more frequent basis. She noted rather severe pain and flatus when she ate foods that normally gave her gas, like navy beans and cabbage. As the attacks became more frequent and more severe, Mrs. K was also having problems with constipation. This was something that was not a problem previously. She tried taking Ex-Lax (phenolphthalein) but ended up with diarrhea and more cramps.

About a month ago she had a very severe attack with severe pain in the LLQ, tenderness, a temperature of 100°, and diarrhea that continued for three days. Mrs. K decided to go to the doctor. He prescribed amoxicillin (Amoxil) and scheduled her to have a BE on an outpatient basis. The results indicated diverticulitis in the sigmoid and descending colon. The physician continued Mrs. K on amoxicillin for ten

days and placed her on a low-fiber diet. He had her see the clinic dietitian before she went home and asked her to come back to see him in two weeks. If she improved, he would change her diet and discharge her.
****

QUESTIONS:

1. Briefly define the following terms:
    Barium enema:

    Diverticulitis:

    Diverticulosis:

    Diverticula:

2. List the symptoms of diverticulitis.

3. List the function, adverse reactions, and/or nutritional interactions of the following drugs: Vasotec, Ex-Lax, and amoxicillin.

4. Determine Mrs. K's IBW and percent IBW (Appendix A, Tables 7 and 8).

****

Before leaving the clinic, Mrs. K talked with the dietitian who completed a typical day's recall with Mrs. K.

RD: Mrs.K, I want you to take me through a typical day at home when you are feeling well and tell me everything you have to eat or drink. When you get up in the morning, what is the first thing you have to eat or drink?

Mrs. K: Generally, I get up about 7 A.M. and have some toast and coffee, a few hash browns, and a little piece of scrapple.

RD: Do you put anything on your toast?

Mrs. K: Yes, a little margarine and occasionally jelly.

RD: What kind of bread do you use?

Mrs. K: I use only white bread. The other is too heavy for me; I don't like it.

RD: I see, and do you put anything in your coffee?

Mrs. K: A little bit of cream and some sugar.

RD: Mrs. K, could you be a little more specific for me and tell me amounts, like the number of spoons of sugar, etc.?

Mrs. K: Oh sure! I use about two tablespoons of cream and two teaspoons of sugar.

RD: Thank you. Anything else for breakfast?

Mrs. K: No, that's all.

RD: What is the next thing you have to eat or drink?

Mrs. K: Well the noon meal is my biggest meal. I don't eat much at night; it doesn't settle well with me if I try to sleep with a full stomach.

RD: Alright, what do you have at the noon meal?

Mrs. K: I may fix a small pork roast, a pork chop, a hamburger, or a nice piece of blood sausage, if I can get it. You can't get good blood sausage any more, ever since my husband died. . . .

RD: And how do you usually fix this meat?

Mrs. K: I broil all my meats except for scrapple, of course; I fry that.

RD: What else do you have with the meat?

Mrs. K: Maybe some boiled potatoes, kohlrabi, navy beans, maybe some carrots, and sauerkraut. Oh, I love my sauerkraut.

RD: Would you ever have a salad?

Mrs. K: No, I'm not much for salads.

RD: Anything else? What would you have to drink?

Mrs. K: Coffee . . . with my cream and sugar.

RD: Do you eat anything else during the day?

Mrs. K: Sometimes in the evening I will have another cup of coffee and some toast, maybe with a little bit of tapioca pudding.

The RD completed the interview with a food frequency and instructed Mrs. K on her diet. It was evident that

Mrs. K did not get much fiber in her diet on most days. The inflammation cleared up so Mrs. K decided not to return.
****

QUESTIONS CONTINUED:

5. Discuss this interview by noting the good points, the bad points, and what you would do differently.

6. What are the principles of the diet recommended for diverticulitis?

7. Contrast the principles of the diet for diverticulitis with those for diverticulosis.

8. Based on her recall, what would you recommend that Mrs. K eat during one of her attacks? Compare this to what you would recommend after the attack is over.

9. Briefly, write out how you would explain diverticulosis and diverticulitis to Mrs. K.

10. Based on her interview, evaluate Mrs. K's diet by listing deficiencies or excesses in her diet.

11. Identify the following food items:
    Scrapple:

Blood sausage:

Kohlrabi:

Tapioca pudding:

12. Assume you are the clinic dietitian that completed the interview of Mrs. K and you had to record the results of your observations in her medical record. Compose a chart note using the SOAP format.

S:

O:

A:

P:

****

PART II: TREATMENT WITH SURGERY

Mrs. K followed her diet for a while but, after she felt better, she did not see any reason to continue. She was supposed to take a stool volume expander daily and drink plenty of fluids. She did not like the taste or consistency of the two different brands of stool volume expanders she tried, so she did not take any. The fluids made her go to the bathroom too much, so she did not do them either. Mrs. K continued to have problems with pain in the LLQ on occasion but it would go away in a few days. She started to have increased instance and severity of constipation followed by diarrhea. She did not associate that problem with diverticulitis. She thought it was something she ate.

Last week she had another severe attack with considerable pain and diarrhea. During these attacks she did not eat much because of the discomfort. One evening, after having suffered with the symptoms for two days, Mrs. K was watching television and feeling much better. She was hungry but did not feel like fixing herself anything. A commercial on television for popcorn reminded her that she had some microwave popcorn. She prepared and ate the contents of the whole package. She awoke that night with severe cramps, flatus, and felt very weak. The cramps got worse and diarrhea started. When she went to the bathroom, she passed a lot of bright red blood. This frightened her so much she called her physician. He had her go to the emergency room where, upon examination, she was found to be experiencing slight rectal bleeding. She was admitted for observation and tests. Mrs. K's labs taken in the ER were as follows:

BASIC METABOLIC PACKAGE							
TEST	RESULT	REFERENCE UNITS Conventional	SI	TEST	RESULT	REFERENCE UNITS Conventional	SI
Glu	80 mg/dl	70-110 mg/dl	3.8-6.1 mmol/L	Na	134 mEq/L	136-145 mEq/L	136-145 mmol/L
BUN	145 mg/dl	6-20 mg/dl	2.1-7.1 mmol/L	K	3.5 mEq/L	3.5-5.2 mEq/L	3.5-5.2 mmol/L
Cr	0.9 mg/dl	0.6-1.1 mg/dl	53-97 µmol/L	Cl	95 mEq/L	96-106 mEq/L	96-106 mmol/L
Ca	9.0 mg/dl	8.8-10.0 mg/dl	2.20-2.60 mmol/L	Mg	2.0 mEq/L	1.8 - 2.6 mEq/L	136-145 mmol/L
Ser alb	3.7 g/dl	3.5-4.8 g/dl	39-50 g/dl	P	2.8mg/dl	2.7-4.5 mg/dl	4.7-6.0 kPa

CBC							
TEST	RESULT	REFERENCE UNITS Conventional	SI	TEST	RESULT	REFERENCE UNITS Conventional	SI
Hgb	11 g/dl	12-16 g/dl	120-160 g/L	WBC	13 x 10^3/µl	4.5-10.5 x 10^3/cells/mm^3	4.5-10.5 x10^9/L
Hct	33 %	36-48%		% Lymph	23%	25 – 40% of total WBC	1500-4000 cells/mm^3
RBC	4.2x10^6/µ	3.6-5.0x10^6/L	3.6-5.0 x10^{12}/L	MCH	25 pg/cell	26-34 pg/cell	0.40-.53 fmol/cell
MCV	80 µm^3	82-98µm^3	82-98 fL	MCHC	33 g/dl	32-36 g/dl	320-360 g/L

The next morning Mrs. K felt worse. She was weaker and had chills. Her T was 101°. The doctor had written a diet order for NPO and started I.V. fluids and antibiotics the previous night. A stool test was still positive for blood. After the diarrhea stopped, a colonoscopy was done and severely inflamed diverticula were found in the sigmoid and descending colon. The MD speculated that Mrs. K had been bleeding slightly for some time because of erosion taking place in her sigmoid colon. He suspected that the heavier bleeding was due to the breaking of a very small blood vessel. His recommendation was removal of the sigmoid colon and a small part of the descending colon. Mrs. K had a partial colectomy with a resulting colostomy. She survived the

surgery without incident and her post-op recovery went well.
****

QUESTIONS CONTINUED:

13. Refer to the table of lab values above and note the abnormal values. Explain these abnormalities in light of her symptoms.

14. Define the following terms:
    Colonoscopy:

    Colostomy:

    Colectomy:

15. List the functions of the descending and sigmoid colon.

16. Give some examples of stool volume expanders.

17. Discuss the possible effects of constipation on Mrs. K's condition.

18. Give a possible explanation for the diarrhea Mrs. K was experiencing.

19. Explain how the stool volume expander, water, and high-fiber diet could possibly have helped prevent this surgery.

20. What kind of diet should Mrs. K be on after she recovers from surgery? Explain your answer.

21. How can diet help with the functioning of a descending colostomy?

22. What would be the differences in diet between someone with a colostomy and an ileostomy? What nutrients would be most affected?

ADDITIONAL OPTIONAL QUESTIONS:

SOAP Drill:

23. Assume you are the clinical dietitian responsible for Mrs. K's nutritional care. Add another SOAP entry in her chart (on the following page), continuing your note from Part I of this case study.

S:

O:

A:

P:

Tube Feeding Drill:

24. Suppose Mrs. K required a long-term hospitalization post surgery and needed to be fed via tube feeding into her stomach. Using the table below, compare several of the enteral nutritional supplements that would be appropriate for Mrs. K.

Product	Producer	Form	Cal/ ml	Non-pro cal/g N	g/L			Na mg	K mg	mOsm /kg water	Vol to meet RDA in ml	g of fiber /L	Free H$_2$O /L in ml
					Pro	CHO	Fat						

25. Suppose Mrs. K required a long-term hospitalization post surgery and needed to be fed via tube feeding into her small intestines. Would you use a different feeding than above? Explain.

26. If so, using the table below, compare several of the enteral nutritional supplements that would be appropriate for Mrs. K.

| Product | Producer | Form | Cal/ ml | Non-pro cal/g N | g/L | | | Na mg | K mg | mOsm /kg water | Vol to meet RDA in ml | g of fiber /L | Free H$_2$O /L in ml |
					Pro	CHO	Fat						

RELATED REFERENCES

1. Aldoori, W.H. (1997). The protective role of dietary fiber in diverticular disease. *Adv. Exp.Med. Biol.* 427:291-308.

2. Aldoori, W.H., Giovannucci, E.L., Rockett, H.R., Sampson, L., Rimm, E.B., & Willett, W.C. (1998). A prospective study of fiber types and symptomatic diverticular disease in men. *J.Nutr.*128(4):714-9.

3. Bennett, W.G., & Cerda, J.J. (1996). Benefits of dietary fiber. Myth or medicine? *Postgrad. Med.* 99(2):153-6, 166-8, 171-2.

4. Cheskin, L.J. & Lamport, R.D. (1995). Diverticular disease. Epidemology and pharmacological treatment. *Drugs Aging.* 6(1):55-63.

5. Cummings, J.H. (1996). Diverticular disease and your mother's diet. *Gut.* 39(3):489-90.

6. Elfrink, R.J. & Miedema, B.W. (1992). Colonic diverticula. When complications require surgery and when they don't. *Postgrad Med.* 92(6):97-8, 101-2, 105, 108.

7. Fischbach, F.T. (2003). *A Manual of Laboratory & Diagnostic Tests.* 7th Ed. Philadelphia. J.B. Lippincott Company.

8. Makapugay, L.M. & Dean, P.J. (1996). Diverticular disease-associated chronic colitis. *Am .J. Surg. Pathol.* 20(1):94-102.

9. Prendergast, A. & Fulton, F.L. (1997) *Medical terminology: A Text/Workbook.* 4th Ed. Redwood City, California. Addison-Wesley Nursing.

10. Pronsky, Z.M., Redfern, C.M., Crowe, J. & Epstein, S. (2003) *Food Medication Interactions*, 13th Ed Phoenix, Arizona. Food-Medications Interactions, Publishers and Distributors.

11. Rolfes, S.R., Pinna, K. & Whitney, E. (2006). *Understanding Normal and Clinical Nutrition*, 7th Ed. West/Wadsworth.

12. Spratto, G.R. & Woods, A.L. (2005). *PDR Nurse's Drug Handbook.* Thompson Delmar Learning, NY.

13. Yun, A.J., Bazar, K.A., & Lee, P.Y. (2005). A new mechanism for diverticular diseases: aging-related vagal withdrawal. *Med Hypotheses.* 64(2):252-5.

CASE STUDY #16
NUTRIGENOMICS
β^+-THALASSEMIA MINOR AND IRON OVERLOAD

INTRODUCTION

β^+-thalassemia minor is a genetic disease that is not uncommon. It usually is asymptomatic and does not require treatment. This is a study of someone with this disease who is improperly treated. This is corrected by another physician and iron overload is prevented. A good review of anemia, β^+-thalassemia, and the dangers of iron overload are presented. Lab values for anemia are introduced. This study requires a considerable amount of critical thinking.
****

SKILLS NEEDED

ABBREVIATIONS:
There are no new abbreviations in this case study.

LABORATORY VALUES:
You will need to be able to interpret the nutritional significance of the following laboratory values for this case study: Ferritin, hct, hgb, lymph, MCH, MCHC, MCV, RBC, serum iron, TIBC, transferrin, transferrin saturation, and WBC (Appendix B).

FORMULAS:
The formulas used in this case study include the calculation of TIBC and transferrin saturation. The formulas can be found in Appendix A, Tables 20 and 21. Growth percentile charts are also needed.

MEDICATIONS:
Become familiar with the following medication before reading the case study. Note the diet-drug interactions, dosages and methods of administration, gastrointestinal tract reactions, etc.
1. Ferrous sulfate.
****

RG is a 13 YOWF of Greek decent who has been healthy all of her childhood. She attends a large middle school in her home town and is a good student. She likes sports but has never participated in organized sports. For some time now it has been her desire to play basketball for her school team. Recently, tryouts for the team were announced and she talked her parents into allowing her to go out for the team. A physical was required before tryouts began. The students were sent to a Female Clinic that had an association with the school to complete physical exams for the students. RG's exam revealed her height to be 5'2" and her weight 110 lbs. She was found to be in good health the day of the physical. Blood was drawn for basic lab values and the results were to be received in two or three days. The results of the labs can be found in Table 1.

Table 1

CBC							
TEST	RESULT	REFERENCE UNITS Conventional	SI	TEST	RESULT	REFERENCE UNITS Conventional	SI
Hgb	10 g/dl	10.3-14.9 g/dl	103-149 g/L	WBC	5.2 10³/µl	5-10³/µl	5-10⁹/L
Hct	30 %	32-42%		% Lymph	18%	20 – 40% of total WBC	1000-4000/mm³
MCV	57 µm³	82-98µm³	82-98 fL	RBC	5.3x10⁶/µ	4.0-5.2x10⁶mm³	4.0-5.2 x10¹²/L
MCH	19 pg/cell	26-34 pg/cell	0.40-.53 fmol/cell	MCHC	33 g/dl	32-36 g/dl	320-360 g/L

When the physician saw the lab values, she had her nurse contact RG and obtained additional information. The RN found out that RG had no complaints of being tired or short of breath. RG established menarche about a year ago but, until recently, it had been very irregular. Lately, her periods were becoming more regular. The RN also asked her about her diet and determined that RG did not consume much meat and did not take vitamins.

****

QUESTIONS:

1. What percentile is RG for her height and weight for her age?

2. What do the abnormal lab values in Table 1 indicate? Be specific and explain each of the abnormal lab values.

****

The physician decided that the labs indicating anemia were the result of menses and not to be greatly concerned about. However, since RG was just beginning to go on a regular cycle and was losing more blood, and since she did not eat much meat or take vitamins and was getting ready to start a heavy exercise regimen, the physician thought it to be prudent to give RG an iron supplement just to be safe. She ordered ferrous sulfate tablets, 325 mg once a day, and told RG to take the iron after eating with a glass of orange juice. RG began taking the iron supplement daily.

After several days of taking the iron, RG began to complain of having nausea in the evening. This occurred every day until a friend suggested that it may be the iron supplement. RG's mom called their pharmacist and he agreed that iron supplements could cause nausea. RG was taking the iron with the evening meal. RG stopped taking the supplement for a few days and the nausea went away. She began taking it again and it returned, so she stopped it altogether and called the doctor. The physician that ordered the iron was out of town and instead of talking to another that did not know the case, RG's father decided to send her to her regular physician. He obtained a copy of the labs and he disagreed with the treatment. He ran some additional tests, the results of which can be found in Table 2.

Table 2

CBC							
TEST	**RESULT**	**REFERENCE UNITS** Conventional	SI	**TEST**	**RESULT**	**REFERENCE UNITS** Conventional	SI
Serum Fe	180 µg/dL	50-120 µg/dl	9.0-21.5 µmol/L	Ferritin	160 ng/ml	7-140 ng/ml	7-140 µg/L
TIBC	?	250-450 µg/dl	44.8-76.1 µmol/L	Trans-ferrin sat	?	15 – 50%	
Trans-ferrin	360 mg/dl	203-360 mg/dl	2.0-3.6 g/L				
RBC morphology: leptocytosis, microcytic, hypochromic, with small numbers of target cells							

Based on the new labs, RG's physician made a new diagnosis of β^+-Thalassemia minor, a genetic disease that directly affects nutrition in that it is concerned with iron metabolism. He D/C'd the iron tablets.
****

QUESTIONS CONTINUED:

3. Describe the interactions and complications possible with po iron.

4. Why did the physician tell RG to take the iron with orange juice?

5. Distinguish between the ferrous and ferric forms of iron in relation to where they are found, how they are absorbed, interfering factors, and the aids in absorption.

6. Distinguish between heme and non-heme iron in relation to where they are found, how they are absorbed, interfering factors, and the aids in absorption.

7. RG did not eat much meat. How does meat affect iron status?

8. The physician saw something in the first set of lab values that caused him to look further for β+-thalassemia minor. Hgb, hct were slightly down while MCV and MCH were down to a greater degree. These lab values with two other values triggered his suspicions. What two other labs values would have done this and why?

9. Define the following terms:
   leptocytosis:

   microcytic, hypochromic anemia:

10. Describe what the following tests indicate:

    Serum Fe:

    TIBC:

    Transferrin:

    Ferritin:

    Transferrin saturation:

11. Calculate RG's TIBC (Appendix A, Table 20).

12. Calculate RG's % saturation (Appendix A, Table 21).

13. Define β^+-thalassemia and explain how it is genetically transmitted. Describe the types of people most often affected.

14. Did RG fit the profile? Explain from a physical and a clinical point of view.

15. How serious is β+-thalassemia compared to its genetic counterpart β+-thalassemia major?

16. β+-thalassemia minor presents as a mild anemia, usually symptom free. This type of anemia is different than an anemia caused by bleeding or iron deficiency. Explain the differences.

17. If a mild anemia is detected but is not recognized as the genetic disorder β+-thalassemia minor, and it is attempted to be corrected nutritionally with increased iron consumption, as in this case, what serious side effects *will* result?

18. Explain what was discovered with the second set of lab values that enabled the physician to make the correct diagnosis.

19. Describe the effects of iron overload.

20. If a dietitian observes a situation in real life that is similar to this case and wants to alert the physician, it should be done in a diplomatic way. Use this SOAP note to indicate how you would do this.

S:	
O:	
A:	
P:	

21. Nutrition's relationship to genetics is a new frontier. There are many genetic diseases that can be helped or made worse by interaction with nutrition and the environment. PKU, diabetes, prostrate cancer, and hypertension are a few examples. There is a center to study this as it relates to minorities, the National Center of Excellence in Nutritional Genomics at the University of California, Davis, and the Children's Hospital Oakland Research Institute (CHORI). Visit their web sites at http://nutrigenomics.ucdavis.edu/ and http://nutrigenomics.ucdavis.edu/pressarticles.htm and define nutrigenomics

RELATED READINGS

1. Bauer, M., Hamm, A., & Pankratz, M.J. (2004). Linking nutrition to genomics. *Biol Chem.* Jul;385(7):593-6.

2. Cohen, A.R., Galanello, R., Pennell, D.J., Cunningham, M.J., and Vichinsky, E. (2004). Thalassemia. *Hematology* (Am Soc Hematol Educ Program). (1):14-34.

3. Desiere, F. (2004). Towards a systems biology understanding of human health: Interplay between genotype, environment and nutrition. *Biotechnol Annu Rev*. 10:51-84.

4. Ebert, P.R. (2004). Genomic strategies in the study of nutrition. *Asia Pac J Clin Nutr*. 13(Suppl):S13.

5. Fischbach, F.T. (2003). *A Manual of Laboratory & Diagnostic Tests*. 7th Ed. Philadelphia. J.B. Lippincott Company.

6. Ommen, B. & Groten, J.P. (2004). Nutrigenomics in efficacy and safety evaluation of food components. *World Rev Nutr Diet*. 93:134-52

7. Papanikolaou, G. and Pantopoulos, K. (2005). Iron metabolism and toxicity *Toxicol Appl Pharmacol*. Jan 15;202(2):199-211.

8. Pietrangelo, A. (2005). Non-invasive assessment of hepatic iron overload: are we finally there? *J Hepatol*. Jan;42(1):153-4.

9. Prendergast, A. & Fulton, F.L. (1997) *Medical terminology: A Text/Workbook*. 4th Ed. Redwood City, California. Addison-Wesley Nursing.

10. Pronsky, Z.M., Redfern, C.M., Crowe, J. & Epstein, S. (2003) *Food Medication Interactions*, 13th Ed Phoenix, Arizona. Food-Medications Interactions, Publishers and Distributors.

11. Ravindran, M.S., Patel, Z.M., Khatkhatay, M.I., and Dandekar, S.P. (2005). beta-thalassaemia carrier detection by ELISA: A simple screening strategy for developing countries. *J Clin Lab Anal*. 19(1):22-5.

12. Rolfes, S.R., Pinna, K. & Whitney, E. (2006). *Understanding Normal and Clinical Nutrition*, 7th Ed. West/Wadsworth.

13. Roche, H.M. (2004). Dietary lipids and gene expression. *Biochem Soc Trans*. Dec;32(Pt 6):999-1002.

14. Ruden, D.M., De Luca, M., Garfinkel, M.D., Bynum, K.L., & Lu, X. (2004). Drosophila Nutrigenomics can Provide Clues to Human Gene-Nutrient Interactions. *Annu Rev Nutr*. May 21.

15. Schrier, S.L. and Angelucci, E. (2005). New strategies in the treatment of the thalassemias. *Annu Rev Med*. 56:157-71.

16. Spratto, G.R. & Woods, A.L. (2005). *PDR Nurse's Drug Handbook*. Thompson Delmar Learning, NY.

17. van der Meer-van Kraaij, C., Kramer, E., Jonker-Termont, D., Katan, M.B., van der Meer, R., & Keijer, J. (2005). Differential gene expression in rat colon by dietary heme and calcium. *Carcinogenesis*. Jan;26(1):73-9. Epub 2004 Nov 11.

18. Voskaridou, E., Douskou, M., Terpos, E., Papassotiriou, I., Stamoulakatou, A., Ourailidis, A., Loutradi, A., and Loukopoulos, D. (2004). Magnetic resonance imaging in the evaluation of iron overload in patients with beta thalassaemia and sickle cell disease. *Br J Haematol*. Sep;126(5):736-42.

CASE STUDY #17
CYSTIC FIBROSIS

INTRODUCTION
This is a study of the genetic disease cystic fibrosis, which usually manifests during infancy or early childhood. The life expectancy for individuals with this disease is about twenty-plus years. The disease involves the mucus-producing glands in the pancreas, bronchi, intestines, and bile ducts. It is more common in whites than blacks, and more common in blacks than Asians.

****

SKILLS NEEDED

ABBREVIATIONS:
There is only one new abbreviation for this case study: CF (Appendix C).

LABORATORY VALUES:
You will need to be able to interpret the nutritional significance of the following laboratory values for this case study: Cl, Na, and the iontophoretic sweat test (Appendix B).

MEDICATIONS:
Become familiar with the following medications before reading the case study. Note the diet-drug interactions, dosages and methods of administration, gastrointestinal tract reactions, etc.
1. bronchodilators; 2. corticosteroids; 3. potassium iodine; 4. Viokase (pancrelipase).

****

RM is a 10 YOWM who has been suffering from CF since he was four years old. His height is 4'3" and he weighs 57 lbs. RM has frequent upper respiratory tract infections and usually has copious secretions of mucous. His parents take excellent care of him, but in spite of their attempts to keep RM healthy, he has recurring respiratory problems. When he was four years old, the disease manifested with abdominal pain, distention, steatorrhea, and a persistent cough that produced copious amounts of sputum. At that time, an iontophoretic sweat test was conducted and the results were:

➤ Na 90 mEq/L
➤ Cl 60 mEq/L

As RM grew older, the symptoms became severe, with respiratory tract infections being the predominant manifestation. RM's medications include bronchodilators, corticosteroids, and potassium iodide daily. When RM has a respiratory attack, he also receives the appropriate antibiotics and respiratory treatments (daily). His physicians are hoping to prevent bronchiectasis, atelectasis, and pneumonia, fatal complications for most CF patients. To help the digestion of his food, RM is receiving pancrelipase (Viokase). His digestion has not been as much of a problem as the respiratory attacks. Steatorrhea is no longer a problem with RM as long as he takes his enzymes. He has a ravenous appetite and does very well with his diet. When RM has respiratory distress, he gets very anxious and this affects his digestion and requires an increase in the dosage of pancrelipase.

****

QUESTIONS:
1. What should RM's height and weight be for his age?

2. What percentile is he in now for height and weight?

131

3. Define the following terms:

    Steatorrhea:

    Bronchiectasis:

    Atelectasis:

4. Discuss the genetic possibility of being born with CF based on gender and race.

5. Explain the effects of CF on the body.

6. What are the goals for nutritional therapy for CF?

7. What information about RM would be helpful in order to determine the percentages of energy that should come from carbohydrates, fats, and proteins?

8. What is a source of fat that would be helpful in the diet of a person with CF?

9. What are the mechanism of action and nutritional complications of the following drugs?

    pancrelipase (Viokase):

    potassium iodide:

    corticosteroid:

10. Explain the iontophoretic sweat test.

ADDITIONAL OPTIONAL QUESTIONS:

Tube Feeding Drill:

11. If RM were to become seriously ill, require hospitalization, and need to be fed via a feeding tube, what characteristics would be appropriate for the tube feeding you would use?

12. Using the table below, compare several of the enteral nutritional supplements that would be appropriate for a seriously ill CF patient (Appendix E).

| Product | Producer | Form | Cal/ml | Non-pro cal/g N | g/L | | | Na mg | K mg | mOsm /kg water | Vol to meet RDA in ml | g of fiber /L | Free H₂O /L in ml |
					Pro	CHO	Fat						

RELATED READINGS

1. Adde, F.V., Rodrigues, J.C., & Cardoso, A.L. (2004). Nutritional follow-up of cystic fibrosis patients: the role of nutrition education. *J Pediatr* Nov-Dec;80(6):475-82.

2. Anthony, H., Bines, J., Phelan, P., & Paxon, S. (1998). Relation between dietary intake and nutritional status in cystic fibrosis. *Arch. Dis. Child.* 78(5):443-7.

3. Benabdeslam, H., Garcia, I., Bellon, G., Gilly, R., & Revol, A. (1998). Biochemical assessment of the nutritional status of cystic fibrosis patients traeted with pancreaticenzyme extracts. *Am. J. Clin. Nutr.* 67(5):912-8.

4. Dorlochter, L., Roksund, O., Helgheim, V., Rosendahl, K., & Fluge, G. (2002). Resting energy expenditure and lung disease in cystic fibrosis. *J Cyst Fibros.* Sep;1(3):131-6.

5. Fischbach, F.T. (2003). *A Manual of Laboratory & Diagnostic Tests.* 7th Ed. Philadelphia. J.B. Lippincott Company.

6. Jelalian, E., Stark, L.J., Reynolds, L., & Seifer, R. (1998). Nutrition intervention for weight gain in cystic fibrosis: a meta analysis. *J. Pediatr.* 132(3):486-92.

7. Quirk, P.C., Ward, L.C., Thomas, B.J., Holt, T.l., Shepherd, R.W., & Cornish, B.H. (1997). Evaluation of bioelectrical impedance for prospective nutritional assessment in cystic fibrosis. *Nutrition.* 13(5):412-6.

8. Murphy, J.L. & Wootton, S.A. (1998). Nutritional managemant in cystic fibrosis—an alternative perspective in gastrointestinal function. *Disabil. Rehabil.* 20(6-7):226-34.

9. Prendergast, A. & Fulton, F.L. (1997) *Medical terminology: A Text/Workbook.* 4th Ed. Redwood City, California. Addison-Wesley Nursing.

10. Pronsky, Z.M., Redfern, C.M., Crowe, J. & Epstein, S. (2003) *Food Medication Interactions,* 13th Ed Phoenix, Arizona. Food-Medications Interactions, Publishers and Distributors.

11. Rendina, E.A., Venuta, F., DeGiacomo, T., Guarino, E., Ciccone, A.M., Quattrucci, S., Rocca, G.D., Antonelli, M., Ricci, C., & Coloni, G.F. (1998). Lung transplantation for cystic fibrosis. *Eur. J. Pediatr. Surg.* 8(4):208-11.

12. Spratto, G.R. & Woods, A.L. (2005). *PDR Nurse's Drug Handbook.* Thompson Delmar Learning, NY.

13. Stallings, V.A., Fung, E.B., Hofley, P.M., & Scanlin, T.F. (1998). Acute pulmonary exacerbation is not associated with increased energy expenditure in children with cystic fibrosis. *J. Pediatr.* 132(3):493-9.

14. Wagener, J.S., Sontag, M.K., Sagel, S.D., & Accurso, F.J. (2004). Update on newborn screening for cystic fibrosis. *Curr Opin Pulm Med.* Nov;10(6):500-4.

15. Wilson, D.C. & Pencharz, P.B. (1998). Nutrition and cystic fibrosis. *Nutrition.* 14(10):792.

CASE STUDY #18
DIETARY MANAGEMENT OF ATHEROSCLEROSIS
RESULTING IN OPEN-HEART SURGERY

INTRODUCTION

This is a three-part study of a patient with atherosclerosis who is treated with diet and balloon dilatation in PART I. In PART II the patient is sent home with a diet and follows the diet with various herbal and antioxidant supplements for a while but rationalizes himself out of it after a few years. In Part III open-heart surgery is required. For class study purposes, three different students or groups of students could each be given a part to present. A review of the foods that are high in cholesterol and saturated fat and basic information about cardiovascular disease is important for the understanding of this case study. Several medical terms and abbreviations are introduced.
****

SKILLS NEEDED

ABBREVIATIONS:
Knowledge of the following abbreviations is required in order to understand this case. You should learn these abbreviations before you begin to read the study (Appendix C).
ALT, AST, BEE, BMI, CABG, cath, Chol, C/O, CRP, C x R EKG, HDL, hs, LDL, sat, TG, and WNL.

LABORATORY VALUES:
You will need to be able to interpret the nutritional significance of the following laboratory values for this case study: BUN, Ca, Chol, Cl, Cr, Glu, HDL, homocysteine K, LDL, Mg, Na, P, ser alb, and TG (Appendix B).

FORMULAS:
The formulas used in this case study include ideal body weight, adjusted body weight, percent ideal body weight, basal energy expenditure, calorie and protein needs, the formula for calculating LDL and an appropriate stress factor (Appendix A).

MEDICATIONS:
Become familiar with the following medications before reading the case study. Note the diet-drug interactions, dosages and methods of administration, gastrointestinal tract reactions, etc.
1. Lipitor (atorvastatin calcium) and 2. Altace (ramipril).
****

PART I: DIET AND BALLOON DILATATION

Mr. F is a 54 YOWM who is a businessman in Ohio. His weight is 235 lbs and he is 6' tall. He has been gradually increasing in weight, about two pounds a year since his 31st birthday. He takes pride in the fact that he eats anything he wants. He does not have a family history of cardiovascular disease or diabetes, but none of his family members have been overweight. He is married and has three children. He has a pleasant job and is not under any particular kind of stress. He has been healthy all his life with only three hospitalizations for minor reasons: an appendectomy when he was a teenager, a hernia repair ten years ago, and two broken ribs from an automobile accident several years ago. Mr. F's job requires him to be on his feet all day but he does little in the way of exercise. A few weeks ago, after a heavy snow, Mr. F was clearing the sidewalk in front of his house with a snow shovel. After about 15 to 20 minutes of shoveling, he felt a sharp pain toward the center of his chest below the sternum. He got light-headed, weak, and his respirations increased. He rested for a while and it passed. He thought he had overworked himself in the cold and did nothing about it.

The next week he was visiting a friend on the fourth floor of a hospital. Because of the large crowd waiting for the elevator, he decided to take the stairs. He was going up the stairs at a brisk pace, partly to see if he would have chest pain again. The fact that he was in a hospital may have psychologically influenced him to make the decision to take this self-test. When he reached the top of the stairs, he had slight chest pain behind the sternum in the center of his chest. He now knew that this could be serious, so he made an appointment with his family physician.

The physician ran the usual tests, EKG, blood work, and CxR. His blood pressure was 144/84. Mr. F's physician agreed with him that his situation could be serious, so he sent him to see a cardiologist. The cardiologist completed a treadmill stress test. Mr. F was not able to finish the test. He was admitted to the hospital for further evaluation. A cardiac cath revealed that Mr. F had 50 percent blockage in two arteries and 80 percent blockage in a third artery. The cardiologist believed that this could be corrected with angioplasty. This procedure was attempted and was successful in opening the 80 percent blocked vessel. The physician recommended that Mr. F go on a weight reduction diet, low in saturated fat, low in cholesterol, and high in fiber with no more than two grams of sodium, and an energy level as recommended by the RD. A more aggressive physician would have started Mr. F on a statin and perhaps an ace inhibitor, but this physician, because of Mr. F's education and lack of family history of cardiovascular disease, decided to take a more conservative approach and try diet first. Mr. F's lab values were as follows:

BASIC METABOLIC PACKAGE							
TEST	RESULT	REFERENCE UNITS Conventional SI		TEST	RESULT	REFERENCE UNITS Conventional SI	
Glu	130 mg/dl	70-110 mg/dl	3.8-6.1 mmol/L	Na	145 mEq/L	136-145 mEq/L	136-145 mmol/L
BUN	12 mg/dl	6-20 mg/dl	2.1-7.1 mmol/L	K	4.2 mEq/L	3.5-5.2 mEq/L	3.5-5.2 mmol/L
Cr	1.0 mg/dl	0.9-1.3 mg/dl	80-115 μmol/L	Cl	102 mEq/L	96-106 mEq/L	96-106 mmol/L
Ca	9.0 mg/dl	8.8-10.0 mg/dl	2.20-2.60 mmol/L	Mg	2.2 mEq/L	1.8 - 2.6 mEq/L	136-145 mmol/L
Ser alb	3.6 g/dl	3.5-4.8 g/dl	39-50 g/dl	P	3.1mg/dl	2.7-4.5 mg/dl	4.7-6.0 kPa

LIPID PROFILE							
TEST	RESULT	REFERENCE UNITS Conventional SI		TEST	RESULT	REFERENCE UNITS Conventional SI	
Chol	300 mg/dl	140-199 mg/dl	3.63-5.15 mmol/L	HDL	35 mEq/L	45-65 mEq/L	1.17-1.68 mmol/L
TG	285 mg/dl	<-150 mg/dl	<1.70 mmol/L	LDL	185 mg/dl	<130 mg/dl	<3.4 mmol/L

****

QUESTIONS:

1. Determine Mr. F's IBW and percent of IBW (Appendix A, Tables 7 and 8).

2. Calculate Mr. F's BMI (Appendix A, Tables 10 and 11).

3. Calculate Mr. F's adjusted body weight (Appendix A, Table 9).

4. Define the following terms:
   Balloon Dilation:

   Cardiac Cath:

   Treadmill Stress Test:

   ACE inhibitor:

   Statin:

5. Using the Harris-Benedict equation, calculate Mr. F's BEE and total energy needs (Appendix A, Table 17).

6. What goals would you set for weight reduction for Mr. F?

7. How many kcals would you recommend he consume daily to meet those goals?

8. List the principles of his heart disease prevention diet (the most recent TLC diet recommended by the American Heart Association, http://www.americanheart.org/presenter.jhtml?identifier=4764 and http://circ.ahajournals.org/cgi/content/full/102/18/2284). Include in your list recommendations for: foods to be avoided, total calories coming from fat, ratio of polyunsaturated to monounsaturated to saturated fat, and total grams of cholesterol, sodium, and fiber per day.

9. What are the latest recommendations for blood pressure? What can be said about Mr. F's blood pressure?

10. What is the relationship between blood pressure and dietary sodium? Do you think Mr. F needs a 2 g sodium restriction? Explain.

11. What are the latest recommendations for lipid profile for those at risk and not at risk of CVD?
    a. Cholesterol:

    b. Triglycerides:

    c. LDL:

    d. HDL:

12. What do statins have to do with preventing atherosclerosis?

13. Describes the side effects of statins and any drug/drug interactions and diet/drug interactions.
    a.   Side effects:

    b.   Drug/drug interactions:

    c.   Diet/drug interactions:

****

The RD went in to visit Mr. F to discuss his diet with him. She did a typical day's recall and obtained the following information. For breakfast, Mr. F enjoyed scrambled eggs with hash browns, one slice of toast with margarine, juice, and coffee with sugar. At work, his only snack was coffee with one sugar. For lunch, he usually ate a sandwich, frequently a dressed hamburger with french fries and coffee with sugar. Sometimes he had a piece of pie or cake for dessert, depending on what was available. At home, he had what he described as a typical dinner consisting of meat at every evening meal (chicken, beef, pork, sometimes fish), potatoes, and usually a boiled vegetable (carrots, green beans, and cabbage are some of his favorites). A salad was seldom eaten at night. Sometimes he had dessert, such as pudding, ice cream, or Jell-o (something soft and sweet). Before bedtime, he frequently had a large snack consisting of cheese and crackers, ice cream, or a sandwich of any meat that was left over from dinner. He usually had a regular soft drink with this snack. The registered dietitian emphasized the importance of keeping his intake of saturated fat low and increasing his polyunsaturated and monounsaturated fats. She also encouraged him to increase his fiber intake.

****

QUESTIONS CONTINUED:

14. List the foods that are high in cholesterol, saturated fat, and sodium in Mr. F's diet.

FOOD	CHOL	SAT FAT	Na

15. Explain the relationship of each of the three types of fat and cholesterol intake to cardiovascular disease.

16. Explain the role of dietary fiber in cardiovascular disease.

PART II: DIET WITH SUPPLEMENTS

Mr. F went home from the hospital feeling that he had a new lease on life. He was encouraged by the doctor's report and was looking forward to trying his new lifestyle and diet. He was also encouraged by a report a friend brought him while he was in the hospital. His friend has become convinced that most diseases can be avoided by the use of herbal medicine. For atherosclerosis, she recommended Mr. F concentrate on taking antioxidants and other supplements. The antioxidants and supplements she recommended included garlic, coenzyme Q, vitamins E, B_{12}, B_6, and folic acid. She also recommended that Mr. F take a baby aspirin each day. Another friend gave him a summary of an article he found that indicated eating almonds, margarines with plant sterols, and psyhelium fiber can lower cholesterol as well as drugs. Before leaving the hospital, Mr. F had some questions for the dietitian, the content of which are included in the questions that follow.
****

17. Define:
    antioxidant:

    free radicals:

    psyhelium fiber:

18. Describe the effect of antioxidants on free radicals and show how this relates to atherosclerosis.

19. What role, if any, does coenzyme Q have with cardiovascular disease?

20. Is it true that taking statins increases the need for coenzyme Q? Explain.

21. What relationship do the vitamins folic acid, B_{12}, and B_6 have with atherosclerosis?

22. What is the purpose of taking a baby aspirin every day? Does it help prevent heart attacks?

23. Describe the possible relationship between garlic and atherosclerosis.

Information Box 21 - 1

While the literature indicates that garlic has the potential to help in the prevention of several diseases, the processing of the garlic is critical to its effectiveness. See the discussion in reference 42, pg. 104.

---

24. Have all preparations and forms of garlic been found to produce a favorable effect? Explain

25. Can you describe a potential problem with taking aspirin, garlic, and vitamin E?

26. Describe the effects of plant sterols (like those in Benecol, Take Control, and Minute Maid Heart Wise orange juice) on cholesterol.

27. What effect, if any, does psyhelium have on atherosclerosis?

28. How would you address Mr. F's willingness to take supplements recommended by a person without professional training in nutrition or medicine?

29. Vitamin, mineral, and herbal supplements are regulated by the:
    a. USDA.
    b. FDA.
    c. state the product is sold in.
    d. none of the above

30. To declare an herbal supplement unsafe, the burden of proof for its lack of safety is on the:
    a. producer of the herb.
    b. USDA.
    c. FDA.
    d. state the herb is sold in.

31. If a product is "all natural," it means:
    a. it is perfectly safe for human consumption.
    b. it has been tested and found to be non-toxic.
    c. it is probably safe.
    d. it is "natural" and nothing else.

32. Describe the process by which a drug is approved for sales.

33. Describe the process by which an herb is approved for sales.

34. Write a SOAP note based on all of the above information.

S:	
O:	
A:	
P:	

ADDITIONAL OPTIONAL QUESTIONS:

35. If Mr. F were to take supplements of aspirin, coenzyme Q, folic acid, vitamins E, B_{12}, and B_6, what doses would you recommend?

36. On a separate sheet of paper, plan a day's menu for Mr. F that will include all of the appropriate diet recommendations.

PART III: OPEN-HEART SURGERY

Mr. F followed his diet and took his nutritional supplements for about a year after he left the hospital and he lost 20 pounds. He also started an exercise program at the recommendation of his cardiologist. He started walking at a slow pace for 15 minutes a day. He gradually increased his pace and the length of time of his exercise. Several weeks after his discharge from the hospital, he was losing weight and was feeling a lot better. His exercise routine was improving. He had increased his walking to 45 minutes per day and was at a faster pace. He felt confident that he was well. His exercise program continued as long as he was following his diet. Things got very busy at work as winter approached and the cold weather kept Mr. F from exercising outside. His walking decreased and his diet changed with the start of the Christmas holidays. There were so many nutritional supplements he had to take that it was expensive and difficult to keep up with. His weight slowly increased but he felt fine, so he did not pay attention to the weight gain. When he went back to the doctor for a check-up, another lipid profile was completed and the physician added some additional lab tests. His lipid profile was still unacceptable.

LIPID PROFILE							
TEST	**RESULT**	**REFERENCE UNITS** Conventional	SI	**TEST**	**RESULT**	**REFERENCE UNITS** Conventional	SI
Chol	330 mg/dl	140-199 mg/dl	3.63-5.15 mmol/L	HDL	36 mEq/L	45-65 mEq/L	1.17-1.68 mmol/L
TG	315 mg/dl	< 150 mg/dl	< 1.7 mmol/L	LDL	? mg/dl	<130 mg/dl	<3.4 mmol/L
hs-CRP	1.3 mEq/L	<0.8 mg/dL	<8 mg/L	Homo-cysteine	25 μmol/L	4 – 17 μmol/L	0.54-2.3 mg/L

****

QUESTIONS:

37. Calculate Mr. F's LDL using the formula in Appendix A, Table 19.

38. What does an elevated CRP and homocysteine indicate in general?

39. What does an elevated CRP and homocysteine indicate in relation to atherosclerosis?

****

The doctor decided that diet and exercise would not work in Mr. F's case and prescribed medication to help lower his cholesterol, triglycerides, and LDL, and raise his HDL. He put Mr. F on Lipitor (atorvastatin calcium), 20 mg/d and Altace (ramipril), 10 mg/d. He also ordered 1 mg of folate, 250 μg of B_{12} and 50 mg of

B$_6$. He instructed Mr. F to take the medication for three months and to come back to check his lipid profile and liver enzymes. Mr. F did this and in three months had the following profile:

LIPID PROFILE							
TEST	RESULT	REFERENCE UNITS Conventional	SI	TEST	RESULT	REFERENCE UNITS Conventional	SI
Chol	179 mg/dl	140-199 mg/dl	3.63-5.15 mmol/L	HDL	42 mEq/L	45-65 mEq/L	1.91-1.68 mmol/L
TG	90 mg/dl	<-150 mg/dl	<1.70 mmol/L	LDL	? mg/dl	<130 mg/dl	<3.4 mmol/L
hs-CRP	0.5 mEq/L	<0.8 mg/dL	<8 mg/L	Homo-cysteine	11 μmol/L	4 – 17 μmol/L	0.54-2.3 mg/L
ALT	36 U/L	10-40 U/L	0.17-0.68 μkat/L	AST	16 U/L	14-20 U/L	0.23-0.33 μkat/L

****

QUESTIONS CONTINUED:

40. Calculate Mr. F's LDL and compare the results of this lipid profile with the previous one (Appendix A, Table 19).

41. What are the side effects or contraindications of Lipitor? (*Hint: Why were ALT & AST checked?*)

****

The physician rechecked Mr. F's lipid profile in three months with the same favorable results. Mr. F was extremely pleased and continued to take his medication faithfully but he conducted a test of his own. He began to eat high-fat foods again, though not as much as he used to. He also decreased his exercise because his work load increased again and he was pressed for time. The winter months helped provide an additional excuse. After a high-fat meal, he obtained a cholesterol test kit from the drugstore and tested his own cholesterol. It was acceptable. He figured that if his cholesterol was acceptable, then the rest of the profile was also. His avoidance of exercise continued as did his diet noncompliance. If the medication worked so well, Mr. F did not see why he had to stay on such a strict diet. He ever so gradually began to include some of his old foods in his diet. He gained 10 pounds. He still felt good and was pleased with his weight and conditioning. He did not restart his exercise and diet program that spring. As time passed, Mr. F continued to gain weight and started to skip his medication to save money. He would take it before he went for a lipid profile to fool the doctor. In a few years, he gained to 235 lbs. He was not doing any exercise and was back to his old routine.

One summer day he was cutting his grass in mid-afternoon. It was very hot and he was perspiring profusely but was not drinking fluids. He started to get tired and his breathing became very fast. He also started having some slight chest pain again. This scared Mr. F and he began to panic. As he panicked, he started to hyperventilate; as he hyperventilated, his anxiety grew worse. With increased anxiety, his chest pain increased. He slowly made his way back into the house and rested on the couch. His wife found him there and called his cardiologist. As Mr. F cooled off, his perspiring and his chest pain stopped, and his anxiety eased. He refused to go to the doctor then but promised he would see a doctor the following week, which he did. The physician completed extensive tests, including an EKG and blood tests. His lab values were normal except for his lipid profile. Cholesterol was 340 mg/dl and triglycerides were 270 mg/dl. The cardiologist suggested that Mr. F be admitted to the hospital and have another cardiac cath done. Mr. F reluctantly agreed. The results showed that the blood vessel that had been 80 percent blocked was now 90 percent blocked. The two blood vessels that were 50 percent blocked were now 70 percent blocked. The cardiologist told Mr. F that, in his opinion, he should have open heart surgery for a CABG x 3. Again, Mr. F reluctantly agreed.

Mr. F's surgery was a complete success. He spent two days in the open heart recovery unit and was then admitted to the surgical floor. While in the recovery unit, he was started on cl liqs and tolerated them well. Within a few days he was on a 2g Na diet. His first tray of solid food was breakfast and it shocked him. On his tray were scrambled eggs, toast, two pats of margarine, whole milk, hash browns, and orange juice. There was no salt on the tray. Mr. F called the nurse and requested to see the dietitian. Later, the RD came to talk to Mr. F. He explained to her his concern. He just had open-heart triple by-pass surgery because of elevated cholesterol levels and received eggs, whole milk, fried potatoes, and margarine for breakfast. Mr. F also C/O not being hungry and said that "things just didn't taste right."

The RD who went to see Mr. F had just finished school and was being oriented to the cardiovascular surgical unit. Since Mr. F asked to consult a dietitian about a complaint, she went to see him to determine the problem. She would later confer with the RD in charge of that floor. She told him that a lack of ability to taste and a lack of appetite were common after open-heart surgery. She also explained that the sodium restriction was to prevent the accumulation of fluid and explained clearly how that worked. The RD stated that she had not yet been oriented to the hospital's policy on post-CABG diets. Thus, she was not sure why Mr. F had so much cholesterol and saturated fat on his tray, and did not attempt to offer an explanation. She told him that she would check to see if he should be receiving a modified diet.

The RD returned the same day with an answer to Mr. F's question about the saturated fat and cholesterol on his tray. She explained that hospital policy allowed open-heart surgical patients to receive eggs on the breakfast tray with a liberal fat intake for the purpose of encouraging intake. She further explained that right after surgery, as she previously mentioned, patients usually do not feel like eating, especially when they are on a restricted diet. Therefore, to encourage caloric intake and to promote healing, eggs and saturated fat were allowed for five days after surgery. During that time, the patients were taught the diet they were expected to follow at home. The RD said that five days of moderate cholesterol and saturated fat intake would not cause harm. Mr. F said that he understood, but since a poor diet may have been the cause of his need for surgery, he would prefer to start his diet right away. The RD agreed and said that he would receive the same diet that he would be expected to follow at home.

QUESTIONS CONTINUED:

42. Calculate Mr. F's energy and protein needs right after surgery and six weeks later. Show your work (Appendix A, Table 17).

43. Mr. F received scrambled eggs, hash browns, whole milk, and margarine for breakfast on his first day on a 2g Na diet. The RD was not sure why this was so but found the answer for Mr. F the same day. Did the RD handle this encounter appropriately? The outcome was that the RD changed his diet to a low-cholesterol, low-saturated fat diet. Do you agree with this or should the RD have insisted upon following hospital policy? Explain your answer.

44. In school, the RD was not introduced to the practice of allowing open heart surgery patients to eat what they want the first few days after surgery. Some hospitals allow this but most probably do not. Discuss the pros and cons of this policy, and offer your feelings about this practice.

45. What are the dietary principles Mr. F should be following after he fully recovers from surgery?

46. What goals should be set for Mr. F's exercise program?

47. Explain what is meant by aerobic exercise. Show how it promotes weight loss.

48. As a health care professional who is not an exercise physiologist, how should you counsel a patient about exercise?

49. What would you tell someone like Mr. F about testing their own cholesterol levels and making a diagnosis?

50. If the "statins" (a family of very effective drugs to which Lipitor belongs) work so well, why do we not tell patients to eat what they want and take their medication?

****

Mr. F's recovery post-op went as well as could be expected. Within a week of his surgery he was discharged from the hospital.

****

QUESTIONS CONTINUED:

51. Briefly describe the procedure for open-heart surgery. In your description, explain how the blocked arteries are bypassed, where the bypass veins come from, and the extent of the surgery, i.e., minor, moderate, major, etc.

<u>**ADDITIONAL OPTIONAL QUESTIONS:**</u>

52. Some may argue that a more aggressive approach should have been taken with Mr. F. Namely, the physician should have measured his hs-CRP and homocysteine at the onset of symptoms and immediately prescribed a statin and an ace inhibitor with the diet; the argument being that the additional expense may pay off in the long run with reduced cost by preventing a cardiovascular event. The other side may argue that the additional blood tests are overkill and are not cost advantageous. On a separate sheet of paper, discuss your thoughts on this matter.

53. Write a SOAP note by continuing with your note from the previous section.

S:

O:

A:

P:

RELATED REFERENCES

1. Aejmelaeus, R., Metsa-Ketela, T., Laippala, P., Solakivi, T., & Alho, H. (1997). Ubiquinol-Q and total peroxyl radical trapping capacity of LDL lipoproteins during aging: the effects of Q-10 supplementation. *Mol. Aspects Med.* 18 Suppl:S113-20.

2. AHA Scientific Statement: AHA Dietary Guidelines: Revision 2000, #71-0193 *Circulation.* 2000; 102:2284-2299; Stroke. 2000;31:2751-2766. http://circ.ahajournals.org/cgi/content/full/102/18/2284

3. AHA Conference Proceedings: Summary of the Scientific Conference on Dietary Fatty Acids and Cardiovascular Health, #71-0200 *Circulation.* 2001;103:1034-1039.

4. Blomhoff, R. (2005). Dietary antioxidants and cardiovascular disease. *Curr Opin Lipidol.* Feb;16(1):47-54.

5. Bonow, R. O. (2002). Primary Prevention of Cardiovascular Disease, *Circulation*. 106:3140-3141.

6. Brosnan, J.T. (2004). Homocysteine and cardiovascular disease: interactions between nutrition, genetics and lifestyle. *Can J Appl Physiol*. Dec;29(6):773-80.

7. Bordia, A., Verma, S.K., & Srivastava, K.C. (1998). Effect of garlic (Allium sativum) on blood lipids, blood sugar, fibrinogen and fibrinolutic activity in patients with coronary artery disease. *Prostaglandins Leukot. Essent. Fatty Acids*. 58(4):257-63.

8. Brown, A.S., Bakker-Akema, R.G., Yellen, L., Henley, R.W., Jr., Guthrie, R., Campbell, C.F., Koren, M., Woo, W., McLain, R., & Black, D.M. (1998). Treating patients with documented atherosclerosis to National Cholesterol Education Program-recommended low-density-lipoportein cholesterol goals with atorvastatin, fluvastatin, lovastatin and simvastatin. *J. Am. Coll. Cardiol*. 32(3):665-72.

9. Brown, B.G., Zhao, X.Q., Chait, A., Frohlg, M., Heise, N., Dowdy, A., DeAngelis, D., Fisher, L.D., & Albers, J. (1998). Lipid altering or antioxidant vitamins for patients with coronary disease and very low HDL cholesterol? The HDL-Atherosclerosis Treatment Study Design. *Can. J. Cardiol*. 14 Suppl. A:6A-13A.

10. Cattaneo, D. & Remuzzi, G. (2005). Lipid oxidative stress and the anti-inflammatory properties of statins and ACE inhibitors. *J Ren Nutr*. Jan;15(1):71-6.

11. Chahoud, G., Aude, Y.W., & Mehta, J.L. (2004). Dietary recommendations in the prevention and treatment of coronary heart disease: do we have the ideal diet yet? *Am J Cardiol*. Nov 15;94(10): 1260-7.

12. Craig, W.J. (1997). Phytochemicals: guardians of our health. *J. Am. Diet. Assoc*. 97(10 Suppl 2): S199-204.

13. De Caterina, R., Zampolli, A., Madonna, R., Fioretti, P., & Vanuzzo, D. (2004). New cardiovascular risk factors: homocysteine and vitamins involved in homocysteine metabolism. *Ital Heart J*. Jun;5 Suppl 6:19S-24S.

14. de Jong, S.C., van den Berg, M., Rauwerda, J.A., & Stehouwer, C.D. (1998). Hyperhomocysteinemia and atherothromobotic disease. *Semin. Thromb. Hemost*. 24(4):381-5.

15. Durak, I., Aytac, B., Atmaca, Y., Devrim, E., Avci, A., Erol, C., & Oral, D. (2004). Effects of garlic extract consumption on plasma and erythrocyte antioxidant parameters in atherosclerotic patients. *Life Sci*. Sep 3;75(16):1959-66.

16. Ehrenstein, M.R., Jury, E.C., & Mauri, C. (2005). Statins for atherosclerosis—as good as it gets? *N Engl J Med*. Jan 6;352(1):73-5.

17. Fischbach, F.T. (2003). *A Manual of Laboratory & Diagnostic Tests*. 7th Ed. Philadelphia. J.B. Lippincott Company.

18. Franco, O.H., Bonneux, L., de Laet, C., Peeters, A., Steyerberg, E.W. & Mackenbach, J.P. (2004). The Polymeal: a more natural, safer, and probably tastier (than the Polypill) strategy to reduce cardiovascular disease by more than 75%. *BMJ*. Dec 18;329(7480):1447-50.

19. Frishman, W.H. & Zuckerman, A.L. (2004). Amlodipine/atorvastatin: the first cross risk factor polypill for the prevention and treatment of cardiovascular disease. *Expert Rev Cardiovasc Ther*. Sep;2(5):675-81.

20. *Health News*. (2004) Oct;10(10):6. How low should your cholesterol go? Even lower may be better. For those at highest risk, very low cholesterol levels may help prevent a second heart attack or stroke.

21. Heber, D. (2004). Vegetables, fruits and phytoestrogens in the prevention of diseases. *J Postgrad Med*. Apr-Jun;50(2):145-9.

22. Hercberg, S., Galan, P., Preziosi, P., Alfarez, M.J., & Vazquez, C. (1998). The potential of antioxidant vitamins in preventing cardiovascular diseases and cancers. *Nutrition*. 14(6):513-20.

23. Homma, Y., Ikeda, I., Ishikawa, T., Tateno, M., Sugano, M., & Nakamura, H. (2003). Decrease in plasma low-density lipoprotein cholesterol, apolipoprotein B, cholesteryl ester transfer protein, and oxidized low-density lipoprotein by plant sterol ester-containing spread: a randomized, placebo-controlled trial. *Nutrition*. Apr;19(4):369-74.

24. Jenkins, D.J., Kendall, C.W., Marchie, A., Faulkner, D., Vidgen, E., Lapsley, K.G., Trautwein, E.A., Parker, T.L., Josse, R.G., Leiter, L.A., & Connelly, P.W. (2003). The effect of combining plant sterols, soy protein, viscous fibers, and almonds in treating hypercholesterolemia. *Metabolism*. Nov;52(11):1478-83.

25. Katan, M.B., Grundy, S.M., Jones, P., Law, M., Miettinen, T., & Paoletti, R. (Stresa Workshop participants). (2003). Efficacy and safety of plant stanols and sterols in the management of blood cholesterol levels. *Mayo Clin Proc*. Aug;78(8):965-78.

26. Kendall, C.W. & Jenkins, D.J. (2004). A dietary portfolio: maximal reduction of low-density lipoprotein cholesterol with diet. *Curr Atheroscler Rep*. Nov;6(6):492-8.

27. Kojda, G. (2004). Direct vasoprotection by aspirin: a significant bonus to antiplatelet activity? *Cardiovasc Res*. Nov 1;64(2):192-4.

28. Lamarche, B., Desroches, S., Jenkins, D.J., Kendall, C.W., Marchie, A., Faulkner, D., Vidgen, E., Lapsley, K.G., Trautwein, E.A., Parker, T.L., Josse, R.G., Leiter, L.A., & Connelly, P.W. (2004). Combined effects of a dietary portfolio of plant sterols, vegetable protein, viscous fibre and almonds on LDL particle size. *Br J Nutr*. Oct;92(4):657-63.

29. Lopez-Sendon, J., Swedberg, K., McMurray, J., Tamargo, J., Maggioni, A.P., Dargie, H., Tendera, M., Waagstein, F., Kjekshus, J., Lechat, P., & Torp-Pedersen, C. (2004). Expert Consensus Document on Angiotensin Converting Enzyme Inhibitors in Cardiovascular Disease. *Rev Esp Cardiol*. Dec;57(12): 1213-1232.

30. Luoto, R., Simojoki, M., Uutela, A., Boice, J.D. Jr., McLaughlin, J.K., & Puska, P. (2004). Consistency of use of plant stanol ester margarine in Finland. *Public Health Nutr*. Feb;7(1):63-8.

31. Magorien, R.D., O'Shaughnessy, C., & Ganz, P. Reversal of Atherosclerosis with Aggressive Lipid Lowering (REVERSAL) Investigators.. (2005) Statin therapy, LDL cholesterol, C-reactive protein, and coronary artery disease. *N Engl J Med*. Jan 6;352(1):29-38.

32. Orekhov, A.N., Tertov, V.V., Sobenin, I.A., & Pivovarova, E.M. (1995). Direct anti-atherosclerosis-related effects of garlic. *Ann. Med.* 27(1):63-5.

33. Prendergast, A. & Fulton, F.L. (1997) *Medical terminology: A Text/Workbook*. 4th Ed. Redwood City, California. Addison-Wesley Nursing.

34. Pietrzik, K. & Bronstrup, A. (1997). The role of homocysteine, folate and other B-vitamins in the development of atherosclerosis. *Arch. Latinoam. Nutr.* 47(2 Suppl 1):9-12.

35. Pincus, J. (1998). Comparative dose efficacy study of atorvastatin versus simvastatin, pravastatin, lovastatin, and fluvastatin in patients with hypercholesterolemia. *Am. J. Cardiol.* 82(3):406-7.

36. Pronsky, Z.M., Redfern, C.M., Crowe, J. & Epstein, S. (2003) *Food Medication Interactions*, 13th Ed Phoenix, Arizona. Food-Medications Interactions, Publishers and Distributors.

37. Robinson, K., Arheart, K., Refsum, H., Brattstrom, L., Boers, G., Ueland, P., Rubba, P., Palma-Reis, R., Meleady, R., Daly, L., Witteman, J., & Graham, I. (1998). Low circulating folate and vitamin B_6 concentrations: risk factors for stroke, peripheral vascular disease, and coronary artery disease. European COMAC Group. *Circulation.* 97(5):437-43.

38. Rolfes, S.R., Pinna, K. & Whitney, E. (2006). *Understanding Normal and Clinical Nutrition*, 7th Ed. West/Wadsworth.

39. Samson, R.H. (2002). Miscellaneous medications for the management of atherosclerosis: mayhem or miracle? *Semin Vasc Surg.* Dec;15(4):275-87.

40. Simons, L.A. (1998). Comparison of atorvastatin alone versus simvastatin +/- cholestyramine in the management of severe primary hypercholesterolaemia (the six cities study). *Aust. N. Z. J. Med.* 28(3):327-33.

41. Spratto, G.R. & Woods, A.L. (2005). *PDR Nurse's Drug Handbook.* Thompson Delmar Learning, NY.

42. Superko, H.R. (1998). Did grandma give you heart disease? The new battle against coronary artery disease. *Am J Cardiol.* Nov 5;82(9A):34Q-46Q.

43. Third Report of the NCEP Expert Panel on Detection, Evaluation, and Treatment of High Blood Cholesterol in Adults (Adult Treatment Panel III), *Circulation.* (2002);106:3143-3421.

44. Thomas, S.R., Neuzil, J., & Stocker, R. (1997). Inhibition of LDL oxidation by ubiquinol-10. A protective mechanism for coenzyme Q in atherogenesis? *Mol. Aspects Med.* 18 Suppl:S85-103.

45. Tran, H. & Anand, S.S. (2004). Oral antiplatelet therapy in cerebrovascular disease, coronary artery disease, and peripheral arterial disease. *JAMA.* Oct 20;292(15):1867-74.

46. Tyler, V.E. (1994). *Herbs of Choice.* Binghamton, NY. Pharmaceutical Products Press.

47. Tyler, V.E. (1993). *The Honest Herbal.* 3rd ED. Binghamton, NY. Pharmaceutical Products Press.

48. van Rosendaal, G.M., Shaffer, E.A., Edwards, A.L., & Brant, R. (2004). Effect of time of administration on cholesterol-lowering by psyllium: a randomized cross-over study in normocholesterolemic or slightly hypercholesterolemic subjects. *Nutr J.* Sep 28;3(1):17.

49. Vogel, R. (1998). Angiotensin-converting enzyme inhibitors, calcium blockers, estrogen and antioxidants in secondary prevention of coronary disease. *Can. J. Cardiol.* 14 Suppl D:8D-10D.

50. Welch, G.N. & Loscalzo, J. (1998). Homocysteine and atherothrombosis. *N.Engl. J. Med.* 338(15):1042-50.

51. Wolffenbuttel, B.H., Mahla, G., Muller, D., Pentrup, A. & Black, D.M. (1998). Efficacy and safety of a new cholesterol synthesis inhibitor, atorvastatin, in comparison with simvastatin and pravastatin, in subjects with hypercholesterolemia. *Neth. J. Med.* 52(4):131-7.

CASE STUDY #19
MYOCARDIAL INFARCTION RESULTING IN CONGESTIVE HEART FAILURE

INTRODUCTION

PART I of this study concerns the nutritional implications of someone who has a myocardial infarction but does not have hypercholesterolemia. The nutritional modifications involve a sodium restricted diet. Another ethnic group is introduced. In **PART II** of the study, the patient's condition worsens and results in congestive heart failure. The patient becomes too sick to eat and a feeding tube has to be placed. Review notes on congestive heart failure and basics about concentrated tube feedings.

****

SKILLS NEEDED

ABBREVIATIONS:

Knowledge of the following abbreviations is required in order to understand this case. You should learn these abbreviations before you begin to read the study.

BEE, BS, CCU, CHF, CPK, CPK_{1-3}, EKG, LD_{1-5}, LDH, MI, N/G, NTG, and PVCs (Appendix C).

LABORATORY VALUES:

You will need to be able to interpret the nutritional significance of the following laboratory values for this case study: BUN, Cl, Ca, Mg, CPK, CPK_1 (CPK-BB), CPK_2 (CPK-MB), CPK_3 (CPK-MM), Cr, Glucose, Hct, Hgb, K, LDH, LD_1, LD_2, LD_3, LD_4, LD_5, MCV, Na, ALT, AST, ALP, and WBC (Appendix B).

FORMULAS:

The formulas used in this case study include total calorie and protein needs using appropriate stress factor (Appendix A, Table 17).

MEDICATIONS:

Become familiar with the following medications before reading the case study. Note the diet-drug interactions, dosages and methods of administration, gastrointestinal tract reactions, etc.

1. Lactated Ringer's; 2. morphine sulfate; 3. Inderal (propranodol; 4. Slow-K (potassium chloride); 5. nitroglycerin; 6. Barbita (phenobarbital); 7. Dobutrex (dobutamine hydrochlorine); 8. Lasix (furosemide).

****

PART I: MYOCARDIAL INFARCTION WITHOUT HYPERCHOLESTEROLEMIA

Mr. Y is a 52 YO Japanese-American who came to the United States as a college student 34 years ago. He is married and has two children. Mr. Y is a very successful computer programmer for a major firm. He has worked his way up to a high level of management and is now in a very stressful position. He is very good at what he does but is in a highly competitive market. His division must produce in order for the company to survive and he feels that it is largely his responsibility to see that this is accomplished. Because great emphasis was placed on excellence in his upbringing, he has always been an over-achiever. He must not only do well, he must be the best. He is married to a woman from Japan. Though he has been in this country for 34 years, he still follows many of the practices of his homeland. His diet is greatly Americanized but many aspects of the Japanese diet are still evident. In his work he has the opportunity to fly to Japan on occasion, so he maintains strong ties with his homeland. He is 5'5" and weighs 155 lbs. There is no family history of cardiovascular disease but he has a family history of intestinal cancer. He has been treated for ulcers twice.

It is very important to him that he continues to be a success in his work. He has become a model for his family in America and in Japan. This places additional stress on him and he stays at the office late at night and brings work home with him in the evenings and on weekends. One day at work he had a heart attack.

He began to feel very weak, turned pale, and felt like he had pressure pushing in on his chest. It was difficult to breathe. There was severe pain in the sternum area that radiated to his left shoulder and down his arm, almost to the elbow. He also had pain radiate up his neck to his jaw. He collapsed to the floor and was rushed to the hospital. He was admitted to the CCU with a Dx of MI. When Mr. Y was admitted, he still felt a crushing sensation on his chest with some burning and pain in the sternum area. He was diaphoretic, pale, was having PVCs, and was very anxious. His temperature was 99.9°. His initial treatment included O_2, morphine sulfate, and lactated Ringer's. He was NPO. The EKG suggested Mr. Y had an MI and that he was in ventricular tachycardia. Mr. Y was given Inderal (propranodol) and nitroglycerin prn. Phenobarbital was used to keep Mr. Y calm. Blood was drawn eight hours after admission and analyzed. The results were as follows:

TABLE 1

BASIC METABOLIC PACKAGE							
TEST	RESULT	REFERENCE UNITS Conventional	SI	TEST	RESULT	REFERENCE UNITS Conventional	SI
Glu	160 mg/dl	70-110 mg/dl	3.8-6.1 mmol/L	Na	141 mEq/L	136-145 mEq/L	136-145 mmol/L
BUN	16 mg/dl	6-20 mg/dl	2.1-7.1 mmol/L	K	4.2 mEq/L	3.5-5.2 mEq/L	3.5-5.2 mmol/L
Cr	1.0 mg/dl	0.9-1.3 mg/dl	80-115 µmol/L	Cl	101 mEq/L	96-106 mEq/L	96-106 mmol/L
Ca	9.4 mg/dl	8.8-10.0 mg/dl	2.20-2.60 mmol/L	Mg	1.9 mEq/L	1.8 - 2.6 mEq/L	136-145 mmol/L
Ser alb	3.6 g/dl	3.5-4.8 g/dl	39-50 g/dl	P	3.3mg/dl	2.7-4.5 mg/dl	4.7-6.0 kPa

TABLE 2

LDH and CPK Isoenzymes							
TEST	RESULT	REFERENCE UNITS Conventional	SI	TEST	RESULT	REFERENCE UNITS Conventional	SI
Total LDH	423 U/L	313-618 U/L	313-618 U/L	CPK	193 U/L	38-174 U/L	0.63-2.90 µkat/L
LD_1	26%	17-27%	0.17-0.27	CPK_1	0 %	0 %	
LD_2	30%	29-39%	0.29-0.39	CPK_2	15 %	0-6%	
LD_3	20%	19-27%	0.19-0.27	CPK_3	95 %	96-100%	
LD_4	14%	8-16%	0.08-0.16	LD_5	8.3%	6-16%	0.06-0.16

TABLE 3

LIVER FUNCTION							
TEST	RESULT	REFERENCE UNITS Conventional	SI	TEST	RESULT	REFERENCE UNITS Conventional	SI
AST	34 U/L	14-20 U/L	0.23-0.33 µkat/L	ALP	53 U/L	25-100 U/L	17-142 U/L
ALT	36 U/L	10-40 U/L	0.17-0.68 µkat/L	Amylase	62 U/L	25–125 U/L	0.4-2.1 µkat/L

****

QUESTIONS:
1. List the lab values for the labs drawn at 8 hrs (TABLES 1-3) that indicate that Mr. Y had had a MI.

****

After 25 hours blood was drawn again and the 24 hr labs were as follows:

TABLE 4

LDH and CPK Isoenzymes							
TEST	**RESULT**	**REFERENCE UNITS** Conventional SI		**TEST**	**RESULT**	**REFERENCE UNITS** Conventional SI	
Total LDH	420 U/L	313-618 U/L	313-618 U/L	CPK	250 U/L	38-174 U/L	0.63-2.90 μkat/L
LD$_1$	50%	17-27%	0.17-0.27	CPK$_1$	0 %	0 %	0
LD$_2$	37%	29-39%	0.29-0.39	CPK$_2$	35 %	0-6%	0-.6
LD$_3$	21%	19-27%	0.19-0.27	CPK$_3$	77 %	96-100%	.96-1.0
LD$_4$	13%	8-16%	0.08-0.16	LD$_5$	8.5%	6-16%	0.06-0.16

TABLE 5

LIVER FUNCTION							
TEST	**RESULT**	**REFERENCE UNITS** Conventional SI		**TEST**	**RESULT**	**REFERENCE UNITS** Conventional SI	
AST	160 U/L	14-20 U/L	0.23-0.33 μkat/L	ALP	54 U/L	25-100 U/L	17-142 U/L
ALT	44 U/L	10-40 U/L	0.17-0.68 μkat/L	Amylase	68 U/L	25–125 U/L	0.4-2.1 μkat/L

****

2. List the lab values for the labs drawn at 24 hrs (**TABLES 4 AND 5**) that indicate that Mr. Y had had a MI.

3. Explain the variance between the two sets of labs. In your explanation, tell how the various enzymes are used to distinguish between MI, liver disease, pulmonary disease, etc.

4. Give the mechanisms of action of the following drugs:

Inderal (propranodol):

nitroglycerin:

Barbita (phenobarbital):

morphine sulfate:

5. What nutritional complications could occur with the listed medications? List any adverse reactions.

Inderal (propranodol):

nitroglycerin:

Barbita (phenobarbital):

morphine sulfate:

6. List the symptoms of a MI.

7. Define the following terms:
   Lactated Ringer's:

   Ventricular Tachycardia:

   Diaphoretic:

****
Mr. Y started to feel better by the next day, but he had occasional chest pain that required morphine sulfate and nitroglycerin. This continued for the first two days of his hospitalization. By the third day, he was feeling much better. Clear liquids, with no hot or cold liquids, were ordered but he did not feel like eating. He said that his stomach felt bloated and the liquids just stayed there. He was still receiving nitroglycerin for chest pain but much less frequently. He continually C/O a distended abdomen. By the fourth day, he tried to drink more of the clear liquids. He gradually advanced to a full liquid diet and then to a 2g Na, low-fat diet. He did not have a fluid restriction, but he was not allowed hot or cold beverages.
****

QUESTIONS CONTINUED:
8. What does a distended abdomen mean? List the possible causes of this.

9. What medications may be having an effect on Mr. Y's distended, bloated feeling?

10. Why would Mr. Y not be allowed to have any hot or cold liquids with his meals?

****

Mr. Y continued to improve and was moved out of CCU to a cardiac floor. During his rehabilitation in the hospital the dietitian started teaching him his diet. When the dietitian interviewed him, she found that Mr. Y ate the following types of foods: His intake of dairy products such as, milk, cheese, and ice cream was satisfactory. Among the protein foods, he ate a variety of fish and shellfish, beef, pork, and chicken. He ate tofu occasionally. As part of his Japanese culture, he also ate whole dried fish, including the bones, and raw fish on occasion. His diet included large quantities of rice and rice products. Among the rice products were mochiko (a flour used to make rice cakes). He and his wife also frequently ate other breads and crackers, somen, millet, and barley. A large variety of vegetables, including eggplant, cucumbers, mushrooms, bamboo shoots, and seaweed, were part of his diet. These products were cooked with soy sauce, salt, horseradish, dried celery, parsley, and onions. He did not mention fruit or bread products. Mr. Y was advised to follow the American Heart Association's TLC diet (http://www.americanheart.org/presenter.jhtml?identifier=4764).

****

QUESTIONS CONTINUED:

11. If you were the dietitian who was going to counsel Mr. Y, list the foods mentioned above that would need to be eliminated from his diet.

12. Give examples of foods that he might substitute for those that are not suggested on his 2 g Na, low-fat diet.

13. Determine Mr. Y's IBW and percent of IBW (Appendix A, Tables 7 and 8).

14. Calculate Mr. Y's BMI (Appendix A, Tables 10 and 11).

15. Calculate Mr. Y's energy and protein needs post MI and recommend a caloric intake level for him. Show what stress factor you would use (Appendix A, Table 17).

16. Define the following foods and list the main nutrients they contribute to the diet:

   tofu:

   somen:

   mochiko:

   seaweed:

   bamboo shoots:

   millet:

   mushrooms:

17. The kinds of food eaten by Mr. Y have been listed but not the amounts. Based on the information given, evaluate Mr. Y's diet.

18. Is the 2 g Na diet prescription too strict? Discuss the reasoning behind your answer.

19. Describe the American Heart Association's TLC diet.

<u>**ADDITIONAL OPTIONAL QUESTIONS:**</u>

20. If Mr. Y had to have a tube feeding, list several appropriate low-sodium tube feedings that could be used.

Product	Producer	Form	Cal/ml	Non-pro cal/g N	Pro	CHO	Fat	Na mg	K mg	mOsm /kg water	Vol to meet RDA in ml	g of fiber /L	Free H$_2$O /L in ml

21. Prepare a SOAP note for Mr. Y.

S:

O:

A:

P:

22. Considering Mr. Y's diet order, and his known dietary habits, plan a day's menu on a separate sheet of paper.

****

PART II: CONGESTIVE HEART FAILURE

Mr. Y continued to do well over the next several days, but then had another episode of severe chest pain. He required morphine sulfate and NTG. He was nauseous, pale, cold, and very anxious. He had some chest pain but it was not as severe as it was in his first attack. He was readmitted to CCU. The chest pain reoccurred frequently and required several doses of morphine sulfate. He was made NPO and C/O a distended abdomen. The tests conducted indicated that Mr. Y had had another MI. His renal output decreased greatly and Mr. Y was diagnosed with CHF and had to be intubated. His new orders included the following:

➤ NPO
➤ furosemide (Lasix)
➤ 1000 cc total fluid every day including I.V.

****

QUESTIONS CONTINUED:

23. Describe the mechanism of action and possible nutritional complications of furosemide.

24. What does intubation mean?

****

Mr. Y improved over the next few days but was still having problems with CHF. He could not talk because of the endotracheal tube but still indicated that he felt distended, even though a N/G tube was in place to low suction. Mr. Y has been in the hospital for 14 days and had solid food for 5 of those days. He has been NPO for the last 4 days. Mr. Y has very faint BS and an abdominal radiographic study suggests that he has a gastric ileus. The physician decided to place a feeding tube into the small bowel and started a TF.

****

Information Box 19 - 1
When a patient requires a feeding tube, in most cases, the optimum placement of the feeding tube is into the small bowel. This is done for the following reasons: First, if an ileus were to occur in a patient after surgery or trauma (including an MI), the ileus would usually be gastric or colonic. The small intestines are usually still functioning during this time. Therefore, a feeding entering the small bowel could be effective without as much of a chance of aspiration. Second, if something were to happen to allow too much tube feeding to flow into the patient, there is less of a chance of aspiration if the tube is in the small bowel.

> The strength and flow rate of the feeding depends on a number of factors: the osmolality of the feeding, the position of the tip of the feeding tube, the length of time since the patient has eaten, the edematous state of the patient's gut, and any disease state affecting digestion or absorption. The more concentrated the feeding and the longer it has been since the patient has eaten, the slower the rate of administration and the greater the dilution of the feeding.

QUESTIONS CONTINUED

25. Explain the reasoning behind the placement of the feeding tube into the small intestines in Mr. Y's case.

26. Calculate Mr. Y's IBW (Appendix A, Tables 7 and 8).

27. Calculate Mr. Y's BEE using the Harris-Benedict equation. Calculate his total daily energy expenditure using the appropriate stress factor (Appendix A, Table 17).

28. What are the goals of nutritional therapy for someone with CHF?

29. Did any of Mr. Y's requirements change with the new Dx? If so, list the changes and explain the factors that caused the changes.

30. What would be an appropriate kind of TF to start for Mr. Y? Remember that Mr. Y is in CHF and is on restricted fluids and remember where the tip of the feeding tube is.

31. At what rate and strength would you start Mr. Y's TF? Explain.

32. What final rate and strength would you try to achieve? Show the progression that you would use each day from your initial rate and strength to your final rate and strength.

33. Define an ileus.

34. Speculate on the possible cause of Mr. Y's gastric ileus. Can you give a suggestion that could help alleviate this ileus?

****

Because of the Lasix, Mr. Y's urinary output has increased considerably, and he is gradually getting over CHF. However, the Lasix has also caused his K to drop. Since K given by I.V. is painful, could cause phlebitis, and is required to be given slowly with lots of fluid, the physician decided to give a K supplement via feeding tube. He ordered the patient to have Slow-K (potassium chloride) t.i.d. The next day, Mr. Y's K was in the normal range and the physician continued the Slow-K. By the next day, Mr. Y started to experience some diarrhea and his serum K dropped again. The physician increased the Slow-K by feeding tube. The diarrhea increased and the serum K dropped further.

****

<u>QUESTIONS CONTINUED:</u>

35. Explain the physiological results of giving Slow-K via Mr. Y's feeding tube.

36. Define the following terms:

Endotracheal tube:

Radiographic:

Phlebitis:

N/G to low suction:

<u>ADDITIONAL OPTIONAL QUESTIONS:</u>

Tube Feeding Drill:

37. If Mr. Y had to have a tube feeding, list several appropriate feedings that could be used. Remember the fluid restriction and the sodium restriction.

Product	Producer	Form	Cal/ml	Non-pro cal/g N	g/L			Na mg	K mg	mOsm/kg water	Vol to meet RDA in ml	g of fiber /L	Free H$_2$O /L in ml
					Pro	CHO	Fat						

38. Prepare a SOAP note for Mr. Y, continuing where you left off in **PART I.**

S:	
O:	
A:	
P:	

RELATED REFERENCES:

1. AHA Scientific Statement: AHA Dietary Guidelines: Revision 2000, #71-0193 *Circulation*. 2000;102:2284-2299; *Stroke*. 2000;31:2751-2766

2. AHA Conference Proceedings: Summary of the Scientific Conference on Dietary Fatty Acids and Cardiovascular Health, #71-0200 *Circulation*. 2001;103:1034-1039

3. Albert, C.M., Hennekens, C.H., O'Donnell, C.J., Ajani, U.A., Carey, V.J., Willett, W.C.,Ruskin, J.N., & Manson, J.E. (1998). Fish consumption and risk of sudden cardiac death. *JAMA*. 279(1):23-8.

4. Bonow, R. O. (2002). Primary Prevention of Cardiovascular Disease, *Circulation*. 106:3140-3141.

5. Fischbach, F.T. (2003). *A Manual of Laboratory & Diagnostic Tests*. 7th Ed. Philadelphia. J.B. Lippincott Company.

6. Fleet, J.C. (1995). Are low-sodium diets appropriate for treated hypertensive men? *Nutr Rev*. Oct;53(10):296-8.

7. Fukuoka, Y., Dracup, K., Kobayashi, F., Ohno, M., Froelicher, E.S., & Hirayama, H. (2004). Illness attribution among Japanese patients with acute myocardial infarction. *Heart Lung*. May-Jun;33(3):146-53.

8. Hellermann, J.P., Jacobsen, S.J., Redfield, M.M., Reeder, G.S., Weston, S.A., & Roger, V.L. (2005). Heart failure after myocardial infarction: clinical presentation and survival. *Eur J Heart Fail.* Jan;7(1):119-25.

9. Kim, K.K., Yu, E.S., Liu, W.T., Kim, J., & Kohrs, M.B. (1993). Nutritional status of Chinese-, Korean-, and Japanese-American elderly. *J. Am. Diet. Assoc.* 93(12):1416-22.

10. Kinsella, A. (2002). American Heart Association issues new dietary guidelines. *Home Healthc Nurse.* Feb;20(2):86-8.

11. Kirsten, R., Nelson, K., Kirsten, D., & Heintz, B. (1998). Clinical pharmacokinetics of vasodilators. Part II. *Clin. Pharmacokinet.* 35(1):9-36.

12. Kojda, G. (2004). Direct vasoprotection by aspirin: a significant bonus to antiplatelet activity? *Cardiovasc Res.* Nov 1;64(2):192-4.

13. Lappalainen, R., Kiokkalainen, M., Julkunen, J., Saarinen, T., & Mykkanen, H. (1998). Association of sociodemographic factors with barriers reported by patients receiving nutrition counseling as part of cardiac rehabilitation. *J.Am. Diet. Assoc.* 98(9):1026-9.

14. Manunta, P. & Bianchi, G. (2004). Low-salt diet and diuretic effect on blood pressure and organ damage. *J Am Soc Nephrol.* Jan;15 Suppl 1:S43-6.

15. Morton, N.E., Gulbrandsen, C.L., Rao, D.C., Rhoads, G.G., & Kagan, A. (1980). Determinants of blood pressure in Japanese-American Families. *Hum. Genet.* 53(2):261-6.

16. Prendergast, A. & Fulton, F.L. (1997) *Medical terminology: A Text/Workbook.* 4th Ed. Redwood City, California. Addison-Wesley Nursing.

17. Pronsky, Z.M., Redfern, C.M., Crowe, J. & Epstein, S. (2003) *Food Medication Interactions*, 13th Ed Phoenix, Arizona. Food-Medications Interactions, Publishers and Distributors.

18. Rolfes, S.R., Pinna, K. & Whitney, E. (2006). *Understanding Normal and Clinical Nutrition*, 7th Ed. West/Wadsworth.

19. Shiba, N., Watanabe, J., Shinozaki, T., Koseki, Y., Sakuma, M., Kagaya, Y., & Shirato, K. (2005). Poor prognosis of Japanese patients with chronic heart failure following myocardial infarction. *Circ J.* Feb;69(2):143-9.

20. Spratto, G.R. & Woods, A.L. (2005). *PDR Nurse's Drug Handbook.* Thompson Delmar Learning, NY.

21. Third Report of the NCEP Expert Panel on Detection, Evaluation, and Treatment of High Blood Cholesterol in Adults (Adult Treatment Panel III), *Circulation.* 2002;106:3143-3421.

22. Vesely, D.L., Dietz, J.R., Parks, J.R., Baig, M., McCormick, M.T., Clinton, G., & Schocken, D.D. (1998). Vessel dilator enhances sodium and water excretion and has beneficial hemodynamic effects in persons with congestive heart failure. *Circulation.* 98(4):323-9.

CASE STUDY #20
OPEN-HEART SURGERY PRECEDED BY CHOLECYSTECTOMY AND COMPLICATED BY COPD

INTRODUCTION

This study involves a smoker that develops atherosclerosis and requires open-heart surgery. Complications set in as a result of COPD, and what would have been routine turns into a life threatening situation. He was warned about COPD earlier in his life when he had cholecystitis that resulted with a cholecystectomy. All three conditions are reviewed in three separate parts. Home health care is involved with recovery. You may use this case study as a brief review of cholecystectomy or you may skip PART I and go directly to PART II, open-heart surgery with COPD complications. PART III is concerned with COPD and home health care.
****

SKILLS NEEDED

ABBREVIATIONS:

Knowledge of the following abbreviations is required in order to understand this case. You should learn these abbreviations before you begin to read the study (Appendix C).
ABGs, cap, CICU, FiO_2, OR, PRN, q6h, q8h, RUQ, SOB, and TPN.

LABORATORY VALUES:

You will need to be able to interpret the nutritional significance of the following laboratory values for this case study: ABGs (HCO^-_3, $PaCO_2$, PaO_2, and pH), BUN, Ca, Cl, CO_2, Cr, glu, hct, hgb, K, lymph, MCH, MCHC, MCV Mg, Na, P, RBC, ser alb, and WBC (Appendix B).

FORMULAS:

The formulas used in this case study include ideal body weight and percent usual body weight. The formulas can be found in Appendix A, Tables 7 and 8.

MEDICATIONS:

Become familiar with the following medications before reading the case study. Note the diet-drug interactions, dosages and methods of administration, gastrointestinal tract reactions, etc.
1. Combivent (ipratropium bromide and albuterol sulfate); 2. Technesium Tc 99m Sestamibi (Cardiolite); 3. Klonopin (clonazepam); 4. Zocar (sivastatin); 5. Nitrostat (nitroglycerin sublingual); 6. Altace (ramipril); 7. Allegra (fexofenadine hydrochloride); 8. Tylox (oxycodone and acetaminophen); 9. Sonata (zaleplon); 10. Xanax (alprazolam); 11. Duoneb (ipratropium bromide and albuterol sulfate)
****

PART I: CHOLECYSTECTOMY

CJ is a 58 YOWM who been relatively healthy most of his life. He is 5'10" and usually weighs 185. He works in a mall in a large department store as a salesman. CJ is not married and lives alone. Since he was 17 he smoked at least one pack of cigarettes per day except for a short time five years ago post-cholecystectomy. At that time he had been suffering from sharp pains in the RUQ and in his left upper back and shoulder blade. The pain was usually accompanied by abdominal discomfort and nausea. The pain would be so severe at times that he could not move and lost sleep when it occurred at night. After several bouts of this pain occurring once or twice weekly, he saw his physician. An ultra sound and a cholecystography revealed cholecystitis with multiple stones in the gallbladder and surgery was scheduled. CJ was hospitalized for a routine laparoscopic cholecystectomy. He went through the usual preps with lab work, and a chest X-ray. It is routine the day of surgery for an anesthesiologist to meet patients that are to have anesthesia prior to entering the OR to discuss the surgery. The questions most frequently asked concern any previous reactions to anesthesia, medications, breathing problems, allergies, etc. The day of CJ's surgery the anesthesiologist met with him. In the conversation, he asked CJ if he smoked and how much per day. After CJ told him 1 pack/d, the physician explained that was probably why he had signs of emphysema. This shocked CJ severely. "Emphysema?" he responded. "Yes, you did not know you had emphysema?" the physician asked. He seemed as shocked as CJ that he did not know. The physician asked him about symptoms and CJ admitted to a nagging cough with SOB on occasion after exertion. He did not realize these were symptoms of emphysema. He thought it was because of his age and his lack of being in shape. The anesthesiologist told him that if he quit smoking, it probably would not get any worse; he did not think any permanent damage was done. CJ said that he would.

The surgery did not go as smoothly as expected. The gallbladder was badly inflamed and filled with stones. In addition, during surgery a choledochography was completed and revealed several small stones in the common bile duct. The surgeons considered it best not to remove the gall bladder through the trocars and conventional surgery was employed. CJ recovered quickly and was out of the hospital in a few days with no special diet.

After the surgery, CJ related the story about emphysema to his brother and said that he learned his lesson; he was going to quit smoking for good. CJ's brother had been trying to get him to quit smoking for years but he would not listen. Like most people that smoke, he admitted it was not good for him, but since he felt fine, he did not have a "real" reason to quit. His cessation lasted for about a month. CJ would visit his brother about once a week and, after a few weeks, his brother noticed the smell of cigarette smoke on him but he could not see cigarettes in his pocket. CJ would leave them in the car before entering his brother's house because he did not want to receive a sermon. Several years passed and CJ continued with his smoking, coughing and frequent bouts of bronchitis. He had to know that the smoking was contributing to his respiratory problems, but it was as if he lived in a state of denial. He kept blaming his problem on something else; for instance, he was under an air conditioning/heating vent at his workplace and it was the draft on him that was causing the problem. Other times he said it was allergies that were giving him a breathing problem; or that a co-worker had a very bad cold and gave it to him, or it was his sinuses.
****

QUESTIONS:

1. Determine CJ's IBW and current percent of his IBW (Appendix A, Tables 7 and 8).

2. Define the following terms:

   Cholecystectomy:

   Cholecystitis:

   Cholecystography:

   Choledochography:

   Trocors:

   Emphysema:

Laproscopic:

3. What are gallstones made of?

4. What relationship, if any, does sex, age, fertility, and weight have on cholecystitis?

5. After surgery, CJ was sent home without a specific diet. Why would someone not be placed on a low-fat diet post-op cholecystectomy?

6. Sketch the location of the GB and identify the hepatic duct, cystic duct, and common bile duct.

****
PART II: OPEN-HEART SURGERY WITH COPD COMPLICATIONS

Recently, CJ has been bothered more by SOB upon exertion. This is not like the occasional SOB he had in the past. Now it takes less and less exertion to cause a greater amount of SOB. One day at work he had to help unload a truck and could not work very long without stopping to breathe and it was very hard to catch his breath. He experienced no chest pain with exertion, but he went to his physician and explained his problem. After a routine exam, the physician decided to give him a pulmonary function test and sent him to a pulmonologist. His physician also told him to lose a few pounds but was not specific. The pulmonary function test revealed emphysema. ABGs were completed to see how serious this was and the results can be found in Table 1.

Table 1 – Initial ABGs

TEST	RESULT	NORM	TEST	RESULT	NORM
PaO_2	50mm Hg	80-90 mm Hg	$PaCO_2$	60mm Hg	35-45 mm Hg
HCO_3^-	40 mEq/L	24-28 mEq/L	pH	7.35	7.35-7.45

CJ was started on combivent inhaler, two inhalations q6h. His blood pressure at this visit was 150/80. Usually it was not that high and the physician decided it was elevated due to the excitement of the current condition and did not do anything about it. The inhaler helped a lot over the next couple of weeks, but the SOB continued to a degree greater than his physician wanted. He sent CJ to a cardiologist to have a treadmill test done because of the symptoms and his age. CJ was not able to make it through the treadmill test. The physician's goal was to get CJ's heart rate to 140 beats/min but at 120 beats he started having pain in his chest and the SOB was too great. The physician rescheduled CJ to have Cardiolite Imaging.

The procedure was performed in the Department of Nuclear Cardiology. CJ reported at 8:00 A.M. and after receiving the appropriate instructions about the risks of the test, signed a consent form. He was then injected I.V. with Technesium Tc 99m Sestamibi (Cardiolite). This is a radioactive isotope that enables a gamma camera to record images of the heart. After the injection, there was a minimum waiting period of one hour before he was placed on a special table and the heart was scanned with a gamma camera for sixteen minutes. The results were recorded in a computer and could be viewed from a computer screen. At that point CJ was injected with I.V. Persantine. This stressed the heart with the equivalent effects of having done exercise. CJ was again injected with Technesium Tc 99m Sestamibi (Cardiolite http://www.bms.com/static/pdf/cardlt.pdf). After a minimum waiting period of thirty minutes, he was again placed on the special table and a gamma camera took images of his heart for sixteen minutes. The results showed "something on the back of the heart" that the physician could not be sure about. This test was very uncomfortable for CJ and caused considerable chest pain. The physician sent him to have another test, a sonogram of the heart. The sonogram did not show anything unusual. The physician scheduled CJ for a cardiac cath the next week. All of this had CJ so concerned about his health that he lost his appetite and lost to 178 lbs.

****

QUESTIONS CONTINUED:

7. What are the ranges for normal and abnormal blood pressure?

8. Describe what the "measurement of blood pressure" means.

9. What are the effects of elevated BP on cardiovascular disease?

10. Define:

    Cardiolite Imaging:

    Sonogram:

    Pulmonary function test:

11. Acording to CJ's ABGs, you can say he is in:
    a. compensated metabolic acidosis.
    b. compensated respiratory acidosis.
    c. compensated respiratory alkalosis.
    d. compensated metabolic alkalosis.

12. Briefly explain your answer to the previous question.

****

CJ reported to the hospital to have a cardiac cath done. After the procedure was complete and he fully recovered from the medication, he was moved to a room and informed that he should be admitted and have open-heart surgery the next morning. They found a blockage of 90% in one artery and 75% in two others. CJ consented and was admitted. The surgery went without a problem and CJ was moved to CICU where open-heart patients are usually kept for a day or so post-op. Open-heart patients are intubated before surgery and arrive at CICU on a ventilator. After a day or two in CICU, they are extubated, and sent to a room. Patients are extubated when their ABGs are normal. CJ's ABGs were very poor and indicative of COPD. His CICU ABGs can be found in Table 2

Table 2 – CICU ABGs

TEST	RESULT	NORM	TEST	RESULT	NORM
PaO_2	98mm Hg	80-90 mm Hg	$PaCO_2$	88mm Hg	35-45 mm Hg
HCO_3^-	43 mEq/L	24-28 mEq/L	pH	7.23	7.35-7.45

His FiO_2 initially was 55% but had to be raised to 100%. CJ initially had an I.V. of D_5 Lactated Ringers infusing at 125 cc/h. Under the conditions this was too much for CJ and precipitated right side heart failure. His second day in CICU, his right lung began filling up with fluid and a chest tube had to be placed. After one day, his condition worsened and his left lung began collecting fluid and a second chest tube had to be placed. It was obvious at this point that CJ was not going to be weaned any time soon. It took two days in this condition before CJ's ABGs began to improve and the first chest tube was removed. A day later a second chest tube was removed. His ABGs were improving. It took two more days before CJ could be extubated and another two days before he left CICU and returned to a room. Thus CJ was in CICU for ten days, eight of those days intubated. His ABGs when he left CICU can be found in Table 3.

Table 3 – ABGs when leaving CICU.

TEST	RESULT	NORM	TEST	RESULT	NORM
PaO_2	60mm Hg	80-90 mm Hg	$PaCO_2$	55mm Hg	35-45 mm Hg
HCO_3^-	34 mEq/L	24-28 mEq/L	pH	7.38	7.35-7.45

During intubation a patient cannot eat. His only nourishment was D_5Lactated now infusing at 75 cc/h. CJ came into the hospital to have a cardiac cath completed and had not eaten for 12 hours prior to the catheterization. Post-catheterization, he was made NPO for open-heart surgery. He has now been without nourishment for almost two weeks. Typically this happens to a lot of patients. The physicians know they need to feed, but they think and hope that they can extubate in just one more day and then the patient will be able to eat. They understandably do not want to start I.V. nutrition for one day, but one day leads to another, and to another, and so on. It would not have hurt CJ to have TPN infusing for several days after extubation to help him get his strength back. Once he was extubated, clear liquids were ordered. By this time CJ was very frightened, in a lot of pain, and did not feel like eating. His throat was sore from the intubation tube and his chest hurt from the surgery. Also, as soon as he was extubated, breathing treatments began to help keep his lungs expanded. This was accomplished by breathing into an inspirometer. This is a small hand-held device with a mouthpiece through which you inhale and hold your breath before exhaling. A floating ball in a tube measures the amount of air your lungs inhale in liters. The procedure was called a Voldyne breathing treatment. At first CJ could only do 500 ml, which is not

much at all. The inspirometer can measure up to 5000 ml. The surgery had his chest so sore, he could not expand. He also had to cough and deep breathe frequently. They gave him a bright red heart-shaped pillow to hold across his chest while he coughed, but it did not help much. Finally, he complained of a bad taste in his mouth. Consequently, he did not feel like eating or drinking very much. When he was moved to his room, he was advanced to a full liquid diet.
****

13 Define:
    chest tube:

    intubated:

    extubated:

    ventilator:

    FiO_2:

14. What are normal ABGs?

15. How many kcals was CJ receiving with D_5Lacted Ringers infusing at 75 cc/h? Please show all work.

16. Describe the adequacy of a clear liquid and a full liquid diet as it pertains to kcals, protein, and vitamins and minerals needed by CJ to heal.

17. CJ's weight is now down to 168. Calculate his total caloric needs by calculating his BEE and an appropriate energy expenditure factor. Use the Harris-Benedict equation and appropriate factor found in Appendix A or use a formula of your own choosing.

18. What recommendation would you give for feeding CJ at this time?

19. Describe right side heart failure.

****

Shortly after in his room, CJ was advanced to a soft 2g Na diet. The dietitian came to visit CJ and encouraged him to eat. One of CJ's fears was that, since he was not hungry and filled up quickly, if he ate or drank too much at one time he would become bloated and may become nauseous. He could not imagine how much it would hurt if he had to throw up. The RD recommended to the physician that his meals be supplemented with _____ (in question #20, name one of the supplemental feedings that would be appropriate for CJ). The physician agreed and wrote the order. CJ tried to sip on the supplement throughout the day. Chest X-rays were done every other day to monitor his lungs and a small amount of fluid was still evident. The physician did not want to have to put in another chest tube so he stuck with a 2g Na restriction. CJ slowly began to eat more each day. They wanted him to get out of bed and walk down the hall and he tried but became so exhausted that he had to come back in a wheelchair. CJ continued with his breathing treatments but still was not able to get much above 500 ml of air. He was also on 2 L of oxygen via nasal cannula. With the O_2 running constantly, they could not get his O_2 saturation (measured by puls oximetry) above 88%. The head nurse told CJ's brother that normally open-heart patients leave the hospital by five days post-op. It took almost three weeks after leaving CICU before CJ left the hospital. At that time his weight was down to 160.

****

20. What nutritional supplement(s) would you recommend for CJ at this stage of recovery and why? Using the table below, compare several of the enteral nutritional supplements that would be appropriate for CJ.

Product	Producer	Form	Cal/ml	Non-pro cal/g N	g/L			Na mg	K mg	mOsm /kg water	Vol to meet RDA in ml	g of fiber /L	Free H_2O /L in ml
					Pro	CHO	Fat						

****

CJ was discharged from the hospital but was not able to go home by himself. He went to stay with his brother and his family until he could get along on his own.

PART III: COPD AND HOME HEALTH CARE

CJ went home on the following orders:

- Zocar 40 mg once every day at hs
- Klonopin 0.5 mg bid
- Nitrostat 0.4 mg prn for chest pain
- Altace 10 mg once daily
- Allegra 60 mg bid prn to help with breathing
- Tylox 500 mg 1 to 2 cap 4 – 6 hrs
- Sonata 10 mg 1 cap at hs for sleep
- DuoNeb one 3 ml vial containing 0.5 mg of ipratropium bromide and 3 mg albuterol sulfate to be used in a nebulizer q4h for breathing
- Combivent (hand held nebulizer that delivers the same medication as DuoNeb but in individual puffs and smaller doses); each actuation of the aerosol delivers a *puff* of medication containing 18 µg of ipratropium bromide and 103 µg of albuterol sulfate, to be used in between the DuoNeb treatments prn, no sooner than 1 hr after the DuoNeb treatment
- Oxygen via nasal cannula, 2 L
- Use inspirometer q4h
- Regular diet
- Home health care to visit patient

CJ had to obtain an oxygen machine from a home health care agency. The machine ran 24 hours a day and was very noisy. It had a long plastic tube that delivered the oxygen so CJ could move around the room and even go to the bathroom while still receiving oxygen. The home health care agency sent an RN to see him three times a week to help him wash, check his BP and vital signs, check his wound area, and maintain records of his progress. At first, a registered dietitian did not come to see him, but as time went on and his nutritional state continued to deteriorate, a registered dietitian went to visit him.

CJ was still in pain from the surgery and still could not cough as deep as they wanted him to. When he left the hospital, he was up to 1000 ml with the inspirometer, still far below his goal. Even with the oxygen, he took short choppy breaths through his mouth. It sounded like he was trying to whistle. This nullified to a degree the effects of the oxygen going into his nose, but he thought it was easier to breathe that way. His difficulty breathing made it even more difficult to eat. It was next to impossible to take continuous short choppy breaths and chew and swallow at the same time. His sister-in-law fixed him high-calorie soft foods but he did not feel like eating. After about ten days he made a visit to his doctor. He was not able to walk to the doctor's office from the parking lot and had to be brought in a wheelchair. His weight was down to 158 and he was beginning to look very skinny. He was still at just 1000 ml of air with the inspirometer and it took a lot of work to reach that. Lab work was completed and the results were as listed below:

CJ could have done more on his own, but his anxiety was increasing. He was concerned that he may never be able to get off of oxygen. He was fearful of trying to do too much and not be able to breathe. He was told to try leaving his oxygen off for a while but he was uncooperative. Xanax 0.25 mg q8h for anxiety and sleep was added to his list of meds.
****

21. Why is it so important for CJ to breathe deeply? Explain the physiology of the events that would occur if he did not.

BASIC METABOLIC PACKAGE							
TEST	RESULT	REFERENCE UNITS Conventional	SI	TEST	RESULT	REFERENCE UNITS Conventional	SI
Glu	103 mg/dl	70-110 mg/dl	3.8-6.1 mmol/L	Na	138 mEq/L	136-145 mEq/L	136-145 mmol/L
BUN	20 mg/dl	6-20 mg/dl	2.1-7.1 mmol/L	K	5.4 mEq/L	3.5-5.2 mEq/L	3.5-5.2 mmol/L
Cr	1.2 mg/dl	0.9-1.3 mg/dl	80-115 µmol/L	Cl	95 mEq/L	96-106 mEq/L	96-106 mmol/L
Ca	8.2 mg/dl	8.8-10.0 mg/dl	2.20-2.60 mmol/L	Mg	1.6 mEq/L	1.8 - 2.6 mEq/L	136-145 mmol/L
Ser alb	2.3 g/dl	3.5-4.8 g/dl	39-50 g/dl	P	2.3mg/dl	2.7-4.5 mg/dl	4.7-6.0 kPa

CBC							
TEST	RESULT	REFERENCE UNITS Conventional	SI	TEST	RESULT	REFERENCE UNITS Conventional	SI
Hgb	12 g/dl	14 - 17.4 g/dl	140-174 g/L	WBC	5.7 10^3/µl	4.5-10.5 x 10^3/cells/ mm^3	4.5-10.5 x 10^9/L
Hct	38%	42 – 52%		% Lymph	21%	25 – 40% of total WBC	1500-4000 cells/mm^3
RBC	4.7x10^6/µ	3.6-5.0x10^6/L	3.6-5.0x10^{12}/L	MCH	25 pg/cell	26-34 pg/cell	0.40-.53 fmol/cell
MCV	80 µm^3	82-98µm^3	82-98 fL	MCHC	32 g/dl	32-36 g/dl	320-360 g/L

22. Give the functions of the medications CJ had to take at home and describe any nutritional complications, associations, or interactions:

➢ Zocar:

➢ Klonopin:

➢ Nitrostat:

➢ Altace:

➢ Allegra:

➢ Tylox:

➢ Sonata:

➢ Xanax:

➢ ipratropium bromide:

➢ albuterol sulfate:

23. Using CJ's new weight, recalculate his percent of IBW and UBW and his percent loss of weight (Appendix A, Tables 7 and 8).

24. Calculate CJ's new total caloric requirement from his BEE and activity factor. Consider his work of breathing (Appendix A, Table 17).

25. If you were the home health RD, outline what your home health care visit would be like to completely access CJ's nutritional status.

26. In interpreting CJ's lab values, indicate those that suggest a nutrition problem and explain why.

27. If CJ smoked a pack of cigarettes a day, and paid $3.00 a pack (change the price to fit you area), how much would he spend a month? This would increase his chances for developing various diseases. List the diseases that can be precipitated or worsened by smoking.

28. CJ is also recovering from open-heart surgery. Explain what you would do about recommending a diet to help lower cholesterol and be appropriate for COPD.

29. Are there any supplements CJ could add to his diet to help with both conditions, as ω3 fatty acids and antioxidants? Explain how they would help.

30. Based on all of the previous information, create a SOAP note that you would write if you were the home health care RD. Include in your note the recommendations you would give to CJ and his care takers.

S:

O:

A:

P:

31. There are tube feedings available for ventilated patients to help them to be weaned more efficiently. In the table below, compare several of the tube feedings on the market for this purpose.

Product	Producer	Form	Cal/ ml	Non-pro cal/g N	g/L			Na mg	K mg	mOsm /kg water	Vol to meet RDA in ml	g of fiber /L	Free H$_2$O /L in ml
					Pro	CHO	Fat						

32. Would there be any advantage to using one of those feeding as a supplement for CJ in his present condition? Explain.

33. Define respiratory quotient.

34. Give the respiratory quotients for the following conditions.
    a. carbohydrate burned as sole fuel source:
    b. fat burned as sole fuel source:
    c. protein burned as sole fuel source:
    d. ketones burned as sole fuel source:
    e. if fat were being deposited:
    f. if a mixture were being burned of CHO, fat, and protein:

35. On a separate sheet of paper, describe how you would use RQ to choose a diet regimen.

EPILOGUE

Since this is based on a real case, it would be good to say that CJ finally started eating and regaining his strength. His brother had to trick him to wean him off of oxygen by gradually turning down the concentration and flow rate of oxygen. When CJ finally realized he was breathing room air, he began to move about more and started eating better. He went to cardio-pulmonary rehab three times a week for three months. This probably helped him more than anything else. Now, two years after surgery, CJ still has to complete two breathing treatments a day at home and is up to 3000 ml on the inspirometer, but he has gained all of his weight back plus some and is back at work living close to a normal life.

RELATED READING

1. AHA Scientific Statement: AHA Dietary Guidelines: Revision 2000, #71-0193 *Circulation.* 2000; 102:2284-2299; Stroke. 2000;31:2751-2766. http://circ.ahajournals.org/cgi/content/full/102/18/2284

2. Brown, A.S., Bakker-Akema, R.G., Yellen, L., Henley, R.W., Jr., Guthrie, R., Campbell, C.F., Koren, M., Woo, W., McLain, R., & Black, D.M. (1998). Treating patients with documented atherosclerosis to National Cholesterol Education Program-recommended low-density-lipoportein cholesterol goals with atorvastatin, fluvastatin, lovastatin and simvastatin. *J. Am. Coll. Cardiol.* 32(3):665-72.

3. Cai, B., Zhu, Y., Ma, Y., Xu, Z., Zao, Y., Wang, J., Lin, Y., & Comer, G,M. (2003). Effect of supplementing a high-fat, low-carbohydrate enteral formula in COPD patients. *Nutrition.* Mar;19(3):229-32.

4. Cattaneo, D. & Remuzzi, G. (2005). Lipid oxidative stress and the anti-inflammatory properties of statins and ACE inhibitors. *J Ren Nutr.* Jan;15(1):71-6.

5. de Leeuw, P.W. & Dees, A. (2003). Fluid homeostasis in chronic obstructive lung disease. *Eur Respir J* Suppl. Nov;46:33s-40s.

6. Fischbach, F.T. (2003). *A Manual of Laboratory & Diagnostic Tests.* 7th Ed. Philadelphia. J.B. Lippincott Company.

7. Gosker, H.R., Bast, A., Haenen, G.R., Fischer, M.A., van der Vusse, G.J., Wouters, E.F., & Schols, A.M. (2005). Altered antioxidant status in peripheral skeletal muscle of patients with COPD. *Respir Med.* Jan;99(1):118-25.

8. Lai, K.H., Peng, N.J., Lo, G.H., Lin, C.K., Chan, H.H., Hsu, P.I., Cheng, J.S., & Wang, Y.Y. (2002). Does a fatty meal improve hepatic clearance in patients after endoscopic sphincterotomy? *J Gastroenterol Hepatol.* Mar;17(3):337-41.

9. Lobato, D. S., Lorenzo, G. F., Mendieta, G. M., Alises, M. S., Arechabala, M. I., & Fernandez-Montes, V. C. (2005). Evaluation of a Home Hospitalization Program in Patients With Exacerbations of Chronic Obstructive Pulmonary Disease. *Arch Bronconeumol.* Jan;41(1):5-10.

10. Lopez-Sendon, J., Swedberg, K., McMurray, J., Tamargo, J., Maggioni, A.P., Dargie, H., Tendera, M., Waagstein, F., Kjekshus, J., Lechat, P., & Torp-Pedersen, C. (2004). Expert Consensus Document on Angiotensin Converting Enzyme Inhibitors in Cardiovascular Disease. *Rev Esp Cardiol.* Dec;57(12):1213-1232.

11. Mackay, S. & Dillane, P. (2004). Biliary pain. *Aust Fam Physician.* Dec;33(12):977-81.

12. Naeije, R. (2003). Pulmonary hypertension and right heart failure in COPD. *Monaldi Arch Chest Dis*. Jul-Sep;59(3):250-3.

13. Prendergast, A. & Fulton, F.L. (1997) *Medical terminology: A Text/Workbook*. 4th Ed. Redwood City, California. Addison-Wesley Nursing.

14. Pronsky, Z.M., Redfern, C.M., Crowe, J. & Epstein, S. (2003) *Food Medication Interactions*, 13th Ed Phoenix, Arizona. Food-Medications Interactions, Publishers and Distributors.

15. Rolfes, S.R., Pinna, K. & Whitney, E. (2006). *Understanding Normal and Clinical Nutrition*, 7th Ed. West/Wadsworth.

16. Spratto, G.R. & Woods, A.L. (2005). *PDR Nurse's Drug Handbook*. Thompson Delmar Learning, NY.

17. Third Report of the NCEP Expert Panel on Detection, Evaluation, and Treatment of High Blood Cholesterol in Adults (Adult Treatment Panel III), *Circulation*. 2002;106:3143-3421.

18. Zaher, C., Halbert, R., Dubois, R., George, D., & Nonikov, D. (2004). Smoking-related diseases: the importance of COPD. *Int J Tuberc Lung Dis*. Dec;8(12):1423-8.

CASE STUDY #21
HYPOGLYCEMIA

INTRODUCTION

This study is designed to help the student understand the various reasons why someone may experience hypoglycemia. This disease could be an early indication of diabetes, but most people who experience hypoglycemia usually do so as a result of poor nutrition. Many think they have hypoglycemia but actually have nothing more than poor eating habits.

****

SKILLS NEEDED

ABBREVIATIONS:
Knowledge of the following abbreviations is required in order to understand this case. You should learn these abbreviations before you begin to read the study.
CHO, FBS, GTT, and gtt (Appendix C).

LABORATORY VALUES:
You will need to be able to interpret the nutritional significance of the following laboratory values for this case study: FBS and GTT (Appendix B).

****

Mrs. J is a 30 YOBF who is married and has four children, ages 5, 6, 8, and 10. Her husband is unemployed and has been for several months. The only work that Mrs. J has been able to obtain is cleaning or cooking in someone's home. Mrs. J works two or three days a week while her husband takes care of the children. They have to depend on food stamps, city subsistence programs, and their family to meet their needs. They are trying hard to make it but times are difficult and they cannot do any better right now. They are embarrassed about their situation and do not like having to depend on anyone else to meet their needs.

Mrs. J has been feeling dizzy and weak. Recently, while grocery shopping, she got so weak she had to sit down. Someone gave her a soda and in a little while she felt better. Her husband convinced her that she should see a doctor, in spite of the cost. He was afraid she might have high blood pressure since it runs in her family. Her father died of a stroke and she has a sister with renal failure due to high blood pressure.

She went to the doctor who examined her and found her blood pressure to be normal. However, her blood sugar was very low, 48 mg/dl. To Mrs. J's knowledge, there is no family history of diabetes or hypoglycemia. She remembers her parents saying that her grandmother had some kind of "blood disease," but she does not know what that meant. The doctor's examination revealed the following: Mrs. J has not been eating as she usually does because of the low cash flow. She has been eating a lot of high-carbohydrate foods that are inexpensive and easy to fix, such as rice, spaghetti, etc. She has also been eating a lot of bread with her meals because it is filling. About two hours after eating she becomes dizzy, weak, and anxious, sweats profusely, and just "does not feel well." If she lies down the symptoms usually pass. Mrs. J also expressed that she is very worried about her family's situation and usually gets upset after one of their "cheap meals" because she believes she is not adequately providing for her family. The MD thought the problem was reactive, functional hypoglycemia based on a high carbohydrate intake accompanied by hyperepinephrinemia due to nervousness. To be sure, he ordered a 5 hour GTT. To prepare for the test, Mrs. J had to be on a diet of at least 150 grams of CHO and had to report early in the morning without eating after midnight. Mrs. J had a hard time drinking the sweet solution (75 g glucose) on an empty stomach. Having blood drawn every hour on an empty and nervous stomach made Mrs. J sick. She started throwing up after about three hours and the test had to be stopped. The results at that time were:

GTT

Time	0 min	30 min	1 hr	2 hr	3 hr
Glucose mg/dl	70	130	160	90	54

The physician felt that this was sufficient to make a diagnosis of reactive functional hypoglycemia. He gave her a sedative and referred her to the dietitian. He assured her that her problem could be resolved by diet and by dealing with her emotions.

The dietitian talked with Mrs. J and determined that she was on a high-carbohydrate, moderate-fat, low-protein diet. The carbohydrate was a mixture of complex carbohydrates and a significant concentration of simple sugars. For the amount of total carbohydrate she was ingesting, the fiber content was low. She consumed three meals per day with frequent high-carbohydrate snacks. The snacks were typically caffeine-containing sodas, candy, cookies, and coffee with sugar. Her total intake of caffeine was high.

The dietitian counseled her and questioned her to see if she understood the diet. When her responses were satisfactory, she sent her home with printed material and a number to call if she had questions.
****

QUESTIONS:
1. Define the following terms:
    Hypoglycemia:

    Hyperepinephrinemia:

2. Describe the effects of hyperepinephrinemia.

3. Mrs. J had a 5 hour GTT. Explain why some GTTs are for 2 h, 3 h, or 5 h.

4. List the symptoms of hypoglycemia.

5. Explain the differences between reactive functional hypoglycemia, reactive hypoglycemia secondary to diabetes, and hypoglycemia secondary to fasting.

6. What are the normal values for a GTT?

7. Explain the results of Mrs. J's GTT in relationship to her family background.

8. What is the difference between GTT and gtt?

9. From the information obtained by the dietitian, list the practices and foods in Mrs. J's lifestyle that could contribute to hypoglycemia.

10. List the principles of a diet to prevent hypoglycemia.

11. What specific points would you try to make to Mrs. J for the prevention of hypoglycemia?

12. The case study indicates three things the dietitian did at the end of her interview that are important. List these three things and explain their importance.

RELATED REFERENCES

1. Blumberg, S. (2005). Should hypoglycemia patients be prescribed a high-protein diet? *J Am Diet Assoc*. Feb;105(2):196-7.

2. Fischbach, F.T. (2003). *A Manual of Laboratory & Diagnostic Tests*. 7th Ed. Philadelphia. J.B. Lippincott Company.

3. Fournet, J.C. and Junien, C. (2004). Genetics of congenital hyperinsulinism *Endocr Pathol*. Fall;15(3):233-40.

4. Gregory, M. (2003). Alcohol-induced hypoglycaemia presenting as drug intoxication. *J Clin Forensic Med*. Sep;10(3):191-2.

5. Prendergast, A. & Fulton, F.L. (1997) *Medical terminology: A Text/Workbook*. 4th Ed. Redwood City, California. Addison-Wesley Nursing.

6. Pronsky, Z.M., Redfern, C.M., Crowe, J. & Epstein, S. (2003) *Food Medication Interactions*, 13th Ed Phoenix, Arizona. Food-Medications Interactions, Publishers and Distributors.

7. Rolfes, S.R., Pinna, K. & Whitney, E. (2006). *Understanding Normal and Clinical Nutrition*, 7th Ed. West/Wadsworth.

8. Rudic, R.D., McNamara, P., Curtis, A.M., Boston, R.C., Panda, .S, Hogenesch, J.B., and Fitzgerald, G.A. (2004). BMAL1 and CLOCK, two essential components of the circadian clock, are involved in glucose homeostasis. *PLoS Biol*. Nov;2(11):e377.

9. Spratto, G.R. & Woods, A.L. (2005). *PDR Nurse's Drug Handbook*. Thompson Delmar Learning, NY.

10. Watson, J and Kerr, D. (1999). The best defense against hypoglycemia is to recognize it: is caffeine useful? *Diabetes Technol Ther*. Summer;1(2):193-200.

CASE STUDY #22
TYPE 1 DIABETES MELLITUS

INTRODUCTION

This is a basic study concerned with insulin-dependent diabetes mellitus. Study the symptoms, treatment (including the types of insulin used for diabetes), and your exchange list for diabetes before you complete this case. A knowledge of carbohydrate counting would also be helpful. Try to understand what is going through this young man's mind. He has never been sick before and has a strong desire to be a professional basketball player. He fears this is no longer going to be possible.
****

SKILLS NEEDED

ABBREVIATIONS:
Knowledge of the following abbreviations is required in order to understand this case. You should learn these abbreviations before you begin to read the study.
CDE, DKA, D_5W, IDDM, JODM, MDI, NPH, and R (Appendix C).

LABORATORY VALUES:
Look up the normal value for glucose and study its relationship to diabetes.

FORMULAS:
The formulas used in this case study include weight for age and total caloric needs.

MEDICATIONS:
Become familiar with the following medications before reading the case study. Note the diet-drug interactions, dosages and methods of administration, gastrointestinal tract reactions, etc.
1. insulin: bovine; porcine; Humulin; NPH, lispro (humulog), and Regular.
****

JJ is a 13 YOWM who has high hopes of being a basketball star. He is tall for his age and is very well coordinated. He loves the game and plays every chance he gets. He has been healthy until recently. He was playing basketball after school with some friends when he became weak and nauseous. His friends noticed that he was sluggish and not himself, but they thought he was having a bad day. He bent over and rested his hands on his knees and then collapsed. When his friends rushed to him, he was disoriented and confused. He had been playing hard but not that hard. They tried to lay him down and give him some water, but he was getting worse. He was perspiring excessively. They called his parents who then called an ambulance.

JJ was rushed to the hospital and was quickly diagnosed with DKA 2° to Type 1 diabetes (formerly called Type I, Juvenile Onset Diabetes Mellitus [JODM] or Insulin Dependent Diabetes Mellitus [IDDM]). His blood sugar was 620 mg/dl. They started an I.V. with D_5W, R insulin, potassium, and phosphorus. Soon JJ was awake and back to his normal self. It was necessary for him to remain in the hospital for a while to regulate his insulin, meal plan, and activity
****

QUESTIONS:

1. Explain the physiology behind the following symptoms:
   Weak, sluggish:

   Nauseous:

   Disoriented and confused:

2. Describe the pathophysiology of DKA.

3. List all of the possible symptoms of Type 1 DM.

4. Explain the use of R Insulin, glucose, potassium, and phosphorous in the I.V. treatment.

****

When the physician talked with JJ's mother, he found out that JJ has a family history of diabetes. His grandfather had diabetes and he has an uncle with diabetes. His mother further explained that JJ had not been as active as usual for the past several days, but he was eating more frequently. She said JJ complained of losing a couple of pounds in two days but she did not believe his weighing was accurate. He was weighing himself daily because he was trying to gain weight to play ball. He is 5'8" and weighs 140 lbs. She did not notice anything else that was unusual. JJ said he had not felt right recently. He tired easily and was always hungry. He thought it was because he had been playing so hard. JJ's blood sugar was down the second day after his admission. He was started on 5 units of Humulin R insulin and 20 units of Humulin N insulin qAM to maintain control. He is to have three meals per day with an AM and hs snack. His energy intake level and snacks for exercise are to be determined by the RD, who is also a CDE. The diabetes teaching nurse is to visit him and instruct him in insulin administration and foot care.
****

QUESTIONS CONTINUED:

5. How do JJ's height and weight compare with the norm for his age?

6. What is/are the difference(s) between lispro, R Insulin and NPH insulin?

7. What are the differences between Humulin, porcine, and bovine insulin?

8. What is the significance of the AM and hs snacks?

9. Why is it important for the RN to teach him foot care?

****

JJ and his mother are now very concerned about his future. JJ has heard horror stories about diabetes and is worried that his basketball career has ended before it started. He knows that his grandfather had to have a leg amputated because of diabetes. Many questions were going through his head when the dietitian came into his room to talk to him about his meal plan. Imagine that you were that dietitian: how would you handle these questions from JJ?

****

QUESTIONS CONTINUED:

10. Will I have to take insulin for the rest of my life?

11. Will I have to go on a special diet and eat diet food?

12. Will I still be able to eat out with my friends, like at the Bigger Burger; and what would I eat at birthday parties and stuff?

13. Why did my grandfather lose a leg? Could that happen to me?

14. Can I still play basketball in high school and college?

15. Will I be able to gain weight and get a lot stronger?

****

JJ will soon be officially starting basketball practice for his junior high school team. This means that for the next several months he will be playing hard almost every day and, assuming he makes the team, will be playing in games once or twice a week. He likes fast food and drinks a lot of sodas. When he goes home from school, he likes to snack on cookies, peanut butter and crackers, etc. He is not a picky eater and will eat anything. The dietitian explained carbohydrate counting to JJ and his mother and encouraged him to start learning the carbohydrate exchanges. She set up an appointment for him in the Out-Patient Diabetes Clinic and told him that the RD, CDE will teach him how to do carbohydrate counting with MDI and the RN, CDE would come and teach him MDI. She told him that the carbohydrate counting is very flexible.

****

QUESTIONS CONTINUED:

16. What energy level would you recommend for JJ? Explain how you arrived at your decision.

17. What would you teach JJ about the kind and amount of snacks he can have?

18. What behavioral changes would you recommend to JJ?

Information Box 22-1

In 1993 the published results of the Diabetes Control and Complications Trial (DCCT) brought about several changes in the nutritional treatment and insulin management of diabetes (there are numerous references to this trial listed at the end of this chapter). Prior to this research, the *Exchange Lists for Meal Planning* was used to teach dietary control of blood sugar. As a result of the DCCT, there is now a second method of teaching meal plan as a means of blood sugar control for people with diabetes known as *Carbohydrate Counting*. The old method is still available but is discouraged because of the simplicity and greater effectiveness of carbohydrate counting used in conjunction with multiple daily injections (MDI). The *Exchange Lists for Meal Planning* has a place in that it is sometimes suitable for the obese because it helps them keep track of total calories from sources other than carbohydrate exchanges. The newer method, *Carbohydrate Counting*, is more flexible and provides a method for calculating insulin dosages. Even with the new method, the user has to be able to keep track of the carbohydrate exchanges.

When counting carbohydrate to balance insulin, the exchange lists are used as a guide but not with the same detail. Example: according to the exchange lists, a bread and fruit exchange are equal to 15 grams of carbohydrate each. A milk exchange is equal to 12 grams of carbohydrate. In the *Carbohydrate Counting* method, the milk exchange is rounded up to 15 grams and all three exchanges, bread, fruit, and milk, are each equal to one *Carbohydrate Counting* exchange of 15 grams. Any food item that contains less than 5 grams of carbohydrate per serving is free if only one serving is eaten at a meal. If more than one serving is eaten, the total amount of carbohydrate in all the servings are added up and compared to the *Carbohydrate Counting* exchange. Example: One vegetable exchange (½ cup) at a meal contains 5 grams of carbohydrate and is considered free. Three vegetable exchanges (1 ½ cups) at a meal contain 15 grams of carbohydrate and are equal to one *Carbohydrate Counting* exchange.[1]

Using the *Carbohydrate Counting* method, there are at least two means to determine the ratio of carbohydrate intake to insulin administered. These are the Carbohydrate Gram Method and the Carbohydrate Choices Method[1]. To teach these methods properly would take more space than allowed here. The references indicated below are good places to look for further instruction.

Assume the energy level you estimated for JJ in question 16 was exactly correct and assume you decided to use the Carbohydrate Counting method to teach JJ his meal plan. Based on the answer in question 16 and the information given about JJ's food preferences, i.e., hamburgers, answer question 19.

19. Using a separate sheet of paper, plan a balanced meal plan for JJ for one day. Include snacks at the appropriate time in accordance with his exercise routine. Make the meal plan realistic for a 13 year-old (a good outside assignment would be to interview an athletic 13 year old and use a "real" meal plan).

20. From this meal plan, on the same sheet of paper, determine the carbohydrate exchanges for each meal and snack.

21. Assume JJ has decided to use intensive insulin control with multiple daily injections (MDI) and he is using 8 units of R insulin in the AM, 4 at lunch, and 6 at the evening meal. Using both methods for determining a carbohydrate/insulin ratio, determine JJ's ratio.

22. The current recommendations allow for the incorporation of sugar into a meal plan for diabetes with caution not to indulge to excess. The assumption is that 15 grams of carbohydrate is 15 grams of carbohydrate regardless of the source. Based on JJ's questions, it would be easy to "scare" him into following a strict or closely controlled meal plan. How would you counsel JJ specifically about sugar in his meal plan without using "scare" tactics?

23. Create a SOAP note for JJ.

S:	**S:**
O:	
A:	
P:	

RELATED REFERENCES

1. American Diabetes Association. (2005). Standards of Medical Care in Diabetes. *Diabetes Care* 2005 28: S4-36

2. American Diabetes Association. (2005). Summary of Revisions for the 2005 Clinical Practice Recommendations. *Diabetes Care* 28: S3.

3. American Diabetes Association. (2005). Diagnosis and Classification of Diabetes Mellitus. *Diabetes Care* 28: S37-42.

4. American Diabetes Association Position Statement: Evidence-based nutrition principles and recommendations for the treatment and prevention of diabetes and related complications. (2002). *J. Am. Diet. Assoc.* 102:109-118.

5. Ahmed, A.B. & Home, P.D. (1998). Optimal provision of daytime NPH insulin in patients using the insulin analog lispro. *Diabetes Care.* 21(10):1707-13.

6. American Diabetes Association. (1993). Implications of the Diabetes Control and Complications Trial. American Diabetes Association. *Diabetes.* 42(11):1555-8.

7. American Diabetes Association. (1994). Nutrition recommendations and principles for people with diabetes mellitus. *J. Am. Diet. Assoc.* 94:504.

8. Anderson, J.W. & Geil, P.B. (1998). New perspectives in nutrition management of diabetes mellitus. *Am. J. Med.* 85(5A):159-65.

9. Current literature in diabetes. (2005). *Diabetes Metab Res Rev.* Jan;21(1):71-78.

10. Davis, D.L. & Gregory, R.P. (1993). Carbohydrate counting alternative in glucose control. *J. Am. Diet. Assoc.* 93(10):1104.

11. Del Sindaco, P., Ciofetta, M., Lalli, C., Perriello, G., Pamanelli, S., Torlone, E., Brunetti, P. & Bolli, G.B. (1998). Use of the short-acting insulin analogue lispro in intensive treatment of type 1 diabetes mellitus: importance of appropriate replacement of basal insulin and time-interval injection-meal. *Diabet. Med.* 15(7):592-600.

12. Diabetes Care. (1995). Implication of treatment protocols in the Diabetes Control and Complications Trial. *Diabetes Care.* 18(3):361-76.

13. Dillinger, Y. & Yass, C. (1995). Carbohydrate counting in the management of diabetes. *Diabetes Edu.* 21(6):547-50, 552.

14. Eastman, R.C., Siebert, C.W., Harris, M., & Gorden, P. (1993). Clinical review 51: Implications of the Diabetes Control and Complications Trial. *J. Clin. Endocrinol. Metab.* 77(5):1105-7.

15. Faro, B. (1995). Students with diabetes: implications of the Diabetes Control and Complications Trial for the school setting. *J. Sch. Nurs.* 11(1):16-21.

16. Fischbach, F.T. (2003). *A Manual of Laboratory & Diagnostic Tests.* 7th Ed. Philadelphia. J.B. Lippincott Company.

17. Franz, M.J. (2001). Carbohydrate and diabetes: is the source or the amount of more importance? *Curr Diab Rep*. 2001 Oct;1(2):177-86.

18. Gregory, R.P. & Davis, D.L. (1994). Use of carbohydrate counting for meal planning in type I diabetes. *Diabetes Educ*. 20(5):406-9.

19. Gillespie, S.J., Kulkarni, K.D., & Daly, A.E. (1998). Using carbohydrate counting in diabetes clinical practice. *J. Am. Diet. Assoc*. 98(8):897-905.

20. Hadden, D.R. (1994). The Diabetes Control and Complications Trial (DCCT): what every endocrinologist needs to know. *Clin. Endocrinol*. 40(3):293-4.

21. Hopkins, D. (2004). Exercise-induced and other daytime hypoglycemic events in patients with diabetes: prevention and treatment. *Diabetes Res Clin Pract*. Sep;65 Suppl 1:S35-9.

22. Kelley, D.E. (2003). Sugars and starch in the nutritional management of diabetes mellitus. *Am J Clin Nutr*. Oct;78(4):858S-864S.

23. Koivisto, V.A. (1998). The human insulin analogue insulin lispro. *Ann. Med*. 30(3):260-6.

24. Leontos, C. (2003). Implementing the American Diabetes Association's nutrition recommendations. *J Am Osteopath Assoc*. Aug;103(8 Suppl 5):S17-20.

25. Mohammed, N.H. and Wolever, T.M. (2004). Effect of carbohydrate source on post-prandial blood glucose in subjects with type 1 diabetes treated with insulin lispro. *Diabetes Res Clin Pract*. Jul;65(1):29-35.

26. Moreland, E.C., Tovar, A., Zuehlke, J.B., Butler, D.A., Milaszewski, K., and Laffel, L.M. (2004). The impact of physiological, therapeutic and psychosocial variables on glycemic control in youth with type 1 diabetes mellitus. *J Pediatr Endocrinol Metab*. Nov;17(11):1533-44.

27. Prendergast, A. & Fulton, F.L. (1997) *Medical terminology: A Text/Workbook*. 4th Ed. Redwood City, California. Addison-Wesley Nursing.

28. Pronsky, Z.M., Redfern, C.M., Crowe, J. & Epstein, S. (2003) *Food Medication Interactions*, 13th Ed Phoenix, Arizona. Food-Medications Interactions, Publishers and Distributors.

29. Rolfes, S.R., Pinna, K. & Whitney, E. (2006). *Understanding Normal and Clinical Nutrition*, 7th Ed. West/Wadsworth.

30. Rabasa-Lhoret, R., Garon. J/, Langelier. H/, Poisson. D., & Chiasson, J.L. (1999). Effects of meal carbohydrate content on insulin requirements in type 1 diabetic patients treated intensively with the basal-bolus (ultralente-regular) insulin regimen. *Diabetes Care*. May;22(5):667-73.

31 Ronnemaa, T. & Viikari, J. (1998). Reducing snacks when switching from conventional soluble to lispro insulin treatment: effects on glycaemic control and hypoglycaemia. *Diabet. Med*. 15(7):601-7.

32. Sjoberg, A., Hallberg, L., Hoglund, D., and Hulthen, L. (2003). Meal pattern, food choice, nutrient intake and lifestyle factors in The Goteborg Adolescence Study. *Eur J Clin Nutr*. Dec;57(12):1569-78.

33. Spratto, G.R. & Woods, A.L. (2005). *PDR Nurse's Drug Handbook.* Thompson Delmar Learning, NY.

34. The American Dietetic Association. (2003). *Basic Carbohydrate Counting.* Chicago, IL.

35. The American Dietetic Association. (2003). *Advanced Carbohydrate Counting.* Chicago, IL.

36. The Diabetes Control and Complications Trial Research Group. (1993). The effect of intensive treatment of diabetes on the development and progression of long-term complications in insulin-dependent diabetes mellitus. The Diabetes Control and Complications Trial Research Group. *N. Engl. J. Med.* 329(14):977-86.

37. Waldron, S., Hanas, R., & Palmvig, B. (2002). How do we educate young people to balance carbohydrate intake with adjustments of insulin? *Horm Res.* 57 Suppl 1:62-5.

CASE STUDY #23
TYPE 2 DIABETES MELLITUS AND METABOLIC SYNDROME

INTRODUCTION

This is a typical account of obesity contributing to diabetes. It is also an introduction to some of the cultural practices of Native Americans, although their eating habits have been greatly influenced by those of the general population. About six percent of the population in the U.S. is said to have diabetes mellitus. The highest recorded incidence is 40 percent seen in the Pima Indians in Arizona of age 45 or older. In PART II Mrs. R's treatment was not effective and her condition worsened. Several new treatments are attempted before one is found that works. The new treatments involve the use of the latest drugs for Type 2 diabetes. This is a long and involved case study but has the potential to teach the student much about lab value, interpretation, diabetes, and behavior.
****

SKILLS NEEDED

ABBREVIATIONS:
Knowledge of the following abbreviations is required in order to understand this case. You should learn these abbreviations before you begin to read the study.
A1c, BP, BS, CDE, D/C'd, NIDDM, R insulin, and UTI (Appendix C).

LABORATORY VALUES:
You will need to be able to interpret the nutritional significance of the following laboratory values for this case study: A1c, ALP, ALT, amylase, AST, BUN, Ca, Chol, Cl, CPK, Cr, DIBL, Glucose, hct, HDL, hgb, K, LDL, lymph, MCH, MCHC, MCV, Mg, Na, P, RBC, ser alb, TIBL, TP, triglycerides, WBC (Appendix B).

FORMULAS:
The formulas used in this case study include ideal body weight, percent of ideal body weight, body mass index, LDL, and total caloric and protein needs (Appendix A, Tables 7, 8, 10, 17, and 19).

MEDICATIONS:
Become familiar with the following medications before reading the case study. Note the diet-drug interactions, dosages and methods of administration, gastrointestinal tract reactions, etc.
1. Glucotrol (glipizide); 2. insulin: Humulin, Regular, and Lantus insulin; 3. Precose (acarbose); 4. Glucophage (metformin); 5. Pravachol (pravastatin).
****

PART I: INITIAL TREATMENT

Mrs. R is a 48 YOF who is a Native American living on a reservation. She has lived there with her family all of her life, is a housewife and has three children. Her husband works in a nearby factory. All of Mrs. R's children have finished high school but one still lives at home and is unemployed. The income for Mrs. R's family is meager and they depend on home-grown vegetables and wild game to supplement their food supply. Government commodities contribute a small amount.

Mrs. R has a pronounced family history of Type 2 diabetes mellitus. Several family members have had severe complications because of poor control of blood glucose. Mrs. R is well aware of the problems in her family's past, but this has not stopped her from eating whatever she wants. She is 5'6" and weighs 210 lbs with a medium frame with a waist of 42". She is not very active but does work in her vegetable garden a lot. Occasionally she goes for long walks on her reservation in the evenings. She has graduated from high school and reads and writes adequately. On several occasions she has been treated for UTIs and has frequent colds. She does not have a history of any major illness. During the past month, Mrs. R noticed some significant changes in the way she feels. She becomes fatigued easily and has to go to the bathroom more frequently, even during the night. She is hungry all the time and is eating more but she lost 10 lbs in the last six weeks and her vision has become blurred. Mrs. R went to the doctor because she developed another bladder infection. She can always tell when she has a bladder infection by the pain in her lower abdomen and the frequency of her urination. She decided to go to the doctor for the infection and, while there, explained the other problems she was having. Her BP was 150/88. The physician obtained some fasting blood tests and found the following:

TABLE 1

CBC							
TEST	RESULT	REFERENCE UNITS		TEST	RESULT	REFERENCE UNITS	
		Conventional	SI			Conventional	SI
Hgb	14 g/dl	12-16 g/dl	120-160 g/L	WBC	10.7 x 10^3/μ	4.5-10.5 x 10^3/cells/mm^3	4.5-10.5 x10^9/L
Hct	42 %	36-48%		% Lymph	26%	25 – 40% of total WBC	1500-4000 cells/mm^3
RBC	3.8x10^6/μ	3.6-5.0x10^6/L	3.6-5.0 x10^{12}/L	MCH	27 pg/cell	26-34 pg/cell	0.40-.53 fmol/cell
MCV	80 μm^3	82-98μm^3	82-98 fL	MCHC	33 g/dl	32-36 g/dl	320-360 g/L

TABLE 2

BASIC METABOLIC PACKAGE							
TEST	RESULT	REFERENCE UNITS		TEST	RESULT	REFERENCE UNITS	
		Conventional	SI			Conventional	SI
Glu	353 mg/dl	70-110 mg/dl	3.8-6.1 mmol/L	Na	148 mEq/L	136-145 mEq/L	136-145 mmol/L
BUN	28 mg/dl	6-20 mg/dl	2.1-7.1 mmol/L	K	4.8 mEq/L	3.5-5.2 mEq/L	3.5-5.2 mmol/L
Cr	1.1 mg/dl	0.6-1.1 mg/dl	53-97 μmol/L	Cl	104 mEq/L	96-106 mEq/L	96-106 mmol/L
Ca	9.1 mg/dl	8.8-10.0 mg/dl	2.20-2.60 mmol/L	Mg	2.0 mEq/L	1.8 - 2.6 mEq/L	136-145 mmol/L
Ser alb	3.7 g/dl	3.5-4.8 g/dl	39-50 g/dl	P	3.1mg/dl	2.7-4.5 mg/dl	4.7-6.0 kPa

TABLE 3

LIPID PROFILE							
TEST	RESULT	REFERENCE UNITS		TEST	RESULT	REFERENCE UNITS	
		Conventional	SI			Conventional	SI
Chol	300 mg/dl	140-199 mg/dl	3.63-5.15 mmol/L	HDL	30 mEq/L	40-85 mEq/L	1.0-2.2 mmol/L
TG	350 mg/dl	<-150 mg/dl	<1.70 mmol/L	LDL	? mg/dl	<130 mg/dl	<3.4 mmol/L

****

QUESTIONS:
1. Determine Mrs. R's IBW and percent of IBW (Appendix A, Tables 7 and 8).

2. Calculate Mrs. R's BMI and interpret the results (Appendix A, Tables 10 and 11).

3. Calculate Mrs. R's LDL in TABLE 3 (Appendix A, Table 19).

4. What is A1c and how is it used with diabetes?

5. List the symptoms of Type 2 diabetes that are manifested in Mrs. R.

6. Explain the pathophysiology of these symptoms.

****
The MD diagnosed Mrs. R with dehydration, obesity with Type 2 diabetes, metabolic syndrome, and anemia. He based his decision on her family history, lab values, anthropometric measurements, elevated BP, and the symptoms he described as polydipsia, polyuria, polyphagia, hyperglycemia, and fatigue. He prescribed a 1000 kcal diet, glipizide (Glucotrol), 5 mg every morning 30 minutes before breakfast, Pravachol (pravastatin sodium), 40 mg once daily at bedtime, and referred her to the clinic's registered dietitian. He also wanted her to start an exercise program, but he wanted her to get her blood glucose down first. He told her it would be all right if she started walking a small amount, even if was just a block a day, and increase her distance as she was able. He told her she had to lose weight and if she did, she may be able to stop taking her medication and be free of the symptoms of diabetes, or at least lessen them. He explained how much of her problem may be due to metabolic syndrome and that diet and exercise could help control those symptoms.
****

7. Define the following terms:
   Polydipsia:

   Polyphagia:

   Polyuria:

   Government commodities:

8. What evidence did the MD have that suggested that Mrs. R was dehydrated?

9. What labs may be elevated due to dehydration?

10. On what basis did the MD decide that Mrs. R was anemic?

11. After Mrs. R's BS is corrected, what changes in other blood values would you expect? Explain your answer.

12. What is considered to be good control for BS for someone with diabetes and what is considered poor control?

13. Why should the physician be concerned about the abnormal lipid profile of a person with diabetes who is out of control like Mrs. R?

14. Describe the function of glipizide and list any nutritional complications.

15. Describe the function of pravastatin sodium and list any nutritional complications. Why did the physician tell Mrs. R to take it at bedtime?

16. Mrs. R's BP was 150/88. What is the current recommended BP for Mrs. R?

17. What is metabolic syndrome and what symptoms of metabolic syndrome does Mrs. R demonstrate?

18. The MD told Mrs. R that if she lost weight, she might not need the medication and could be free of her symptoms. Describe the relationship between obesity, diabetes, and metabolic syndrome.

19. Prepare a SOAP note for Mrs. R up to this point.

S:
O:
A:
P:

****

The RD interviewed Mrs. R and discovered that she ate a high-fat, low-protein, high-carbohydrate diet. She did not follow her traditional tribal eating patterns but ate like any modern American with a few exceptions. She liked fry bread and on rare occasions would fix wojapi. She consumed a large amount of soda, candy, cookies, potato chips, and corn chips, etc. The sodium content of her diet was high. She did not tolerate milk and ate cheese only when it could be obtained through government commodities. The only fresh vegetables she ate were those her family could grow: squash, peppers, a lot of beans, corn, and some greens. There was very little fruit in her diet, and she did not eat meat often. She was used to eating a snack before going to bed at night. She usually got up early in the morning to avoid the heat and had a light snack before going out and working in the garden for a couple of hours. She then came in and ate breakfast; lunch was around 1 PM, and the evening meal was about 6 PM. Sometimes she would take a walk after supper but not specifically for the purpose of getting exercise.

****

PART II: ADJUSTMENTS IN DIET AND MEDICATIONS

QUESTIONS CONTINUED:

20. Approximate Mrs. R's energy needs for weight reduction. Show your work.

21. Would you prescribe a 1000 kcal diet? Why or why not?

22. What recommendations for dietary intervention would you give Mrs. R? Would you use the Carbohydrate Counting method or would you follow the standard Exchange Lists for Meal Planning? Explain your answer.

23. According to the list of likes and dislikes above, Mrs. R consumes a significant amount of sweets. The guidelines for meal plans for people with diabetes allows for a limited amount of sugar to be incorporated into the meal plan. Think about how you would persuade Mrs. R to limit her sugar intake and describe how you would teach her to use sugar in her meal plan. Include in your discussion any possible pitfalls of allowing sugar in the meal plan.

24. Describe the Native-American foods, *fry bread* and *wojapi*.

25. What nutritional deficiencies are likely to result from following the diet Mrs. R described? Explain.

26. What behavioral changes would you recommend to Mrs. R to help her keep her dietary and treatment goals?

27. On a separate sheet of paper, use the kcal levels and the proportions of each major nutrient you recommended (questions 19-22 and 24-25) and plan a day's menu for Mrs. R based on food availability. Unless your instructor tells you otherwise, prepare the meal plan using the exchange method and the carbohydrate method. List the foods you would give her in diabetic exchanges and carbohydrate exchanges. Adjust her meal plan to meet her usual eating habits as much as possible. For example, incorporate a reasonable amount of sweets into Mrs. R's meal plan. If you use

carbohydrate counting, prepare her meal plan based on carbohydrate exchanges. In your meal plan, regardless of the method, Mrs. R will benefit from a consistent intake of grams of carbohydrate at each meal and snack. You also have to remember to take into account activity and when her medications are taken.

****

Mrs. R took her medication and stayed on her meal plan as best she could but many of her symptoms continued. She has not worked in her garden or walked as much as usual because she still did not feel very well. She returned to her doctor for regular checkups, the first being three months later. Her weight had decreased by ten pounds to 200. Her labs were as follows:

TABLE 4

| TEST | RESULT | REFERENCE UNITS | | TEST | RESULT | REFERENCE UNITS | |
		Conventional	SI			Conventional	SI
Chol	224mg/dl	140-199 mg/dl	3.63-5.15 mmol/L	HDL	35 mEq/L	40-85 mEq/L	1.0-2.2 mmol/L
TG	185 mg/dl	<-150 mg/dl	<1.70 mmol/L	LDL	? mg/dl	<130 mg/dl	<3.4 mmol/L
Glu	255 mg/dl	70-110 mg/dl	3.8-6.1 mmol/L	A1c	10.0%	5.5 – 8.5%	

There was not a significant change in her A1c. Her glucose showed slight improvement. The lipid profile was better but still had much room for improvement. Her original dose of Glucotrol was 5 mg in the morning 30 minutes before breakfast. The physician increased her dose to 10 mg and had her report back in two weeks. He also increased the pravastatin to 80 mg once daily and strongly encouraged her to start a walking program. She was supposed to be coming to the clinic weekly to see the CDE dietitian and nurse, but was non-compliant. The physician encouraged her to come weekly and to show them her daily log of BS levels from her finger sticks. Over the next several months, Mrs. R continued to report to her doctor with little success. Her weight stayed about the same with slight changes in her glucose and A1c. Her lipid profile continued to be worrisome. The physician continued to increase her Glucotrol until she was at two doses of 15 mg each. On her last visit her labs were as follows:

TABLE 5

| TEST | RESULT | REFERENCE UNITS | | TEST | RESULT | REFERENCE UNITS | |
		Conventional	SI			Conventional	SI
Chol	200 mg/dl	140-199 mg/dl	3.63-5.15 mmol/L	HDL	40 mEq/L	40-85 mEq/L	1.0-2.2 mmol/L
TG	150 mg/dl	<-150 mg/dl	<1.70 mmol/L	LDL	? mg/dl	<130 mg/dl	<3.4 mmol/L
Glu	225 mg/dl	70-110 mg/dl	3.5-6.1 mmol/L	A1c	9.1%	5.5 – 8.5%	

****

28. Continue with your SOAP note for Mrs. R.

S:
O:

A:
P:

After increasing her Glucotrol, her weight decreased to 193 pounds. Still, with this slow level of improvement, the physician decided to start her on insulin, 15u of Humulin N every morning before breakfast with a sliding scale for Regular insulin if her morning glucose was more than 200.

Information Box 23 - 1

The sliding scale formula the physician used was as follows: if the BS is more than 200, subtract 200 from the actual BS value and divide by two. The final number would be the amount of R insulin used. Example: If the BS was 230:

230 - 200 = 30 → 30/2 = 15 → Mrs. R. would add 15 u of R insulin to her morning dose.

****

QUESTIONS CONTINUED:

29. Determine Mrs. R's LDL level in TABLES 4 and 5 (Appendix A, Table 19).

30. Define Humalin N and R insulin.

31. Research the insulin Lantus and describe how it may help Mrs. R.

32. After injection, when do Humalin N and R insulin begin to have an effect, how long do the effects last, and when do they peak?

Insulin	Onset	Peak	Duration
Humulin N			
R			
Lantus			

****

Mrs. R had to learn how to give herself insulin and did not like it at all. The physician told her that if she got her glucose under control and lost weight, she may not need the insulin. This motivated her to follow her meal plan and her walking routine. However, as time passed, her condition worsened as she refused to follow a special meal plan and did not take her medications as she should because of the cost. The physician did not realize all of the financial problems. Mrs. R gained some of her weight back and her glucose was still elevated and her A1c was back to 10%. Her physician added Precose to her regimen. This immediately had an effect on Mrs. R's BS but too much of an effect. The day she started taking the Precose, she decided to take all of her meds and took the Glucotrol and insulin. It caused her BS to drop below 60 and gave Mrs. R signs of hypoglycemia. She also complained about excessive gas, abdominal cramps and diarrhea. The physician increased her Humulin N to 40 u every morning, left the sulfonylurea the same, and D/C'd the Precose.

Time continued to pass and Mrs. R continued to gain weight. Her BS was going up instead of going down and her A1c was increasing. The physician decided she was having more problems with insulin resistance then he realized. He added Glucophage (metformin) to the regimen.

****

QUESTIONS CONTINUED:

33. What is the action of Precose and what are its side effects?

34. Describe fully the process of insulin resistance.

35. List the aspects of Mrs. R's case that indicate insulin resistance.

36. What is the action of Glucophage and what are its side effects?

****

Mrs. R finally had favorable results with her new regimen but only after she began to follow her meal plan, finally started a walking program, and took her meds as prescribed. The BS levels were coming down along with her A1c. Triglycerides, total cholesterol, LDL and HDL all stayed in an appropriate range.

****

QUESTIONS CONTINUED:

37. This has been a long ordeal for Mrs. R with many opportunities for her to become discouraged. Try to imagine what it would be like to be her dietitian and to be counseling her through this ordeal. What advice would you give Mrs. R?

38. Continue your SOAP note for Mrs. R.

S:
O:
A:
P:

RELATED REFERENCES

1. American Diabetes Association. (2005). Standards of Medical Care in Diabetes. *Diabetes Care* 2005 28: S4-36

2. American Diabetes Association. (2005). Summary of Revisions for the 2005 Clinical Practice Recommendations. *Diabetes Care* 28: S3.

3. American Diabetes Association. (2005). Diagnosis and Classification of Diabetes Mellitus. *Diabetes Care* 28: S37-42.

4. American Diabetes Association Position Statement: Evidence-based nutrition principles and recommendations for the treatment and prevention of diabetes and related complications. (2002). *J. Am. Diet. Assoc.* 102:1, 109-18.

5. Archer, S.L., Greenlund, K.J., Valdez, R., Casper, M.L, Rith-Najarian, S., & Croft, J.B. (2004). Differences in food habits and cardiovascular disease risk factors among Native Americans with and without diabetes: the Inter-Tribal Heart Project. *Public Health Nutr.* Dec;7(8):1025-32.

6. Archer, S.L., Greenlund, K.J., Casper, M.L., Rith-Najarian, S., & Croft, J.B. (2002). Associations of community-based health education programs with food habits and cardiovascular disease risk factors among Native Americans with diabetes: the inter-tribal heart project, 1992 to 1994. *J Am Diet Assoc* Aug;102(8):1132-5.

7. Bell, D.S. (2004). Practical considerations and guidelines for dosing sulfonylureas as monotherapy or combination therapy. *Clin Ther.* Nov;26(11):1714-27.

8. Brown, S.L., Pope, J.F., Hunt, A.E., & Tolman, N.M. (1998). Motivational strategies used by dietitians to counsel individuals with diabetes. *Diabetes Educ.* 24(3):313-8.

9. Bruttomesso, D., Pianta, A., Crazzolara, D., Capparotto, C., Dainese, E., Zurlo, C., Minicuci, N., Briani , G., & Tiengo,. (2001). Teaching and training programme on carbohydrate counting in Type 1 diabetic patients. *Diabetes Nutr Metab.* Oct;14(5):259-67. A

10. Costacou, T., Levin, S., & Mayer-Davis, E.J. (2000). Dietary patterns among members of the Catawba Indian nation. *J Am Diet Assoc.* Jul;100(7):833-5.

11. Current literature in diabetes. (2005). *Diabetes Metab Res Rev.* Jan;21(1):71-78.

12. Delahanty, L.M. & Nathan, D.M. (2004). Research navigating the course of clinical practice in diabetes. *J Am Diet Assoc.* Dec;104(12):1846-53.

13. Diabetes Care. (1995). Implication of treatment protocols in the Diabetes Control and Complications Trial. *Diabetes Care.* 18(3):361-76.

14. Dillinger, Y. & Yass, C. (1995). Carbohydrate counting in the management of diabetes. *Diabetes Edu.* 21(6):547-50, 552.

15. Fagot-Campagna, A., Nelson, R.G., Knowler, W.C., Pettit, D.J., Robbins, D.C., Go, O., Welly, T.K., Lee, E.T., & Howard, B.V. (1998). Plasma lipoproteins and the incidence of abnormal excretion of albumin in diabetic American Indians: The Strong Heart Study. *Diabetologia.* 41(9):1002-9.

16. Feinglos, M.N. & Bethel, M.A. (1998). Treatment of type 2 diabetes mellitus. *Med. Clin.North Am.* 82(4):757-90.

17. Fischbach, F.T. (2003). *A Manual of Laboratory & Diagnostic Tests.* 7th Ed. Philadelphia. J.B. Lippincott Company.

18. Franz, M.J. (2001). Carbohydrate and diabetes: is the source or the amount of more importance? *Curr Diab Rep.* 2001 Oct;1(2):177-86.

19. Gillespie, S.J., Kulkarni, K.D., & Daly, A.E. (1998). Using carbohydrate counting in diabetes clinical practice. *J. Am. Diet. Assoc.* 98(8):897-905.

20. Glasgow, R.E., Nutting, P.A., King, D.K., Nelson, C.C., Cutte,r G., Gaglio, B., Rahm, A.K, Whitesides, H., & Amthauer, H. (2004). A practical randomized trial to improve diabetes care. *J Gen Intern Med.* Dec;19(12):1167-74.

21. Hood, V.L., Kelly, B., Martinez, C., Shuman, S., & Secker-Walker, R. (1997). A Native American community initiative to prevent diabetes. *Ethn. Health.* 2(4):277-85.

22. Isaac, M.B. & Isaac, M.T. (2004). Should diet be a medical intervention? *Lancet.* Dec 11;364(9451):2095.

23. Jonnalagadda, S.S. (2004). Effectiveness of medical nutrition therapy: importance of documenting and monitoring nutrition outcomes. *J Am Diet Assoc.* Dec;104(12):1805-15.

24. Kabadi, U.M. (2004). Cost-effective management of hyperglycemia in patients with type 2 diabetes using oral agents. *Manag Care.* Jul;13(7):48-9, 53-6, 58-9.

25. Kelley, D.E. (2003). Sugars and starch in the nutritional management of diabetes mellitus. *Am J Clin Nutr.* Oct;78(4):858S-864S.

26. Leontos, C. (2003). Implementing the American Diabetes Association's nutrition recommendations. *J Am Osteopath Assoc.* Aug;103(8 Suppl 5):S17-20.

27. Mahoney, M.C. & Michalek, A.M. (1998). Health status of American Indians/Alaska Natives: genera; patterns of mortality. *Fam. Med.* 30(3):190-5.

28. Martin-Lazaro, J.F., & Becerra-Fernandez, A. (2005). The metabolic syndrome: Uncertain criteria. *Pharmacol Res.* Apr;51(4):385-6.

29. Moller, D.E., & Kaufman, K.D. (2005). Metabolic syndrome: A Clinical and Molecular Perspective. *Annu Rev Med.* 56:45-62.

30. Peterson, K.P., Pavlovich, J.G., Goldstrin, D., Little, R., England, J., & Peterson, C.M. (1998). What is hemoglobin A1c? An analysis of glycated hemoglobins by electrospray ionization mass spectrometry. *Clin. Chem.* 44(9):1951-8.

31. Prendergast, A. & Fulton, F.L. (1997) *Medical terminology: A Text/Workbook.* 4th Ed. Redwood City, California. Addison-Wesley Nursing.

32. Pronsky, Z.M., Redfern, C.M., Crowe, J. & Epstein, S. (2003) *Food Medication Interactions*, 13th Ed Phoenix, Arizona. Food-Medications Interactions, Publishers and Distributors.

33. Rendell, M. (2004). The role of sulphonylureas in the management of type 2 diabetes mellitus. *Drugs* 64(12):1339-58.

34. Rizvi, A.A. (2004). Type 2 diabetes: epidemiologic trends, evolving pathogenic concepts, and recent changes in therapeutic approach. *South Med J.* Nov;97(11):1079-87.

35. Robinson, L.E., & Graham, T.E. (2004). Metabolic syndrome, a cardiovascular disease risk factor: role of adipocytokines and impact of diet and physical activity. *J Appl Physiol.* Dec;29(6):808-29.

36. Rolfes, S.R., Pinna, K. & Whitney, E. (2006). *Understanding Normal and Clinical Nutrition*, 7th Ed. West/Wadsworth.

37. Roubicek, M., Vines, G., & Gonzalez, S.A. (1998). Use of HbA1c in screening for diabetes. *Diabetes Care.* 21(9):1577-9.

38. Spratto, G.R. & Woods, A.L. (2005). *PDR Nurse's Drug Handbook.* Thompson Delmar Learning, NY.

39. Sudhakar, M.K. (2004). Ghost of metabolic syndrome. *J Assoc Physicians India.* Apr;52:342.

40. Waldron, S., Hanas, R., &Palmvig, B. (2002). How do we educate young people to balance carbohydrate intake with adjustments of insulin? *Horm Res.* 57 Suppl 1:62-5.

41. Wiener, K. & Roberts, N.B. (1998). The relative merits of haemoglobin A1c and fasting plasma glucose as first-line diagnostic tests for diabetes mellitus in nonpregnant subjects *Diabet. Med.* 15(7):558-63.

42. Yesavage, S. (2004). A possible quick-assessment tool for patients with diabetes. *J Am Diet Assoc.* Dec;104(12):1827.

43. Zieve, F.J. (2004). The metabolic syndrome: diagnosis and treatment. *Clin Cornerstone.* 6 Suppl 3:S5-13.

CASE STUDY #24
COMPLICATIONS OF DIABETES

INTRODUCTION
This is a complicated study involving diabetes, renal problems, cardiovascular problems, obesity, tube feedings, and a surgical procedure. It requires knowledge of several terms, involves practical application of nutrition counseling, and considers some habits of an ethnic group. Study all of the previously mentioned disease states before beginning the case.

****

SKILLS NEEDED

ABBREVIATIONS:
Knowledge of the following abbreviations is required in order to understand this case. You should learn these abbreviations before you begin to read the study.
BMI, BS, DVT, MH, MI, N/G, N/V, PEJ, PVD, R/O, SBO, S/P, and TF (Appendix C).

LABORATORY VALUES:
Look up the normal values for the following parameters: A1c, BUN, Ca, Cl, Cr, Glu, hct, hgb, K, % lymph, MCH, MCHC, MCV, Mg, Na, P, RBC, ser alb, and WBC (Appendix B).

FORMULAS:
The formulas used in this case study include ideal body weight, percent ideal body weight, adjusted body weight, BMI, total energy and protein needs, and percentage calculations of tube feeding constituents based on flow rates (Appendix A, Tables 7-11 and 17).

MEDICATIONS:
Become familiar with the following medications before reading the case study. Note the diet-drug interactions, dosages and methods of administration, gastrointestinal tract reactions, etc.
1. heparin; 2. insulin; 3. potassium supplements; 4. phosphorus supplements; 5. Reglan (metoclopramide).

****

Mrs. M is a 64-year-old Cuban-American who was admitted to the ER with a Dx of DVT in her right leg and hyperglycemia, her fifth admission in the last year. She has a long standing MH that includes: Type 2 diabetes mellitus, PVD, retinopathy, neuropathy, nephropathy, hypertension, and S/P MI. Mrs. M is 5'3" and weighs 252 lbs. She lives with her son, who is also obese, and does not understand the importance of diet. Because of her problems, her son feels sorry for her and goes along with whatever she wants. This solicitousness is usually centered around eating. Her son works as a short-order cook and enjoys making dishes for her that she likes. They live in Miami, where there is a large Cuban population and where many Cuban foods are available. Some of the foods Mrs. M and her son eat on a daily basis are fried plantains, dried black beans, and chick peas. Rice is always eaten with legumes. Arroz con qui is another favorite dish. Yams (yucca) are eaten more often than white potatoes, but french fries are consumed often. Chicken and pork are more frequent choices than beef. Their favorite vegetables include fried eggplant, beets, and greens. The vegetables are cooked with salt pork, ham, or lard. Mrs. M and her son drink several cups of strong coffee per day with sugar. Sugar is also used in cooking; for instance, the plantains are fried in a skillet with a little oil and then sprinkled with sugar. They even add sugar to the yams. Very little fruit is eaten, although they do drink orange juice on a regular basis. They also eat many foods not common to the Cuban culture.

Mrs. M's eyesight is poor, but she is not blind. She enjoys watching her son bowl at the local bowling alley two to three times a week. Whenever her son takes her to the bowling alley he buys her a large hamburger, french fries, and a large soda. She knows it is not good for her, but she does it anyway. Sometimes she will drink a couple of beers while watching her son bowl.

207

Mrs. M's kidney function is not seriously abnormal but it has been affected by her weight and hypertension. Nephrotic syndrome with the concurrent proteinuria and edema is slight, but her nephrologist is concerned that it will become much worse if she does not start following her meal plan. Mrs. M had a slight MI one year ago 2° to atherosclerosis. Angioplasty was successful, and again she was warned that she needed to change her meal plan or she could soon have more severe blockages. A cardiologist explained to her that she would eventually require open-heart surgery if she did not lose weight and follow her meal plan. All the emphasis on meal plan was ignored. After her MI, Mrs. M gained 40 lbs due to the decreased activity. The increased weight caused more inactivity, and hence, a DVT.

****

QUESTIONS:

1. Define the following as they relate to diabetes:

    Hyperglycemia:

    Retinopathy:

    Neuropathy:

    Nephropathy:

    Nephrotic Syndrome:

    Proteinuria:

    Angioplasty:

    Myocardial Infarction:

2. Determine Mrs. M's IBW and percent of IBW (Appendix A, Tables 7 and 8).

3. Calculate Mrs. M's BMI (Appendix A, Tables 10 and 11).

4. Give the pathophysiology of the following:
    Retinopathy:

    Neuropathy:

    Nephropathy:

Nephrotic Syndrome:

5. Describe the following foods and include the amount of carbohydrates per serving:

Plantains:

Yucca:

Chick Peas:

Yams:

Arroz con qui:

6. Some of Mrs. M's food choices are extremely poor for her medical condition. Her intake is complicated by her obese son who cooks for her. The meal plan she should be following is complex because of the multiple problems she has. Each of Mrs. M's problems is listed as a heading below. Under each heading list the foods mentioned in the case study that Mrs. M should avoid. Many foods may be listed more than once.

OBESITY	DIABETES	RENAL	CARDIOVASCULAR

7. For the above mentioned foods that should be avoided, suggest an appropriate substitute.

8. While Mrs. M is hospitalized for DVT, the RD will have a chance to work with her. Outline the steps that you, as the RD, would take to teach Mrs. M her meal plan and the importance of following it.

9. Considering the lifestyle presented, what behavioral changes would you suggest to Mrs. M to help her follow her meal plan?

****

Mrs. M's lab values were as follows:

BASIC METABOLIC PACKAGE							
TEST	RESULT	REFERENCE UNITS Conventional	SI	TEST	RESULT	REFERENCE UNITS Conventional	SI
Glu	203 mg/dl	70-110 mg/dl	3.8-6.1 mmol/L	Na	144 mEq/L	136-145 mEq/L	136-145 mmol/L
BUN	27 mg/dl	6-20 mg/dl	2.1-7.1 mmol/L	K	3.1 mEq/L	3.5-5.2 mEq/L	3.5-5.2 mmol/L
Cr	1.2 mg/dl	0.6-1.1 mg/dl	53-97 μmol/L	Cl	98 mEq/L	96-106 mEq/L	96-106 mmol/L
Ca	9.1 mg/dl	8.8-10.0 mg/dl	2.20-2.60 mmol/L	Mg	1.9 mEq/L	1.8 - 2.6 mEq/L	136-145 mmol/L
Ser alb	3.7 g/dl	3.5-4.8 g/dl	39-50 g/dl	P	4.4mg/dl	2.7-4.5 mg/dl	4.7-6.0 kPa

CBC							
TEST	RESULT	REFERENCE UNITS Conventional	SI	TEST	RESULT	REFERENCE UNITS Conventional	SI
Hgb	13 g/dl	12-16 g/dl	120-160 g/L	WBC	6.8 10^3/μl	4.5-10.5 x 10^3/cells/mm^3	4.5-10.5 x10^9/L
Hct	39 %	36-48%		% Lymph	25%	25 – 40% of total WBC	1500-4000 cells/mm^3
RBC	4.6 x10^6/μ	3.6-5.0x10^6/L	3.6-5.0 x10^{12}/L	MCH	28 pg/cell	26-34 pg/cell	0.40-.53 fmol/cell
MCV	85 μm^3	82-98μm^3	82-98 fL	MCHC	33 g/dl	32-36 g/dl	320-360 g/L

****

QUESTIONS CONTINUED:

10. Mrs. M has hyperglycemia and nephrotic syndrome. How are these conditions going to affect her lab values?

****

Mrs. M was treated with I.V. heparin therapy, insulin, potassium and phosphorus supplementation prn, bed rest, and a 1000 kcal, 2 g Na diet, with a protein intake not to exceed .7 g per kg IBW.
****

11. Calculate Mrs. M's adjusted body weight (Appendix A, Table 11).

12. Why would the MD order a protein restriction of .7 g/kg of IBW? Explain.

13. Why use the IBW weight instead of the adjusted body weight? In your answer, relate how this would affect her protein requirement.

14. Why was it important for Mrs. M to receive potassium and phosphorous I.V. along with insulin?

****

Mrs. M progressed well on her treatment and the clot resolved. The RNs started getting her out of bed and ambulating her 2x daily. They were preparing her for D/C when she developed a new symptom. She C/O not getting enough to eat most of the time, but one day she refused her tray. She said she was still full from the last meal. Later she felt nauseous and began vomiting. She continued with N/V to such a degree that an N/G tube had to be placed. Her abdomen became distended and hard to touch but her BS decreased. Mrs. M had either had a gastric ileus or an obstruction. The physicians had to R/O a SBO. First an esophagogastroduodenoscopy was done and the results were negative. Gastric emptying time was studied and a significant delay was found. Venography studies indicated that ischemia of the gastric arteries was slowing down the blood supply to the stomach and causing a decrease in gastric functioning. This was termed gastroparesis 2° to diabetic gastrovasculitis.

The physicians were not sure if this was a permanent condition or if it would improve enough for Mrs. M to be able to eat again. The GI tract seemed to be functioning well beyond the stomach. All Mrs. M could tolerate po was cl liqs. Therefore, until Mrs. M recovered from this setback, a PEJ was performed and a feeding tube was placed. The MD also prescribed Reglan to aid in gastric emptying when po feedings were resumed.

****

QUESTIONS CONTINUED:
15. Define the following terms:
Ileus:

Venography:

Ischemia:

Esophagogastroduodenoscopy:

Gastroparesis:

Gastrovasculitis:

16. Summarize what has happened to Mrs. M with this latest complication of diabetes and explain what may have caused this.

17. What is the action of Reglan and what are its side effects?

18. Describe the placement and purpose of a PEJ.

19. Considering all of the problems Mrs. M has, what TF would you recommend? Justify your answer.

20. Describe the initial strength and flow rate you would use, the progression to the final flow rate, and the total kcals and protein Mrs. M would be receiving at the final flow rate (in total kcals and total grams and in kcals and grams per kg of IBW).

<u>**ADDITIONAL OPTIONAL QUESTIONS**</u>
Tube Feeding Drill:

21. Using the table below, compare several of the enteral nutritional supplements that would be appropriate for someone with diabetes with Mrs. M's complications (Appendix E).

Product	Producer	Form	Cal/ml	Non-pro cal/g N	Pro	CHO	Fat	Na mg	K mg	mOsm /kg water	Vol to meet RDA in ml	g of fiber /L	Free H₂O /L in ml

22. Complete a SOAP note on Mrs. M.

S:

O:

A:

P:

RELATED REFERENCES

1. American Diabetes Association. (2005). Standards of Medical Care in Diabetes. *Diabetes Care* 2005 28: S4-36

2. American Diabetes Association. (2005). Summary of Revisions for the 2005 Clinical Practice Recommendations. *Diabetes Care* 28: S3.

3. Brown, S.L., Pope, J.F., Hunt, A.E., & Tolman, N.M. (1998). Motivational strategies used by dietitians to counsel individuals with diabetes. *Diabetes Educ.* 24(3):313-8.

4. Caudle, P. (1993). Providing culturally sensitive health care to Hispanic clients. *Nurse Pract.* 18(12):40, 43-6, 50-1.

5. Coronado, G.D., Thompson, B., Tejeda, S., and Godina, R. (2004). Attitudes and beliefs among Mexican Americans about type 2 diabetes. *J Health Care Poor Underserved.* Nov;15(4):576-88.

6. Current literature in diabetes. (2005). *Diabetes Metab Res Rev.* Jan;21(1):71-78.

7. Delahanty, L.M. & Nathan, D.M. (2004). Research navigating the course of clinical practice in diabetes. *J Am Diet Assoc.* Dec;104(12):1846-53.

8. Diabetes Care. (1995). Implication of treatment protocols in the Diabetes Control and Complications Trial. *Diabetes Care.* 18(3):361-76.

9. Enck, P. & Frieling, T. (1997). Pathophysiology of diabetic gastroparesis. *Diabetes.* Suppl2:S77-81.

10. Feinglos, M.N. & Bethel, M.A. (1998). Treatment of type 2 diabetes mellitus. *Med. Clin.North Am.* 82(4):757-90.

11. Fischbach, F.T. (2003). *A Manual of Laboratory & Diagnostic Tests.* 7th Ed. Philadelphia. J.B. Lippincott Company

12. Flegal, K.M., Ezzati, T.M., Harris, M.I., Haynes, S.G., Juarez, R.Z., Knowler, W.C., Perez-Stable, E.J., & Stern, M.P. (1991). Prevalence of diabetes in Mexican Americans, Cubans, and Puerto Ricans from the Hispanic Health and Nutrition Examination Survey, 1982-1984. *Diabetes Care.* 14(7):628-38.

13. Glasgow, R.E., Nutting, P.A., King, D.K., Nelson, C.C., Cutte,r G., Gaglio, B., Rahm, A.K, Whitesides, H., & Amthauer, H. (2004). A practical randomized trial to improve diabetes care. *J Gen Intern Med.* Dec;19(12):1167-74.

14. Hadden, D.R. (1994). The Diabetes Control and Complications Trial (DCCT): What every endocrinologist needs to know. *Clin. Endocrinol.* 40(3):293-4.

15. Hanis, C.L., Hewett-Emmett, D., Bertin, T.K., & Schull, W.J. (1991). Origins of U.S. Hispanics. Implications for diabetes. *Diabetes Care.* 14(7):618-27.

16. James, W.P. (1998). What are the health risks? The medical consequences of obesity and its health risks. *Exp. Clin. Endocrinol. Diabetes.* 106 Suppl 2:1-6.

17. Kelley, D.E. (2003). Sugars and starch in the nutritional management of diabetes mellitus. *Am J Clin Nutr.* Oct;78(4):858S-864S.

18. Khan, L.K., Sobal, J., & Martorell, R. (1997). Acculturation, socioeconomic status, and obesity in Mexican Americans, Cuban Americans, and Puerto Ricans. *Int. J. Obes. Relat. Metab. Disord.* 21(2):91-6.

19. Kim, C.H. & Nelson, D.K. (1998). Venting percutaneous gastrostomy in the treatment of refractory idiopathic gastroparesis. *Gastrointest. Endosc.* 47(1):67-70.

20. Leontos, C. (2003). Implementing the American Diabetes Association's nutrition recommendations. *J Am Osteopath Assoc.* Aug;103(8 Suppl 5):S17-20.

21. Prendergast, A. & Fulton, F.L. (1997) *Medical terminology: A Text/Workbook.* 4th Ed. Redwood City, California. Addison-Wesley Nursing.

22. Pronsky, Z.M., Redfern, C.M., Crowe, J. & Epstein, S. (2003) *Food Medication Interactions*, 13th Ed Phoenix, Arizona. Food-Medications Interactions, Publishers and Distributors.

23. Rolfes, S.R., Pinna, K. & Whitney, E. (2006). *Understanding Normal and Clinical Nutrition*, 7th Ed. West/Wadsworth.

24. Spratto, G.R. & Woods, A.L. (2005). *PDR Nurse's Drug Handbook.* Thompson Delmar Learning, NY.

25. Wen, L.K., Shepherd, M.D., and Parchman, M.L. (2004). Family support, diet, and exercise among older Mexican Americans with type 2 diabetes. *Diabetes Educ.* Nov-Dec;30(6):980-93.

EPILOGUE

This was an unusual case but basically happened as is listed. The major exception was the patient was not Cuban. That was added for cultural diversity.

Case Study #25
Gestational Diabetes

Introduction

In this study the diagnosis and treatment of gestational diabetes are examined. Emphasis is placed on the regulation of insulin in conjunction with nutritional management. The student should review the nutritional implications of pregnancy, the medical nutrition therapy for diabetes, and the use of insulin in managing diabetes prior to studying this case.
****

Skills Needed

Abbreviations:
Knowledge of the following abbreviations is required in order to understand this case. You should learn these abbreviations before you begin to read the study. (Appendix C).
A1c, ABW, ACOG, BS, CDE, DM, Fe, GCT, GDM, GTT, IVGTT, NDDG, NPH, OGTT, and R insulin.

Laboratory Values:
You will need to be able to interpret the nutritional significance of the following laboratory values for this case study: A1c, BUN, Ca, Cl, Cr, glucose, hgb, hct, K, Mg, Na, P, ser alb, and urinary ketones (Appendix B).

Formulas:
The formulas used in this case study include metric conversions, ideal body weight, adjusted body weight, body mass index, and the Harris-Benedict equation (Appendix A, Tables 1, 2, 7, 8, 11 through 13, and 17).

Medications:
Become familiar with the following medications before reading the case study. Note the diet-drug interactions, dosages and methods of administration, gastrointestinal tract reactions, etc.
1. Folate; 2. NPH insulin; 3. Regular insulin; 4. Lispro insulin.
****

Mrs. C is a 31 YOWF who is in the 27th week of her first pregnancy. She is 165.1 cm tall and weighs 81.8 kg. Her weight prior to pregnancy was 72.7 kg. She has not been going to her physician as she should since becoming pregnant, but she was dutiful in making prepregnancy plans. She saw her physician prior to becoming pregnant and followed his advice by taking a prenatal vitamin and 800 µg of folate every day. She was also advised to follow a diet and an exercise plan but Mrs. C has never been able to practice healthy eating habits or exercise regularly. Her family history is positive for diabetes. A grandmother, an aunt, and two cousins were diagnosed with DM during pregnancy. Mrs. C was supposed to see her physician by the 24th week of pregnancy to be screened for GDM but she did not keep her appointment. She is visiting her physician in her 27th week to be screened for GDM.

One hour after consuming 50 g of glucose, Mrs. C's plasma glucose was 165 mg/dL. These results are indicative of GDM and require further testing. Mrs. C agreed to make an appointment to come back to the clinic for an OGTT.
****

Questions:
1. Convert Mrs. C's height and weight from metric and determine her IBW (Appendix A, Tables 1, 2, 7 and 8).

2. Mrs. C gained 9.09 kg by her 24th week of pregnancy. What is the recommended weight gain by the 24th week of gestation?

3. Why is it important to take additional folate daily prior to becoming pregnant?

4. According to the Expert Committee on the Diagnosis and Classification of Diabetes Mellitus, Mrs. C has three risk factors for GDM. What are those risk factors? (See reference # 19.)

5. Pregnant women who are a high risk for GDM are recommended to be screened between the _____ [th] and the _____ [th] week of gestation.

Information Box 25 - 1

The screening test for GDM, or the glucose challenge test (GCT), consists of a venous plasma glucose measurement one hour after the consumption of 50 g of oral glucose. This test does not take into account the time of the last meal or the time of day. A value of 140 mg/dl or greater is a positive screening according to the Second, Third, and Fourth International Workshop-Conferences on GDM. A positive screening requires further testing with a GTT. There are two variations of the GTT used for pregnant women: a 75 g OGTT and a 100 g OGTT. There is an ongoing debate in the literature as to which is best, but a positive result with either is acceptable diagnostic criteria for GDM.

The test is performed in the morning after an overnight fast of at least eight hours but no greater than 14 hours. There should be at least three days of unrestricted diet and activity preceding the test. Venous blood is drawn prior to the oral ingestion of the 75 or 100 g glucose load and analyzed for plasma glucose. This is considered time "0." This procedure is repeated after 1, 2, and 3 hours. According to the National Diabetes Data Group (NDDG), in order to obtain a definitive diagnosis of GDM, two or more of the four venous plasma glucose determinations must exceed the levels listed in the table below.

NDDG Diagnostic Criteria for GDM Using the 100 g OGTT[36]

Time in hrs	mg/dl
0	105
1	190
2	165
3	145

According to Carr and Gabbe[12], there are at least three sets of guidelines in the literature used to diagnose GDM, one of which is the NDDG guidelines listed in the table above. The other two are recommended by O'Sullivan and Mahan[37] and Carpenter and Coustan[11]. The American College of Obstetricians and Gynecologists (ACOG) and the Expert Committee on the Diagnosis and Classification of Diabetes Mellitus recommend that two or more of the NDDG values be met or exceeded to make the diagnosis of

GDM[13]. There are those that question the best way to classify gestational diabetes [43, 46-47] and there are numerous studies that have investigated different methods of screening for gestational diabetes[3, 8-11, 14-15, 24, 31, 36-37].

A fasting plasma glucose level > 126 mg/dl is sufficient to make a diagnosis of GDM and does not warrant a GTT. In fact, it may be dangerous to administer a GTT under such circumstances. The OGTT is considered the most definitive method of making a positive diagnosis of GDM. Some people, particularly during pregnancy, cannot tolerate an oral load of 100 g of glucose on an empty stomach. An IVGTT is available but does not correlate well with the OGTT.

The results of Mrs. C's OGTT are found in Table 1.

TABLE 1 – Results of OGTT

Time in hrs	Plasma Glucose in mg/dL
0	112
1	235
2	195
3	160

Mrs. C was diagnosed with GDM. Prior to Mrs. C's pregnancy, she consulted with her physician in preparation for pregnancy. At that time the dietitian recommended a diet based on her adjusted body weight. If you were the dietitian consulting with Mrs. C, you would have access to this information. The answers to the next eight questions will provide that information.
****

QUESTIONS CONTINUED:

6. Calculate Mrs. C's ABW using her weight prior to pregnancy (Appendix A, Table 9).

7. Calculate Mrs. C's BMI based on her actual body weight prior to pregnancy (Appendix A, Table 10).

8. Based on Mrs. C's BMI, would you classify her as underweight, in her normal weight range, overweight, or obese?

9. Use the Harris-Benedict equation to calculate Mrs. C's basal metabolic rate. Use her ABW prior to her pregnancy in the formula (Appendix A, Table 17).

10. Assume Mrs. C to be lightly active. Choose the appropriate activity factor and determine the daily caloric requirement she would have had prior to pregnancy.

11. How many kcals do you add for pregnancy with a patient like Mrs. C who is overweight? Explain your answer and if you recommended additional calories, describe what should be the source of those kcals.

12. How much of an additional protein intake is recommended during pregnancy?

13. List the RDAs for the following nutrients prior to and during pregnancy.

Nutrient	RDA for Nonpregnant Women	RDA for Pregnancy
Ca		
P		
Fe		
Vitamin D		
Folate		

****

Mrs. C was hospitalized to get her blood glucose under control. Her initial insulin dose was calculated using the following formula: 0.9 U/kg of body weight. During her stay in the hospital, her blood glucose was closely monitored using a capillary glucose meter. The target plasma glucose levels recommended by the ACOG were used as criteria to determine if additional insulin was needed. Those levels are: fasting, 60 - 90 mg/dL; preprandial, 60 - 105 mg/dL; 1-hour postprandial, not > 130 - 140 mg/dL; 2-hours postprandial, < 120 mg/dL[2]. If her plasma glucose was not in one of those ranges, additional insulin was given using the formula, BS -100.20 = U of insulin to be administered. It was also desirable to keep her A1c < 7%. The average BS for Mrs. C 2-hours postprandial was 180 mg/dL. The ultimate goal was to achieve euglycemia to reduce the chances of macrosomia in the newborn.

Mrs. C's initial insulin dosing included R and NPH insulin in three daily injections according to a method adapted from Jovanovic-Peterson and Peterson[26] as reported by Carr and Gabbe[13]. The method consists of administering 4/9 of the total insulin as NPH and 2/9 of the total insulin as R in the morning, 1/6 of the total insulin as R at dinner, and 1/6 of the total insulin as NPH at bedtime.

Mrs. C had a diet order that included three snacks, A.M., P.M., and hs. The dietitian was experimenting with the caloric content of the snacks, trying to find the right combination of kcals and carbohydrate to balance Mrs. C's blood glucose. One of her hs snacks consisted of four graham crackers and 8 oz of skim milk. As part of her new daily routine, Mrs. C is being taught how to measure her urine ketone accumulation in the first voided specimen in the morning. Several lab tests were also conducted. The results of the labs are listed in TABLE 2.

TABLE 2

BASIC METABOLIC PACKAGE							
TEST	RESULT	REFERENCE UNITS Conventional	SI	TEST	RESULT	REFERENCE UNITS Conventional	SI
Glu	80 mg/dl	70-110 mg/dl	3.8-6.1 mmol/L	Na	138 mEq/L	136-145 mEq/L	136-145 mmol/L
BUN	5 mg/dl	6-20 mg/dl	2.1-7.1 mmol/L	K	3.8 mEq/L	3.5-5.2 mEq/L	3.5-5.2 mmol/L
Cr	0.3 mg/dl	0.6-1.1 mg/dl	53-97 μmol/L	Cl	101 mEq/L	96-106 mEq/L	96-106 mmol/L
Ca	8.8 mg/dl	8.8-10.0 mg/dl	2.20-2.60 mmol/L	Mg	1.8 mEq/L	1.8 - 2.6 mEq/L	136-145 mmol/L
Ser alb	3.1 g/dl	3.5-4.8 g/dl	39-50 g/dl	P	2.5mg/dl	2.7-4.5 mg/dl	4.7-6.0 kPa

After reviewing the patient's medical record, the perinatal dietitian, who was also a CDE, interviewed Mrs. C to determine her nutritional intake and daily activity. She determined that Mrs. C was under exercising and overeating, particularly foods high in simple sugars. She calculated a caloric level and protein level for Mrs. C. She advised her to eat more protein-rich foods, complex carbohydrates, and fiber. She discouraged the intake of simple sugars. The dietitian developed a meal plan for Mrs. C that included less than 30 g of CHO for breakfast with none of the CHO coming from juice. The plan included 45% of the kcals from CHO, 25% from protein, and 30% from fat. Mrs. C's urine ketone level that morning was "small," so the RD changed her hs snack to a meat sandwich with skim milk.
****

QUESTIONS CONTINUED:
14. The following terms are in common usage among health professionals working with pregnant women who have gestational diabetes. Give a brief definition of the terms:
Capillary glucose meter:

Pre- and postprandial:

Euglycemia:

Macrosomia:

15. In question 11, you calculated a caloric level for Mrs. C based on her ABW prior to pregnancy. Since she is now in her 27th week of gestation and has gained 20 lbs, would you recommend the same caloric level or a different one? Explain your answer.

16. Based on the information given, calculate Mrs. C's initial insulin dose and divide it into three injections. Indicate the appropriate amount of NPH and R to be given in each of the three doses.

17. In the labs reported for Mrs. C, plasma glucose was 280 mg/dL. Determine the additional insulin to be administered as a result of that lab.

18. Explain why the RD recommended a diet 45% CHO, 25% protein, and 30% fat. Show how you could use the results of her labs and her interview to arrive at this diet prescription.

19. Why did the RD recommend a breakfast that is high in protein and has less than 30 g of carbohydrate with no juice?

20. Why is it important to check ketones?

21. Explain the change in the hs snack.

****

Mrs. C was able to get her blood glucose under control and went home in less than a week.
****

ADDITIONAL OPTIONAL QUESTIONS:

22. On a separate sheet of paper, plan a day's menu with three meals and three snacks for Mrs. C.

23. Prepare a SOAP note for Mrs. C.

S:
O:
A:
P:

RELATED REFERENCES

1. Albert, E., Reece, D.R., Coustan, G., & Gabbe, S. (2004). *Diabetes in Women: Adolescence, Pregnancy, and Menopause.* Lippincott Williams & Wilkins.

2. American College of Obstetricians and Gynecologists (1994): Diabetes and Pregnancy. ACOG Technical Bulletin #200. Washington, DC. *ACOG.*

3. American College of Obstetricians and Gynecologists. (2001). Pregnant Women Should Be Screened for Gestational Diabetes; Though No One Test Is Ideal. http://www.acog.org/from_home/publications/press_releases/nr08-31-01.cfm

4. American Diabetes Association. (2001). *Gestational Diabetes: What to Expect.* 4 Ed. American Diabetes Association.

5. American Diabetes Association (2003). Gestational diabetes mellitus (Clinical Practice Recommendations 2003). Diabetes Care, 26(Suppl 1): S103–S105.

6. American Diabetes Association (2003). Evidence-based nutrition principles and recommendations for the treatment and prevention of diabetes and related complications (Clinical Practice Recommendations 2003). *Diabetes Care,* 26(Suppl 1): S51–S61.

7. Bartha, J.L., Martinez-Del-Fresno, P., & Comino-Delgado, R. (2003). Early diagnosis of gestational diabetes mellitus and prevention of diabetes-related complications. *Eur J Obstet Gynecol Reprod Biol.* Jul 1;109(1):41-4.

8. Bonomo, M., Gandini, M.L., Mastropasqua, A., Begher, C., Valentini, U., Faden, D., & Morabito, A. (1998). Which cutoff level should be used in screening for glucose intolerance in pregnancy? Definition of Screening Methods for Gestational Diabetes Study Group of the Lombardy Section of the Italian Society of Diabetology. *Am. J. Obstet. Gynecol.* 179(1):179-85.

9. Bobrowski, R.A., Bottoms, S.F., Micallef, J.A., & Dombrowski, M.P. (1996). Is the 50-gram glucose screening test ever diagnostic? *J. Matern. Fetal Med.* 5(6):317-20.

10. Brody, S.C. Harris, R., & Lohr, K. (2003). Screening for gestational diabetes: A summary of the evidence for the U.S. Preventive Services Task Force. *Obstetrics and Gynecology*, 101(2): 380–92.

11. Carpenter, M.W. & Coustan, D.R. (1982). Criteria for screening tests for gestational diabetes. *Am. J. Obstet. Gynecol.* 144:768-73.

12. Carr, D.B. & Gabbe, S. (1998). Gestational Diabetes: Detection, Management, and Implications. *Clinical Diabetes.* 16(1):4-11.

13. Carr, S.R. (1998). Screening for gestational diabetes mellitus. A perspective in 1998. *Diabetes Care.* Supp l2:B14-8

14. Coustan, D.R., Widness, J.A., Carpenter, M.W., Rotondo, L., & Pratt, D.C. (1987). The "breakfast tolerance test": screening for gestational diabetes with a standardized mixed nutrient meal. *Am. J. Obstet. Gynecol.* 157(5):1113-7

15. Coustan, D.R. & Carpenter, M.W. (1998). The diagnosis of gestational diabetes. *Diabetes Care.* Supp l2:B5-8

16. Diamond, T. & Kormas, N. (1997). Possible adverse fetal effect of insulin lispro. *N. Engl. J. Med.* 337:1009.

17. Dietitians of Canada, American Dietetic Association. (2001). *Manual of Clinical Dietetics.* 6 Ed. American Dietetic Association.

18. Fischbach, F.T. (2003). *A Manual of Laboratory & Diagnostic Tests.* 7th Ed. Philadelphia. J.B. Lippincott Company.

19. Funnell, M.M. (2001). *A Core Curriculum For Diabetes Educators.* 4 Ed. American Association of Diabetes Educators.

20. Gillen, L.J. & Tapsell, L.C. (2004). Advice that includes food sources of unsaturated fat supports future risk management of gestational diabetes mellitus. *J Am Diet Assoc.* Dec;104(12):1863-7.

21. Gunderson, E.P. (2004). Gestational diabetes and nutritional recommendations. *Curr Diab Rep.* Oct;4(5):377-86.

22 Hamaouil, E. & Hamaoui, M. (1998). Nutritional assessment and support during pregnancy. *Gastroenterol. Clin. North Am.* 27(1):89-121.

23. Innes, K.E., Byers, T.E., Marshall, J.A., Baron, A. Orleans, M. & Hamman, RF. (2002). Association of a woman's own birthweight with subsequent risk for gestational diabetes. *JAMA,* 287(19): 2534–41.

24. Jovanovic, L. (2004). Achieving euglycaemia in women with gestational diabetes mellitus: current options for screening, diagnosis and treatment. *Drugs.* 64(13):1401-17.

25. Jovanovic, L. (2003). Medical Management of Pregnancy Complicated by Diabetes. 3Ed. American Diabetes Asociation.

26. Jovanovic-Peterson, L. & Peterson, C.M. (1996). Review of gestational diabetes mellitus and low-calorie diet and physical exercise as therapy. *Diabetes Metab. Rev.* 12:287-308.

27. Jovanovic, L. (1998). American Diabetes Association's Fourth International Workshop-Conference on Gestational Diabetes Mellitus: Summary and discussion. *Diabetes Care,* 21(Suppl 2): B131–37.

28. Kim, C., Newton, K.M., & Knopp, R.H. (2002). Gestational diabetes and the incidence of type 2 diabetes: a systematic review. *Diabetes Care.* Oct;25(10):1862-8. Review.

29. Kopp, W. (2005). Role of high-insulinogenic nutrition in the etiology of gestational diabetes mellitus. *Med Hypotheses.* 64(1):101-3.

30. Kuhl, C. (1998). Etiology and pathogenesis of gestational diabetes. *Diabetes Care.* Supp l2:B19-26.

31. Lamar, M.E., Kuehl, T.J., Cooney, A.T., Gayle, L.J., Holleman, S., & Allen, S.R. . (1999). Jelly beans as an alternative to a fifty-gram glucose beverage for gestational diabetes screening. *American Journal of Obstetrics and Gynecology.* 181: 1154–57

32. MacNeill, S., Dodds, L, Hamilton, D.C., Armson, B.A., & VandenHof, M. (2001). Rates and risk factors for recurrence of gestational diabetes. *Diabetes Care*, 24(4): 659–62.

33. Magee, M.S., Knoop, R.H., & Benedetti, T.J. (1990). Metabolic effects of a 1200 kcal diet in obese pregnant women with gestational diabetes. *Diabetes*. 39:234-40.

34. Metzger, B.E. & Coustan, D.R. (1998). Summary and recommendations of the Fourth International Workshop-Conference on Gestational Diabetes Mellitus. *Diabetes Care*, 21(Suppl 2): B161–67.

35. Mulcahy, K. & Lumber, T. (2004). *Diabetes Ready Reference Guide for Health Care Professionals*. 2nd Ed. American Diabetes Association.

36. National Diabetes Data Group. (1979). Classification and diagnosis of diabetes mellitus and other categories of glucose intolerance. *Diabetes*. 28:1039-57.

37. O'Sullivan, J.B. & Mahan, C.M. (1964). Criteria for the oral glucose tolerance test in pregnancy. *Diabetes*. 13:278-85.

38. Preece, R. & Jovanovic, L. (2002). New and future diabetes therapies: are they safe during pregnancy? *J Matern Fetal Neonatal Med*. Dec;12(6):365-75. Review.

39. Prendergast, A. & Fulton, F.L. (1997) *Medical terminology: A Text/Workbook*. 4th Ed. Redwood City, California. Addison-Wesley Nursing.

40. Pronsky, Z.M., Redfern, C.M., Crowe, J. & Epstein, S. (2003) *Food Medication Interactions*, 13th Ed Phoenix, Arizona. Food-Medications Interactions, Publishers and Distributors.

41. Reader, D. & Franz, M.J. (2004). Lactation, diabetes, and nutrition recommendations. *Curr Diab Rep*. Oct;4(5):370-6.

42. Rolfes, S.R., Pinna, K. & Whitney, E. (2006). *Understanding Normal and Clinical Nutrition*, 7th Ed. West/Wadsworth.

43. Sacks, D.A., Abu-Fadil, S., Greenspoon, J.S., & Fotheringham, N. (1989). Do the current standards for glucose tolerance testing represent a valid conversion of O'Sullivan's original criteria? *Am. J. Obstet. Gynecol*. 161:638-41.

44. Setji, T.L., Brown, A.J., & Feinglos, M.N. (205). Gestational Diabetes Mellitus. *Clinical Diabetes*; 23(1):17-24.

45. Spratto, G.R. & Woods, A.L. (2005). *PDR Nurse's Drug Handbook*. Thompson Delmar Learning, NY.

46. Sullivan, B.A., Henderson, S.T., & Davis, J.M. (1998). Gestational Diabetes. *J. Am. Pharm. Assoc*. 38(3):364-73.

47. Weiss, P.A., Haeusler, M., Kainer, F., Purstner, P., & Hass, J. (1998). Toward universal criteria for gestational diabetes: relationships between seventy-five and one hundred gram glucose loads and between capillary and venous glucose concentrations. *Am. J. Obstet Gynecol*. 174(4):830-5.

CASE STUDY #26
METABOLIC SYNDROME

INTRODUCTION
This study examines the syndrome X or metabolic syndrome. It promotes an understanding of the relationship of obesity, diabetes, and cardiovascular disease. The student should review the criteria for metabolic syndrome and its relationship to diabetes and cardiovascular disease.
****

SKILLS NEEDED

ABBREVIATIONS:
Knowledge of the following abbreviations is required in order to understand this case. You should learn these abbreviations before you begin to read the study. BP, SOB (Appendix C).

LABORATORY VALUES:
You will need to be able to interpret the nutritional significance of the following laboratory values for this case study: A1c, BUN, Ca, chol, Cl, Cr, glucose, HDL, K, LDL, Mg, Na, P, ser alb and TG (Appendix B).

FORMULAS:
The formulas used in this case study include BMI and waist to hip ratio (Appendix A, Tables 10, 11 and 16).

MEDICATIONS:
Become familiar with the following medications before reading the case study. Note the diet-drug interactions, dosages and methods of administration, gastrointestinal tract reactions, etc.
1. Micardis (telmisartan); 2. HydroDIURIL (hydrochlorothiazide).
****

KB is a 51 YOWF who is 5'1" and weighs 217 lbs. Her waist is 48 inches and her hip circumference is 52". She reported to her doctor with burning and itching upon urination. She has had these symptoms in the past when she had bladder infections. She also C/O frequent urination all the time, even during the night, and is tired. A physical exam revealed a BP of 144 over 84, pulse of 88, and respirations 20. KB has a family history of HTN, diabetes, and cardiovascular disease. A random blood lab analysis revealed the following:

BASIC METABOLIC PACKAGE							
TEST	RESULT	REFERENCE UNITS Conventional	SI	TEST	RESULT	REFERENCE UNITS Conventional	SI
Glu	245 mg/dl	70-110 mg/dl	3.8-6.1 mmol/L	Na	138 mEq/L	136-145 mEq/L	136-145 mmol/L
BUN	8 mg/dl	6-20 mg/dl	2.1-7.1 mmol/L	K	3.9 mEq/L	3.5-5.2 mEq/L	3.5-5.2 mmol/L
Cr	0.9 mg/dl	0.6-1.1 mg/dl	53-97 μmol/L	Cl	101 mEq/L	96-106 mEq/L	96-106 mmol/L
Ca	9.1 mg/dl	8.8-10.0 mg/dl	2.20-2.60 mmol/L	Mg	2.1 mEq/L	1.8 - 2.6 mEq/L	136-145 mmol/L
Ser alb	3.6 g/dl	3.5-4.8 g/dl	39-50 g/dl	P	2.8mg/dl	2.7-4.5 mg/dl	4.7-6.0 kPa

The physician scheduled KB to come back and have a fasting blood analysis which revealed the following:

LIPID PROFILE

TEST	RESULT	REFERENCE UNITS Conventional	SI	TEST	RESULT	REFERENCE UNITS Conventional	SI
Chol	255 mg/dl	140-199 mg/dl	3.63-5.15 mmol/L	HDL	46 mEq/L	40-85 mEq/L	1.17-2.2 mmol/L
TG	257 mg/dl	<-150 mg/dl	<1.70 mmol/L	LDL	192 mg/dl	<130 mg/dl	<3.4 mmol/L
Glucose	146	70-110 mg/dl	3.8-6.1 mmol/L	A1c	7.2.%	5.5-8.5%	

KB's drug history includes Micardis and HydroDIURIL.

****

QUESTIONS:

1. KB complained of being tired and frequent urination and went to the physician for a UTI. What are these symptoms of?

2. What are the values for a normal BP, borderline, and high? Compare these to KB's values.

3. List the normal ranges for cholesterol, triglycerides, LDL, and HDL and compare these to KB's values.

4. Calculate KB's BMI and compare it to the normal ranges.

5. Calculate KB's waist-to-hip ratio and compare to normal.

6. What is a normal A1c? Compare this to KB's A1c.

7. List all the indications of metabolic syndrome that KB displayed.

8. Why did the physician order the second set of labs to be fasting?

9. What are the actions, side effects, and nutritional implications of KB's medications?

    Micardis:

    HydroDIURIL:

10. What diet would you recommend for KB and why?

11. Prepare a SOAP note for KB.

S:
O:
A:
P:

RELATED REFERENCES

1. Fischbach, F.T. (2003). *A Manual of Laboratory & Diagnostic Tests.* 7th Ed. Philadelphia. J.B. Lippincott Company.

2. Martin-Lazaro, J.F., & Becerra-Fernandez, A. (2005). The metabolic syndrome: Uncertain criteria. *Pharmacol Res.* Apr;51(4):385-6.

3. Moller, D.E., & Kaufman, K.D. (2005). Metabolic syndrome: A Clinical and Molecular Perspective. *Annu Rev Med.* 56:45-62.

4. Prendergast, A. & Fulton, F.L. (1997) *Medical terminology: A Text/Workbook.* 4th Ed. Redwood City, California. Addison-Wesley Nursing.

5. Pronsky, Z.M., Redfern, C.M., Crowe, J. & Epstein, S. (2003) *Food Medication Interactions*, 13th Ed Phoenix, Arizona. Food-Medications Interactions, Publishers and Distributors.

6. Roberts, S.S. (2004). Back to basics. Your A1C. *Diabetes Forecast.* 2004 Dec;57(12):31-2.

7. Robinson, L.E., & Graham, T.E. (2004). Metabolic syndrome, a cardiovascular disease risk factor: role of adipocytokines and impact of diet and physical activity. *J Appl Physiol.* Dec;29(6):808-29.

8. Rolfes, S.R., Pinna, K. & Whitney, E. (2006). *Understanding Normal and Clinical Nutrition*, 7th Ed. West/Wadsworth.

9. Spratto, G.R. & Woods, A.L. (2005). *PDR Nurse's Drug Handbook.* Thompson Delmar Learning, NY.

10. Steffes, M., Cleary, P., Goldstein, D., Little, R., Wiedmeyer, H.M., Rohlfing, C., England, J., Bucksa, J., & Nowicki, M. (2005). Hemoglobin A1c Measurements over Nearly Two Decades: Sustaining Comparable Values throughout the Diabetes Control and Complications Trial and the Epidemiology of Diabetes Interventions and Complications Study. *Clin Chem.* Jan 31.

11. Sudhakar, M.K. (2004). Ghost of metabolic syndrome. *J Assoc Physicians India.* Apr;52:342.

12. Zhu, S., Heymsfield, S.B., Toyoshima, H., Wang, Z., Pietrobelli, A., & Heshka, S. (2005). Race-ethnicity-specific waist circumference cutoffs for identifying cardiovascular disease risk factors. *Am J Clin Nutr.* 2005 Feb;81(2):409-15.

13. Zieve, F.J. (2004). The metabolic syndrome: diagnosis and treatment. *Clin Cornerstone.* 6 Suppl 3:S5-13.

CASE STUDY #27
LOW-CARBOHYDRATE WEIGHT REDUCTION DIETS

INTRODUCTION
This study examines multiple side effects of a low-carbohydrate, high-fat, high-protein diet. It introduces the student to some new diagnostic tests and requires some research into the literature to answer some of the questions. It would be better adapted for the advanced student or will require considerable guidance for a less advanced student.

****

SKILLS NEEDED

ABBREVIATIONS:
Knowledge of the following abbreviations is required in order to understand this case. You should learn these abbreviations before you begin to read the study. CT, DEXA, and pDEXA (Appendix C).

LABORATORY VALUES:
You will need to be able to interpret the nutritional significance of the following laboratory values for this case study: ALP, ALT, AST, BUN, Ca, chol, Cl, Cr, DBIL, glucose, HDL, K, LDH, LDL, Na, ser alb, TG, and TBIL (Appendix B).

****

RC, a 43 YOWF, has been plagued all of her life with chronic obesity. Having tried numerous diets without success, she decided to try one of the popular low-carbohydrate, high-protein, high-fat diets. She has been on the diet for a little over a year, longer than she has lasted on a diet previously. It's not because she liked the diet so much as it is she became determined that she was going to lose weight. She probably would have stuck to any diet this time. She has lost 110 pounds and was very proud of it. However, lately she has not been feeing well. She has been nauseous and has had lower back pain on her left side that has been getting worse. She decided to see her doctor. A random blood lab analysis revealed the following:

BASIC METABOLIC PACKAGE							
TEST	**RESULT**	**REFERENCE UNITS** Conventional SI		**TEST**	**RESULT**	**REFERENCE UNITS** Conventional SI	
Glu	125 mg/dl	70-110 mg/dl	3.8-6.1 mmol/L	Na	136 mEq/L	136-145 mEq/L	136-145 mmol/L
BUN	23 mg/dl	6-20 mg/dl	2.1-7.1 mmol/L	K	4.2 mEq/L	3.5-5.2 mEq/L	3.5-5.2 mmol/L
Cr	1.6 mg/dl	0.6-1.1 mg/dl	53-97 µmol/L	Cl	102 mEq/L	96-106 mEq/L	96-106 mmol/L
Ser alb	3.1 g/dl	3.5-4.8 g/dl	39-50 g/dl	TBIL	0.5 mg/dl	0.3-1.0 mg/dl	5-17 µmol/L
AST	80 U/L	10-36 U/L	0.17-0.60 µkat/L	DBIL	0.1 mg/dl	0-0.2 mg/dl	0-3.4 µmol/L
ALT	63 U/L	7-35 U/L	0.12-0.60 µkat/L	LDH	570 U/L	313-618 U/L	313-618 U/L
ALP	196 U/L	25-100 U/L	17-142 U/L				

A fasting profile revealed the following:

LIPID PROFILE							
TEST	RESULT	REFERENCE UNITS Conventional	SI	TEST	RESULT	REFERENCE UNITS Conventional	SI
Chol	240 mg/dl	140-199 mg/dl	3.63-5.15 mmol/L	HDL	45 mEq/L	40-85 mEq/L	1.0-2.28 mmol/L
TG	195 mg/dl	<-150 mg/dl	<1.70 mmol/L	LDL	167 mg/dl	<130 mg/dl	<3.4 mmol/L

The physician's clinical exam exhibited an enlarged palpable liver approximately 3 inches below her right rib cage. An ultrasound of the liver revealed a large homogeneous liver and an ultra sound of the kidneys revealed several small stones in the left kidney. A follow-up CT scan showed a large liver with the density consistent with a fatty liver. The physician also completed a peripheral DEXA and found RC's bone density to be borderline for osteoporosis.

Information Box 27 - 1
In a "normal" body, the end of the liver on the right side just barely protrudes out from under the rib cage. If the liver protrudes out further, it usually indicates a swollen or enlarged liver. This is usually measured by the width of the fingers that it takes to cover the protruded liver. Most physicians know how many inches three of four of their fingers compressed together will be comparable to so they can estimate measurements like the one described here.

****

QUESTIONS:

1. Look up basic information for ultra sound tests and explain what the following tests will reveal:
   Ultrasound of the liver:

   Ultrasound of the kidneys:

2. Look up the basics for a CT scan and describe what a CT scan of the liver will reveal. What does "CT" stand for?

3. Look up a DEXA and describe what a DEXA measures. Compare a DEXA to a peripheral DEXA and explain what a pDEXA will determine. What are the advantages and disadvantages of each?

4. Compare the usefulness, advantages, and disadvantages between an ultrasound, CT scan, and DEXA.

5. List the abnormal lab values found for RC and give the possible reason why they could be out of line.

6. Research the reasons/theories being given for fatty liver formation for people on high-fat, low-carbohydrate diets.

7. Research the relationship between kidney stones and osteoporosis that could occur on high-fat, high-protein, low-carbohydrate diets.

8. Discuss what RC's likely prognosis would be for her fatty liver if she returned to a normal diet low in fat.

9. Research and discuss the implications of the high-fat, high-protein, low-carbohydrate diet and atherosclerosis.

10. Discuss the possible results RC could have obtained had she followed a diet just as low in total calories but with at least 150 g of carbohydrate and 30-35% of her calories from fat. Include the following points in your discussion with more than just a "yes" or "no" answer, but an explanation of the possibilities:

    a. Would she have likely lost as much weight?

    b. Would she have likely had a calcium imbalance with kidney stones and borderline osteoporosis?

    c. Would she likely have elevated cholesterol, LDL, and TG?

    d. Would she likely have a fatty liver and elevated liver enzymes, even though they may be slightly elevated?

    e. Overall, which diet would be the healthiest?

11. Considering all of RC's complications, what diet would you recommend she now follow?

12. Prepare a SOAP note for RC.

S:
O:
A:
P:

RELATED REFERENCES

1. Acheson, K.J. (2004). Carbohydrate and weight control: where do we stand? *Curr Opin Clin Nutr Metab Car*e. Jul;7(4):485-92.

2. Agnew, B. (2004).. Rethinking Atkins. New research suggests that the famous low-carb diet may be safe--at least in the short term. *Diabetes Forecast*. Apr;57(4):64-6, 68-70.

3. Amanzadeh, J., Gitomer, W.L., Zerwekh, J.E., Preisig, P.A., Moe, O.W., Pak, C.Y., & Levi, M. (2003). Effect of high protein diet on stone-forming propensity and bone loss in rats. *Kidney Int*. Dec;64(6):2142-9.

4. Anderson, J.W., Konz, E.C., & Jenkins, D.J. (2000). Health advantages and disadvantages of weight-reducing diets: a computer analysis and critical review. *J Am Coll Nutr.* Oct;19(5):578-90.

5. Astrup, A, Meinert, L.T, & Harper, A. (2004). Atkins and other low-carbohydrate diets: hoax or an effective tool for weight loss? *Lancet.* Sep 4;364(9437):897-9.

6. Bilsborough, S.A. & Crowe, T.C. (2003). Low-carbohydrate diets: what are the potential short- and long-term health implications? *Asia Pac J Clin Nutr.* ;12(4):396-404.

7. Dansinger, M.L., Gleason, J.A., Griffith, J.L., Selker, H.P., & Schaefer, E.J. (2005). Comparison of the Atkins, Ornish, Weight Watchers, and Zone diets for weight loss and heart disease risk reduction: a randomized trial. *JAMA.* Jan 5;293(1):43-53.

8. Fischbach, F.T. (2003). *A Manual of Laboratory & Diagnostic Tests.* 7th Ed. Philadelphia. J.B. Lippincott Company.

9. Fleming, M.E., Sales, K.M., & Winslet, M.C. (2005). Diet and colorectal cancer: implications for the obese and devotees of the Atkins diet. *Colorectal Dis.* Mar;7(2):128-32.

10. Foster, G.D., Wyatt, H.R., Hill, J.O., McGuckin, B.G., Brill, C., Mohammed, B.S., Szapary, P.O., Rader, D.J., Edman, J.S., & Klein, S. (2003). A randomized trial of a low-carbohydrate diet for obesity. *N Engl J Med.* May 22;348(21):2082-90.

11. Harper, A., & Astrup, A. (2004). Can we advise our obese patients to follow the Atkins diet? *Obes Rev.* May;5(2):93-4.

12. Katz, D.L. (2003). Pandemic obesity and the contagion of nutritional nonsense. *Public Health Rev.* 31(1):33-44.

13. Khor, G.L. (2004). Dietary fat quality: a nutritional epidemiologist's view. *Asia Pac J Clin Nutr.* Aug;13(Suppl):S22.

14. Mayo Clin Health Lett. 2004 Low-carb diets. Answers to your questions Nov;22(11):4-5.

15. National Heart, Lung, and Blood Institute. (1998). Clinical Guidelines on the Identification, Evaluation, and Treatment of Overweight and Obesity in Adult. National Institutes of Health. Publication 98-4083. http://www.nhlbi.nih.gov/guidelines/obesity/ob_gdlns.htm

16 NIDDK. Weight-loss and Nutrition Myths: How much do you really know? Diet Myths: Myth: *Fad diets work for permanent weight loss.* Myth: High-protein/low-carbohydrate diets are a healthy way to lose weight. Myth: *Starches are fattening and should be limited when trying to lose weight.* Myth: *Eating red meat is bad for your health and makes it harder to lose weight. NIDDK Weight-control Information Network.* NIH Publication No. 04-4561; March 2004 Posted: April 2004. http://win.niddk.nih.gov/publications/myths.htm

17. Nurs Times. (2003) Oct 28-Nov 3;99(43):20-1. Understanding the implications of adopting the Atkins' diet.

18. Ornish, D. (2004). Was Dr Atkins right? *J Am Diet Assoc.* Apr;104(4):537-42.

19. Physicians Committee for Responsible Medicine: http://www.pcrm.org/ Health Risks of Low Carbohydrate diets: http://www.atkinsdietalert.org/advisory.html; Expert Opinions: http://www.atkinsdietalert.org/expert.html

20. Position paper of the American Dietetic Association. (2002). Weight management *J Am Diet Assoc.* 102:1145-1155.

21. Prendergast, A. & Fulton, F.L. (1997) *Medical terminology: A Text/Workbook.* 4th Ed. Redwood City, California. Addison-Wesley Nursing.

22. Pronsky, Z.M., Redfern, C.M., Crowe, J. & Epstein, S. (2003) *Food Medication Interactions*, 13th Ed Phoenix, Arizona. Food-Medications Interactions, Publishers and Distributors.

23. Reddy, S.T., Wang, C.Y., Sakhaee, K., Brinkley, L., & Pak, C.Y. (2002). Effect of low-carbohydrate high-protein diets on acid-base balance, stone-forming propensity, and calcium metabolism. *Am J Kidney Dis.* Aug;40(2):265-74.

24. Riley, M.D. & Coveney, J. (2004). Atkins and the new diet revolution: is it really time for regimen change? Weight loss occurs in the short term, but not enough is known to recommend long term use. *Med J Aust.* Nov 15;181(10):526-7.

25. Rolfes, S.R., Pinna, K. & Whitney, E. (2006). *Understanding Normal and Clinical Nutrition*, 7th Ed. West/Wadsworth.

26. Spratto, G.R. & Woods, A.L. (2005). *PDR Nurse's Drug Handbook.* Thompson Delmar Learning, NY.

27. Tapper-Gardzina, Y., Cotugna, N., & Vickery, C.E. (2002). Should you recommend a low-carb, high-protein diet? *Nurse Pract.* Apr;27(4):57.

28. Truby, H., Millward, D., Morgan, L., Fox, K., Livingstone, M.B., DeLooy, A., & MacDonald, I. (2004). A randomised controlled trial of 4 different commercial weight loss programmes in the UK in obese adults: body composition changes over 6 months. *Asia Pac J Clin Nutr.* Aug;13 (Suppl): S146.

29. Weight-control Information Network. November, (2001) *Understanding Adult Obesity.* NIH . NIH Publication No. 01-3680, October. http://win.niddk.nih.gov/publications/understanding.htm

30. Weight-control Information Network. March, (2001). *Weight Cycling.* NIH Publication No. NIH Publication No. 01-3901. e-text updated March 2004. http://win.niddk.nih.gov/publications/cycling.htm

31. Weight-control Information Network. May, (2004). *Do you know the health risks of being overweight?* NIH Publication No. 04-4098, e-text posted: November 2004. http//win.niddk.nih.gov/publications/health_risks.htm

CASE STUDY #28
CLOSED HEAD INJURY AND HOME HEALTH CARE

INTRODUCTION

This is a two-part study about a closed head injury. PART I is a good introduction to the use of tube feedings for unconscious patients. It requires a basic knowledge of starting tube feedings and the importance of monitoring tube feedings as the patient's condition improves. In PART II patient is discharged from the hospital but still requires nursing care and nutritional assessment. This case provides an introduction to the use of tube feedings at home as well as home health care consulting.

****

SKILLS NEEDED

ABBREVIATIONS:

Knowledge of the following abbreviations is required in order to understand this case. You should learn these abbreviations before you begin to read the study.

BMR, CHI, ICP, LBM, NSICU, and PEG (Appendix C).

LABORATORY VALUES:

You will need to be able to interpret the nutritional significance of the following laboratory values for this case study: Hgb, Hct, and ICP (Appendix B).

FORMULAS:

The formulas used in this case study include ideal body weight and percent ideal body weight, total caloric needs using the Harris-Benedict equation and appropriate stress factors, total protein needs, and calculation of tube feeding flow rates. The formulas can be found in Appendix A, Tables 7, 8 and 17.

****

PART I: HOSPITAL CARE

RK is a 25 YOWM who was in a MVA nine months ago. He was thrown from his vehicle and received multiple fractures, contusions, and a severe CHI. RK stayed in a NSICU for five weeks. He was unconscious most of the time and had to be fed via a N/G feeding tube. He received normal saline and electrolytes via I.V. It was necessary to monitor his intracranial pressure, so a ventriculostomy cather was put in place. His ICP remained in the 30s for most of the first week and gradually returned to normal. RK's lab values were normal upon admission with the exception of hgb and hct, which were low due to bleeding. Packed cells were administered and RK equilibrated rapidly.

After one week in NSICU, RK began to respond to physical stimuli but not verbal stimuli. In the third week, RK opened his eyes and started responding to sound but still would not obey verbal commands. By the fourth week, he was moving all limbs well but without coordination. At the beginning of the fifth week RK was transferred to a neurosurgical ward and continued to be monitored. He was still receiving a tube feeding but the screw had been removed since his ICP returned to normal.

According to his brother, RK was 5'11" and weighed 180 lbs at the time of the accident. He was not able to be weighed in the ER when admitted. When RK was transferred to a ward, he weighed 135 lbs. While still in NSICU, a feeding tube was placed in the small bowel and he received a 1.5 kcal/cc tube feeding at one-half strength at 30 cc/hr. This was started five days after admission. After one day, the tube feeding was changed to full-strength and gradually increased to 50 cc/hr. The neurosurgeon attending to RK was concerned about fluid overload and CO_2 buildup secondary to feeding. He would not even consider starting a tube feeding prior to 72 hours post injury. After being on the tube feeding for a week, the physician changed it to a 2 kcals/cc feeding for a more concentrated feeding. The 2 kcals/cc feeding was started at one-half-strength at a rate of 30 cc/hr. After 24 hours the feeding was changed to full-strength and was gradually increased to 50 cc/hr. RK tolerated this feeding for his entire stay in the hospital. After he was transferred to the ward, RK received a PEG and was continued on Two Cal HN but by bolus instead of continuous drip. The physician ordered the bolus feedings to be given at full strength in a quantity sufficient to equal the amount given in 24 hours by the continuous drip. The end of the feeding tube was in the stomach.

With RK responding positively to the PEG and maintaining a normal blood pressure and vital signs, he was not monitored as closely as he was during his stay in NSICU. This was particularly true for his weight. Immediately after a CHI, most patients respond with a very high basal metabolic rate and lose weight rapidly. The nutritional treatment for this is high caloric/high protein intake. After recovery, the BMR returns to normal or lower than normal and weight gain begins at a rapid pace. Many victims of CHIs are bed ridden and are unable to exercise, thus requiring fewer kilocalories. This results in excessive weight gain as adipose tissue if the tube feeding is not decreased. This was the case with RK. His mental condition never improved. He still responded to painful stimuli and to sound but could not follow any commands. He was able to move all four limbs on his own but without any coordination and not in response to commands. Posturing of all limbs was moderately severe. He did not appear to respond any differently to the voices of his family members than he did to the voices of the hospital staff. His physician and his parents were pleased to see him gaining weight but did not realize how heavy he was becoming. His tube feeding was reduced to 40 cc/hr.
****

QUESTIONS:
1. Define closed head injury.

2. Determine RK's ideal body weight.

3. Calculate RK's caloric and protein needs at admission and when he was transferred to a ward.

4. Calculate the kilocalories and protein RK was receiving from the 1.5 kcal/cc feeding at 35cc/h half-strength and at 50cc/hr full-strength.

5. Look up two 1.5 kcals/cc and two 2.0 kcals/cc tube feedings and compare using the table below.

Product	Producer	Form	Cal/ml	Non-pro cal/g N	g/L			Na mg	K mg	mOsm /kg water	Vol to meet RDA in ml	g of fiber /L	Free H$_2$O /L in ml
					Pro	CHO	Fat						

6. How many kcals did RK receive with 2 kcals/cc feeding full-strength at 50 cc/hr?

7. What was the reason for starting the 1.5 kcal/cc feeding at half-strength?

8. Would you still start at half-strength if the tip of the feeding tube was in the stomach instead of the small bowel? If not, explain why not.

9. What was the reason for starting the 2 kcal/cc feeding at half-strength?

10. Compare bolus feeding to a continuous drip as to expense, and advantages and disadvantages for the patient and for the nurses.

11. Calculate the amount of 2 kcal/cc feeding needed per bolus feeding, and the frequency of feedings necessary to equal the amount given in 24 hours as a continuous feeding at 50 cc/h. Plan to give the bolus feedings between 7 A.M. and 10 P.M. How much would you reduce each bolus feeding to equal a reduction in the continuous feeding from 50 cc/hr to 40 cc/hr?

12. What is a PEG?

13. Why would this be used instead of a nasogastric tube?

14. What is a ventriculostomy and what does it have to do with a CHI?

15. What relationship does CO_2 have with ICP and feeding rate?

16. Why would the neurosurgeon not even consider a tube feeding until 72 hours post injury?

****

RK was sent home with the following nutritional orders:

➢ 2 kcal/cc bolus feeding via PEG.
➢ Feed full-strength 240 cc qid.
➢ Flush tube with 30 cc of water after each feeding.

****

17. How many kcals and protein and how much free water does this provide?

18. What would be the equivalent flow rate per hour?

19. How much total free water is he receiving with the water being used to flush the tube after feeding?

20. What is the rule of thumb water requirement for an adult receiving a tube feeding?

<u>**ADDITIONAL OPTIONAL QUESTIONS:**</u>
Tube Feeding Drill:

21. Using the table on the following page, compare several of the enteral nutritional supplements that are formulated to help reduce CO_2 production.

Product	Producer	Form	Cal/ml	Non-pro cal/g N	g/L			Na mg	K mg	mOsm /kg water	Vol to meet RDA in ml	g of fiber /L	Free H$_2$O /L in ml
					Pro	CHO	Fat						

22. Prepare a SOAP note below summarizing RK's hospital stay.

S:

O:

A:

P:

****

PART II: HOME HEALTH CARE

RK continued to do well in the hospital from a medical standpoint but did not improve mentally. RK was awake and alert and responded to sound by looking in the direction of the sound but could not obey any commands. The nurses responsible for RK could not tell any difference in his response to family as compared to strangers; yet, his mother insisted that he responded more to her voice than anyone else's. RK's movements were totally spastic and without any coordination. Posturing of both arms and legs was still evident although it was not as bad as previously. The physician did not give the family any hope that RK would improve mentally. As long as someone fed him and kept him clean, he would live a long but unresponsive life.

His mother refused to accept this prognosis. She insisted that he could understand her and was responding to her commands and not just to her voice. No one else shared that opinion. This is frequently the case with a mother and a nonresponsive patient. The physician wanted to discharge RK to a nursing home but his mother insisted on taking him home. She did not work and vowed to become his nurse. The physician agreed. It was necessary for the physician to D/C RK with orders so he asked the attending nurse how he was doing on the hospital orders. The response was "fine" so he ordered her to D/C him to home with the same orders. The nurse failed to tell him that RK's weight was up to 160 lbs. His discharge orders were as follows:

➢ Continue 2 kcals/cc bolus feeding via PEG.
➢ Feed full strength 240 cc qid.
➢ Flush tube with 30 cc of water after each feeding.
➢ Instruct family how to feed patient.
****

QUESTIONS CONTINUED:
23. Define the following terms:
prognosis:

posturing:

24. What does posturing indicate?

25. Would posturing affect RK's caloric needs? Why or why not?

26. Compare RK's weight before the accident, at his discharge from NSICU, and upon his discharge from the hospital. Compare the probable composition of his body prior to the accident and at the time of discharge from the hospital (fat to lean body mass ratio).

27. Calculate RK's caloric and protein requirements at discharge from the hospital. Compare this to the amount of calories and protein he is receiving from the 2 kcals/cc tube feeding at 240 cc qid.

28. What suggestions would you have at this point concerning his nutrition? Consider such factors as inactivity, Ca, trace minerals, fluid, and fiber.

29. What is the purpose of flushing the tube with water after each feeding?

****

RK was discharged home and his mother learned very quickly how to give excellent nursing care. She followed the instructions she received from the nurses exactly. RK continued to tolerate the bolus feedings as far as she could tell but getting up during the night to feed every four hours was really a strain. Her husband and her son helped her to accomplish this, but after a few weeks they were all very tired. RK continued to gain weight. His mother had no way of weighing him but she could tell he was getting considerably heavier and very difficult to move. She did not mention this to the home health care nurse because she assumed that it meant he was doing well. After a short time RK developed another problem: he became constipated. Several days passed without a bowel movement so RK's mother called his physician for help. He sent a lab tech to draw blood for some basic tests and found the following:

BASIC METABOLIC PACKAGE								
TEST	RESULT	REFERENCE UNITS Conventional SI		TEST	RESULT	REFERENCE UNITS Conventional SI	
Glu	145 mg/dl	70-110 mg/dl	3.8-6.1 mmol/L	Na	146 mEq/L	136-145 mEq/L	136-145 mmol/L
BUN	27 mg/dl	6-20 mg/dl	2.1-7.1 mmol/L	K	4.9 mEq/L	3.5-5.2 mEq/L	3.5-5.2 mmol/L
Cr	1.3 mg/dl	0.9-1.3 mg/dl	80-115 µmol/L	Cl	103 mEq/L	96-106 mEq/L	96-106 mmol/L
Ca	9.4 mg/dl	8.8-10.0 mg/dl	2.20-2.60 mmol/L	Ser alb	4.4 g/dl	3.5-4.8 g/dl	39-50 g/dl

CBC							
TEST	RESULT	REFERENCE UNITS Conventional SI		TEST	RESULT	REFERENCE UNITS Conventional SI	
Hgb	20 g/dl	14 - 17.4 g/dl	140-174 g/L	WBC	5.3 10^3/μl	4.5-10.5 x 10^3/cells/ mm^3	4.5-10.5 x 10^9/L
Hct	60%	42 – 52%		% Lymph	27%	25 – 40% of total WBC	1500-4000 cells/mm^3
RBC	$4.8x10^6$/μ	3.6-$5.0x10^6$/L	3.6-$5.0x10^{12}$/ L	MCH	28 pg/cell	26-34 pg/cell	0.40-.53 fmol/cell
MCV	85 $μm^3$	82-98$μm^3$	82-98 fL	MCHC	33 g/dl	32-36 g/dl	320-360 g/L

He then asked her home health care agency to send a dietitian for an assessment. The agency contacted one of their consultants and sent an RD to RK's house. After assessing the patient and reviewing RK's old hospital records and current lab values, the RD found RK to be dehydrated and made the following suggestions:

➢ Change RK's feeding to a 1 kcal/cc with added fiber, 350 cc qid during wakening hours.
➢ Flush feeding tube with 30 cc water before and after each feeding.
➢ Give 60 cc of prune juice bid via PEG.
➢ Obtain bed weight and monitor weight monthly and every three months after weight stabilizes.
➢ RD to assess patient every two weeks until weight stabilizes, then prn.
****

QUESTIONS CONTINUED:
30. What lab values indicated dehydration?

31. Why was RK dehydrated?

32. Choose a 1 kcal/cc tube feeding that has fiber added and compare it to a 2 kcals/cc feeding.

Product	Producer	Form	Cal/ml	Non-pro cal/g N	g/L			Na mg	K mg	mOsm /kg water	Vol to meet RDA in ml	g of fiber /L	Free H_2O /L in ml
					Pro	CHO	Fat						

33. Explain the reasoning behind using the lower kcal fiber tube feeding instead of the 2 kcals/cc.

34. Note the amount of free water in the two different feedings. Explain the physiology of RK's constipation and relate how the fiber and additional free water in the new feeding will help prevent constipation.

35. What is the purpose of prune juice bid?

36. After a bed weight is obtained the RD will be able to calculate a specific caloric and protein need. Considering RK's lack of activity and posturing, estimate his kcal and protein needs per kg of body weight.

37. RK's lack of activity and excessive intake is causing his lean body mass to decrease and his adipose tissue to increase. His LBM to fat ratio is not going to be like that of a person who is active. Suggest a technique the RD could use to determine RK's actual body composition.

38. Update RK's SOAP note.

S:
O:
A:
P:

EPILOGUE

When I was practicing as pat of a nutrition support, I had this patient in my NICU. Just as in this case, he went to a regular unit and I did not see again before he left the hospital. At the time, I was also consulting for a home health care agency. A couple of weeks after discharge, I was sent to this patient's house for the problems mentioned in this case. Most of this is exactly as it occurred.

RELATED REFERENCES

1. Bosscha, K., Nieuwenhuijs, V.B., Vos, A., Samsom, M., Roelofs, J.M., & Akkermans, L.M. (1998). Gastrointestinal motility and gastric tube feeding in mechanically ventilated patients. *Crit. Care Med.* 26(9):1510-7.

2. Falcao de Arruda, I.S. & de Aguilar-Nascimento, J.E. (2004). Benefits of early enteral nutrition with glutamine and probiotics in brain injury patients. *Clin Sci* (Lond). Mar;106(3):287-92.

3. Fertl, E., Steinhoff, N., Schofl, R., Potzi, R., Doppelbauer, A., Muller, C., & Auff, E. (1998). Transient and long-term feeding by means of percutaneous endoscopic gastrostomy in neurological rehabilitation. *Eur. Neurol.* 40(1):27-30.

4. Formisano, R., Carlesimo, G.A., Sabbadini, M., Loasses, A., Penta, F., Vinicola, V., & Caltagirone, C. (2004). Clinical predictors and neuropsychological outcome in severe traumatic brain injury patients. *Acta Neurochir.* May;146(5):457-62.

5. Goff, K. (1998). Enteral and parenteral nutrition transitioning from hospital to home. *Nurs. Case Manag.* 3(2):67-74.

6. Loan, T., Magnuson, B., & Williams, S. (1998). Debunking six myths about enteral feeding. *Nursing.* 28(8):43-9.

7. Moore, R., Najarian, M.P., & Konvolinka, C.W. (1989). Measured energy expenditure in severe head trauma. *J. Trauma.* 29(12):1633-6.

8. O'Keefe, S.J., Foody, W., & Gill, S. (2003). Transnasal endoscopic placement of feeding tubes in the intensive care unit. *J Parenter Enteral Nutr.* Sep-Oct;27(5):349-54.

9. Rhoney, D.H., Parker, D. Jr, Formea, C.M., Yap, C, & Coplin, W.M. (2002). Tolerability of bolus versus continuous gastric feeding in brain-injured patients. *Neurol Res.* Sep;24(6):613-20.

10. Sacks, G.S., Brown, R.O., Teague, D., Dickerson, R.N., Tolley, E.A., & Kudsk, K.A. (1995). Early nutrition support modifies immune function in patients sustaining severe head injury. *JPEN.* 19(5):387-92.

11. Thelan, L.A., Davie, J.K., Urden, L.D., & Lough, M.E. (1994). *Critical Care Nursing. Diagnosis and Management.* 2nd Ed. St. Louis, MO. Mosby.

12. Williams, D.M. (1998). The current state of home nutrition support in the United States. *Nutrition.* 14(4):416-9.

13. Yanagawa, T., Bunn, F., Roberts, I., Wentz, R., & Pierro, A. (2002). Nutritional support for head-injured patients. *Cochrane Database Syst Rev.* (3):CD001530.

14. Young, B., Ott, L., Kasarskis, E., Rapp, R., Moles, K., Dempsey, R.J., Tibbs, P.A., Kryscio, R., & McClain, C. (1996). Zinc supplementation is associated with improved neurologic recovery rate and visceral protein levels of patients with severe closed head injury. *J. Neurotrauma.* 13(1):25-34.

CASE STUDY #29
PANCREATITIS/HEPATITIS RESULTING IN ALCOHOLIC CIRRHOSIS

INTRODUCTION

In PART I of this case study, the patient develops pancreatitis with alcoholic hepatitis. This progresses to Laennec's cirrhosis. In PART II, the patient's condition worsens and he must be fed by a tube feeding. The study reviews the lab values and diet for liver disease. Knowledge of tube feedings for hepatic disease is required. Review the diets for pancreatitis and liver disease and the appropriate lab values before reading this case.
****

SKILLS NEEDED

ABBREVIATIONS:
Knowledge of the following abbreviations is required in order to understand this case. You should learn these abbreviations before you begin to read the study. BRB, DTs, NH_3, PT, and TBIL (Appendix C).

LABORATORY VALUES:
The normal values for the following parameters will be needed for this case study: ALT, ALP, AST, BUN, Cl, CPK, Cr, DBIL, hgb, hct, MCH, MCHC, MCV, glucose, % lymph, Mg, K, Na, P, PT, RBC, ser alb, serum amylase, TBIL, TP, and WBC (Appendix B).

FORMULAS:
The formulas used in this case study include ideal body weight, percent ideal body weight, total lymphocyte count, basal energy expenditure using the Harris-Benedict equation, and an appropriate stress factor (Appendix A, Tables 7 through 10, 15, and 17).

MEDICATIONS:
Become familiar with the following medications before reading the case study. Note the diet-drug interactions, dosages and methods of administration, gastrointestinal tract reactions, etc.
1. Pancrease (lipancreatin); 2. potassium chloride (Slow-K); 3. .spironolactone (Aldactone);
4. furosemide (Lasix); 5. lactulose enema; 6. Neomycin
****

PART I: PANCREATITIS WITH ALCOHOLIC HEPATITIS

Mr. N is a 45-year-old automobile mechanic. He is divorced with two children who are in college. He always believed he was "down on his luck." Every time a misfortune came his way, he had a pity party. He frequently spent time just sitting in a corner feeling sorry for himself. Whenever those periods of depression came upon him, he knew only one way out of them: alcohol. He started drinking beer and whiskey when he was in high school. His intake increased as he grew older. He went to trade school to learn automobile mechanics and then married in his early twenties. Several years ago, after Mr. N drank too much, he awoke with a severe epigastric pain that radiated to his back. He was sweating, felt nauseous, and had to vomit. His abdomen was sore to touch and felt swollen. He could tell that he had an elevated temperature. This continued for a couple of days before he went to a neighborhood treatment center to see a physician. The physician took a medical history and did an examination that included lab values.

The physician told Mr. N that he had acute pancreatitis with an enlarged fatty liver. He told him that his liver enzymes were elevated and that if he continued drinking, he could develop a very severe liver disease. He also told him that if he stopped drinking, his liver could clear up in a matter of weeks. He encouraged Mr. N to follow a low-fat, high-protein diet with absolutely no alcohol. The physician told Mr. N to call him back if the pain and discomfort did not clear up within two or three days. Mr. N's height was 5'11" and he weighed 170 lbs. The physician sent Mr. N home with the following prescriptions:

➢ Pancrease (lipancreatin)--enough for 3 days
➢ potassium chloride (Slow-K)--enough for 3 days

His labs were as follows:

BASIC METABOLIC PACKAGE							
TEST	RESULT	REFERENCE UNITS Conventional	SI	TEST	RESULT	REFERENCE UNITS Conventional	SI
Glu	190 mg/dl	70-110 mg/dl	3.8-6.1 mmol/L	Na	144 mEq/L	136-145 mEq/L	136-145 mmol/L
BUN	18 mg/dl	6-20 mg/dl	2.1-7.1 mmol/L	K	3.1 mEq/L	3.5-5.2 mEq/L	3.5-5.2 mmol/L
Cr	1.2 mg/dl	0.9-1.3 mg/dl	80-115 µmol/L	Cl	103 mEq/L	96-106 mEq/L	96-106 mmol/L
Ca	8.8 mg/dl	8.8-10.0 mg/dl	2.20-2.60 mmol/L	Mg	1.7 mEq/L	1.8 - 2.6 mEq/L	136-145 mmol/L
Ser alb	2.9 g/dl	3.5-4.8 g/dl	39-50 g/dl	P	2.6mg/dl	2.7-4.5 mg/dl	4.7-6.0 kPa

LIVER FUNCTION							
TEST	RESULT	REFERENCE UNITS Conventional	SI	TEST	RESULT	REFERENCE UNITS Conventional	SI
AST	183 U/L	14-20 U/L	0.23-0.33 µkat/L	TBIL	3.2 mg/dl	0.3-1.0 mg/dl	5.0-17.0 µmol/L
ALT	132 U/L	10-40 U/L	0.17-0.68 µkat/L	DBIL	0.1 mg/dl	0-0.2 mg/dl	0-3.4 µmol/L
ALP	253 U/L	25-100 U/L	17-142 U/L	CPK	150 U/L	38–174 IU/L	0.63-2.90 µkat/L
PT	12.2 sec	11-13 secs		Amylase	485 U/L	25–125 U/L	0.4-2.1 µkat/L

The physician advised Mr. N not to take pancreatin with antacids. He also strongly advised him to eat a well-balanced diet with ample protein, and to take a multiple vitamin and mineral supplement daily for the next several months. He emphasized again that Mr. N would absolutely have to avoid alcohol.
****

QUESTIONS:
1. Explain the reasoning behind the diet order Mr. N received: "low fat, high protein with absolutely no alcohol."

2. Did the physician give Mr. N enough information about his diet or the condition of his liver? Outline the instruction you would give Mr. N concerning his diet and liver disease.

3. List the lab values that are indicative of liver disease.

4. What abnormal lab values are indicative of pancreatitis?

5. What was the purpose of the MD giving Mr. N the potassium chloride? Explain your answer.

6. Give the pathophysiology of a fatty liver 2° to alcoholism.

7. After the symptoms of pancreatitis and hepatitis are gone, should Mr. N be on a diet for pancreatitis or for a fatty liver? Explain.

****

Mr. N followed his diet and took his medication and began to feel better. He stayed off the alcohol for three or four days but then began to have the DTs and had to start drinking again. He drank smaller amounts until his next depression period, when he started drinking heavily again. It was around this time that his wife began suing him for divorce. This caused additional depression, and he began to have stomach pains different from the epigastric pain he had experienced earlier. He was diagnosed with an ulcer and had to go on a liberal bland diet. This still did not stop Mr. N from drinking. He started having the kind of epigastric pain again like he had with his previous bout of pancreatitis. When it persisted for several days, he returned to his neighborhood emergency clinic. The physician again drew blood and examined Mr. N. His liver function tests were elevated to a much greater degree.

CBC							
TEST	RESULT	REFERENCE UNITS Conventional	SI	TEST	RESULT	REFERENCE UNITS Conventional	SI
Hgb	12.g/dl	14 - 17.4 g/dl	140-174 g/L	WBC	4.7×10^3/µl	$4.5\text{-}10.5 \times 10^3$/cells/mm³	$4.5\text{-}10.5 \times 10^9$/L
Hct	38%	42 – 52%		% Lymph	23%	25 – 40% of total WBC	1500-4000 cells/mm³
RBC	3.6×10^6/µ	$3.6\text{-}5.0\times10^6$/L	$3.6\text{-}5.0\times10^{12}$/L	MCH	33 pg/cell	26-34 pg/cell	0.40-.53 fmol/cell
MCV	110 µm³	82-98µm³	82-98 fL	MCHC	32 g/dl	32-36 g/dl	320-360 g/L

LIVER FUNCTION							
TEST	RESULT	REFERENCE UNITS Conventional	SI	TEST	RESULT	REFERENCE UNITS Conventional	SI
AST	240 U/L	14-20 U/L	0.23-0.33 µkat/L	TBIL	4.8 mg/dl	0.3-1.0 mg/dl	5.0-17.0 µmol/L
ALT	200 U/L	10-40 U/L	0.17-0.68 µkat/L	DBIL	0.1 mg/dl	0-0.2 mg/dl	0-3.4 µmol/L
ALP	363 U/L	25-100 U/L	17-142 U/L	CPK	145 U/L	38–174 IU/L	0.63-2.90 µkat/L
PT	15.4 secs	11-13 secs		Amylase	685 U/L	25–125 U/L	0.4-2.1 µkat/L

BASIC METABOLIC PACKAGE							
TEST	RESULT	REFERENCE UNITS Conventional	SI	TEST	RESULT	REFERENCE UNITS Conventional	SI
Glu	87 mg/dl	70-110 mg/dl	3.8-6.1 mmol/L	Na	140 mEq/L	136-145 mEq/L	136-145 mmol/L
BUN	14 mg/dl	6-20 mg/dl	2.1-7.1 mmol/L	K	5.1 mEq/L	3.5-5.2 mEq/L	3.5-5.2 mmol/L
Cr	0.6 mg/dl	0.9-1.3 mg/dl	80-115 µmol/L	Cl	102 mEq/L	96-106 mEq/L	96-106 mmol/L
Ca	8.4 mg/dl	8.8-10.0 mg/dl	2.20-2.60 mmol/L	Mg	1.6 mEq/L	1.8 - 2.6 mEq/L	136-145 mmol/L
Ser alb	2.3 g/dl	3.5-4.8 g/dl	39-50 g/L	P	2.3mg/dl	2.7-4.5 mg/dl	4.7-6.0 kPa

The physician advised Mr. N to see a family practice physician or an internist. He believed Mr. N should be hospitalized for more tests and treatment. Mr. N was admitted to the hospital with a Dx of Laennec's cirrhosis with pancreatitis. It was a year and a half since Mr. N had been first treated for pancreatitis. Mr. N's weight was now 150 lbs.
****

QUESTIONS CONTINUED:

8. Determine Mr. N's IBW and percent IBW (Appendix A, Tables 7 and 8).

9. What is the significance of hgb and hct being depressed while MCV is elevated? What nutritional deficiencies do these lab values indicate?

10. Define the following terms:

    Pancreatitis:

    Hyperbilirubinemia:

    Ascites:

    Hepatomegaly:

    Laennec's cirrhosis:

    Hypocalcemia:

11. Calculate Mr. N's BEE using the Harris-Benedict equation. Calculate his total energy needs with the appropriate stress factor (Appendix A).

12. How much protein should Mr. N receive per day?

13. Explain the relationship between alcoholism and ulcers.

<u>ADDITIONAL OPTIONAL QUESTIONS:</u>
Tube Feeding Drill:

14. Using the table below, compare the enteral nutritional supplements suitable for liver disease.

Product	Producer	Form	Cal/ml	Non-pro cal/g N	Pro	CHO	Fat	Na mg	K mg	mOsm /kg water	Vol to meet RDA in ml	g of fiber /L	Free H$_2$O /L in ml

15. Prepare a SOAP note for Mr. N.

S:

O:

A:

P:

****

PART II: TUBE FEEDING

Mr. N's condition seemed to worsen. He developed ascites and pedal edema. His urinary output was decreasing. His diet consisted of the energy and protein levels recommended by the dietitian and a 1 g Na restriction. Mr. N did not like his diet at all. He ate sparingly and was not receiving the nutrients he needed. He continued to lose weight. After a few days without alcohol, he began to have DTs and had to be restrained. During this time he began to hallucinate and use very abusive language. He also started to exhibit asterixis. Blood was drawn and his NH_3 25 µmol/L. His intake dropped to almost nothing. He was receiving only D_5W by I.V. with added vitamins, minerals, and electrolytes. That night he started throwing up large amounts of BRB. A Sengstaken-Blakemore tube had to be placed. Mr. N bled so excessively that whole blood had to be administered. His physician added to his Dx the following:

1. hepatic encephalopathy
2. portal hypertension
3. esophageal varices

Mr. N was now in a semi-comatose state and had to keep the Sengstaken-Blakemore tube in place for another day. After the tube was removed, Mr. N had a N/G tube in place to low intermittent suction. He was NPO and was receiving D_5W by I.V. with electrolytes, vitamins, and minerals. Mr. N continued to have severe ascites and pedal edema with reduced urinary output. He had some blood drawn again and his NH_3 was now up to 92 Fmol/L. His prothrombin time was off by 4 sec. His serum albumin was down to 2.2 g/dl. AST was 2x ALT and GGTP was 800. New orders for Mr. N included the following:

1. spironolactone (Aldactone) I.V.
2. furosemide (Lasix) I.V.
3. lactulose enema
4. Neomycin via N/G tube
5. D_5W at 75 cc/hr

The physician called for the dietitian to recommend an appropriate tube feeding and flow rate.

****

QUESTIONS CONTINUED:

16. What is the mechanism of action of the following drugs:
    Spironolactone (Aldactone):

    Furosemide (Lasix):

17. What are the nutritional implications of these drugs, especially as they pertain to Mr. N's condition?

18. Explain the mechanism of action of lactulose.

19. Explain the mechanism of action of Neomycin.

20. Define the following terms:

    Portal hypertension:

    Esophageal varices:

    Sengstaken-Blakemore tube:

    Hepatic encephalopathy:

    Asterixis:

21. Explain the pathophysiology of esophageal varices and portal hypertension as it relates to liver disease and Mr. N's bleeding.

22. What does it mean to have a N/G tube to low intermittent suction?

23. What is the relationship between prothrombin time and liver disease?

24. Mr. N's AST was 2x ALT and GGTP was 800. What does this tell the physician concerning Mr. N's liver?

25. What is the significance of Mr. N's NH_3 level being elevated prior to his bleeding? What is the significance of it being elevated to an even greater degree after his bleeding?

26. Before his bleeding, what diet would have been appropriate for Mr. N? Be specific for protein, carbohydrate, fat, total energy, Na, fluid, and vitamins and minerals.

27. The tube feeding Mr. N should receive is obviously one designed for liver failure. List the characteristics of a hepatic TF and explain the reasoning behind each characteristic.

28. Are there any vitamins or minerals in particular that need to be added to a hepatic TF? Explain your answer.

29. Calculate Mr. N's total energy needs using the Harris-Benedict formula and the appropriate stress factor.

30. Calculate his protein needs.

31. Mr. N is receiving D_5W at 75 cc/hr. How much fluid, grams of CHO, and kcals is this per day? Show your work.

32. Considering the above, of the available hepatic formulas, which one would you choose and why?

33. How much of this formula will Mr. N need to meet the requirements you previously calculated? Consider the I.V. kcals from D_5W.

34. Give the starting strength and flow rate you would use and the progression to the final strength and flow rate. Explain your rationale.

35. Considering that Mr. N is receiving lactulose and neomycin, can the TF be properly absorbed? Explain your answer.

****

Assume that Mr. N is going to recover from his hepatic encephalopathy; the edema and ascites will diminish significantly, and his renal function will return to normal. He will again be able to resume his diet. Also, assume that Mr. N will be discharged with end stage cirrhosis and will not be able to drink alcohol at all. He will still have some edema and some ascites, his serum albumin will be very low and he will be very weak.

****

36. On a separate sheet of paper assume that Mr. N will go home on a diet and estimate what that diet will be. Include in your estimate the number of kcals he should have, the grams and percent of protein, the grams and percent of carbohydrate, the grams and percent of fat, the cc of fluid, the grams of Na, and any other restrictions or supplements that you feel are necessary.

37. Complete an updated SOAP note on Mr. N.

S	
O:	
A:	
P:	

RELATED REFERENCES

1. Addolorato, G., Capristo, E., Greco, A.V., Stefanini, G.F., & Gasbarrini, G. (1997). Energy expenditure, substrate exidation, and body composition in subjects with chronic alcoholism: new finding from metabolic assessment. *Alcohol Clin. Exp. Res.* 21(6):962-7.

2. Addolorato, G. Capristo, E., Stefanini, G.F., & Gasbarrini, G. (1998). Metabolic features and nutritional status in chronic alcoholics. *Am. J. Gastroenterol.* 93(4):665-6.

3. Addolorato, G., Capristo, E., Greco, A.V., Caputo, F., Stefanini, G.F., & Gasbarrini, G. (1998). Three months of abstinence from alcohol normalizes energy expenditure and substrate oxidation in alcoholics: a longitudinal study. *Am J Gastroenterol.* Dec;93(12):2476-81.

4. Apte, M., Norton, I., Haaber, P., Applegate, T., Korsten, M., McCaughan, G., Pirola, R., & Wilson, J. (1998). The effect of ethanol on pancreatic enzymes—a dietary artifact? *Biochem. Biophys. Acta.* 2;1379(3):314-24.

5. Arteel, G., Marsano, L., Mendez, C., Bentley, F., & McClain, C.J. (2003). Advances in alcoholic liver disease. *Best Pract Res Clin Gastroenterol.* Aug;17(4):625-47.

6. Campillo, B., Richardet, J.P., Scherman, E., & Bories, P.N. (2003). Evaluation of nutritional practice in hospitalized cirrhotic patients: results of a prospective study. *Nutrition.* Jun;19(6):515-21.

7. Cerra, F.B., Cheung, N.K., Fischer, J.E., Kaplowitz, N., Schiff, E.R., Dienstag., J.L., Bower, R.H., Mabry, C.D., Leevy, C.M., & Kiernan, T. (1985). Disease-specific amino acid infusion (F080) in hepatic encephalopathy: a prospective, randomized, double-blind, controlled trial. *JPEN J Parenter Enteral Nutr.* 9(3):288-295.

8. Charlton, M.R. (1996). Branched chains revisited. *Gastroenterology.* 111(1):252-5.

9. Cravo, M.L., & Camilo, M.E. (2000). Hyperhomocysteinemia in chronic alcoholism: relations to folic acid and vitamins B(6) and B(12) status. *Nutrition.* Apr;16(4):296-302.

10. de Ledinghen, V., Beau, P., Mannant, P.R., Borderie, C., Ripault, M.P., Silvain, C., & Beauchant, M. (1997). Early feeding or enteral nutrition in patients with cirrhosis after bleeding from esophageal varices? A randomized controlled study. *Dig Dis Sci.* 42(3): 536-41.

11 Fernandez-Sola, J., Garcia, G., Elena, M., Tobias, E., Sacanella, E., Estruch, R., & Nicolas, J.M. (2002). Muscle antioxidant status in chronic alcoholism. *Alcohol Clin Exp Res.* Dec;26(12):1858-62.

12. Fischbach, F.T. (2003). *A Manual of Laboratory & Diagnostic Tests.* 7th Ed. Philadelphia. J.B. Lippincott Company.

13. Garcia-de-Lorenzo, A., Ortiz-Leyba, C., Planas, M., Montejo, J.C., Nunez, R., Ordonez, F.J.,Aragon, C., & Jimenez, F.J. (1997). Parenteral administration of different amounts of branch-chain amino acids in septic patients: clinical and metabolic aspects. *Crit Care Med.* Mar;25(3):418-24.

14. Halsted, C.H. (2004). Nutrition and alcoholic liver disease. *Semin Liver Dis.* Aug;24(3):289-304.

15. Hill, D.B. & Kugelmas, M. (1998). Alcoholic liver disease. Treatment strategies for the potentially reversible stages. *Postgrad. Med.* 103(4):261-4, 267-8, 273-5.

16. Ichida, T., Shibasaki, K., Muto, Y., Satoh, S., Watanabe, A., Ichida, F. (1995). Clinical study of an enteral branched-chain amino acid solution in decompensated liver cirrhosis with hepatic encephalopathy. *Nutrition.* 11(2 Suppl):238-44.

17. Lee, R.D., Nieman, D.C., & Nieman, D. (2002). *Nutritional Assessment.* 3rd Ed. McGraw-Hill.

18. Lieber, C.S., & Leo, M.A. (1998). Metabolism of ethanol and some associated adverse effects on the liver and stomach. *Recent Dev. Alcohol.* 14:7-40.

19. McEwen, D. (1998). End-stage alcoholism. *A.O.R.N. J.* 68(4):674-7.

20. Nicolas, J.M., Garcia,G., Fatjo, F., Sacanella, E., Tobias E., Badia, E., Estruch, R., & Fernandez-Sola, J. . (2003). Influence of nutritional status on alcoholic myopathy. *Am J Clin Nutr* Aug;78(2):326-33.

21. Prendergast, A. & Fulton, F.L. (1997) *Medical terminology: A Text/Workbook.* 4th Ed. Redwood City, California. Addison-Wesley Nursing.

22. Prakash, S., & Joshi, Y.K. (2004). Assessment of micronutrient antioxidants, total antioxidant capacity and lipid peroxidation levels in liver cirrhosis. *Asia Pac J Clin Nutr.*;13(Suppl):S110.

23. Pronsky, Z.M., Redfern, C.M., Crowe, J. & Epstein, S. (2003). *Food Medication Interactions,* 13th Ed Phoenix, Arizona. Food-Medications Interactions, Publishers and Distributors.

24. Radenkovic, D., & Johnson, C.D. (2004). Nutritional support in acute pancreatitis. *Nutr Clin Care.* Jul-Sep;7(3):98-103

25. Rolfes, S.R., Pinna, K. & Whitney, E. (2006). *Understanding Normal and Clinical Nutrition,* 7th Ed. West/Wadsworth.

26. Roongpisuthipong, C., Sobhonslidsuk, A., Nantiruj, K., & Songchitsomboon, S. (2002). Nutritional assessment in various stages of liver cirrhosis. *Nutrition.* Sep;17(9):761-5.

27. Santolaria, F., Perez-Manzano, J.L., Milena, A., Gonzalez-Reimers, E., Gomez-Rodriguez, M.A., Martinez-Riera, A., Aleman-Valls, M.R., de la Vega-Prieto, M.J. (2000). Nutritional assessment in alcoholic patients. Its relationship with alcoholic intake, feeding habits, organic complications and social problems. *Drug Alcohol Depend.* Jun 1;59(3):295-304.

28. Singh, N., & Saraya, A. (2004). Nutrition support in acute pancreatitis. *Trop Gastroenterol.* Jul-Sep;25(3):108-12.

29. Spratto, G.R. & Woods, A.L. (2005). *PDR Nurse's Drug Handbook.* Thompson Delmar Learning, NY.

30. Windsor, A.C., Kanwar, S., Li, A.G., Barnes, E., Guthrie, J.A., Spark, J.I., Welsh, F., Guillou, P.J., & Reynolds, J.V. (1998). Compared with parenteral nutrition, enteral feeding attenuates the acute phase response and improves disease severity in acute pancreatitis. *Gut.* 42(3):431-5.

CASE STUDY #30
ESOPHAGEAL CANCER AND CHEMOTHERAPY

INTRODUCTION

PART I of this case's two parts is concerned with esophageal cancer. The location of the cancer adds to the nutritional problem since it affects swallowing. This case provides an introduction to the dietary treatment of chemotherapy patients as well as patients who have difficulty swallowing. The interpretation of laboratory values and an understanding of medical terminology are important in this case study. PART II is more advanced and involves TPN formulation and monitoring.
****

SKILLS NEEDED

ABBREVIATIONS:

Knowledge of the following abbreviations is required in order to understand this case. You should learn these abbreviations before you begin to read the study.
BEE, BS, CA, D_5NS, $D_{10}W$, FH, LDH, LES, prn, TLC, and TPN (Appendix C).

LABORATORY VALUES:

You will need to be able to interpret the nutritional significance of the following laboratory values for this case study: ALP, ALT, AST, Bili, BUN, Cl, CPK, Cr, glucose, hct, hgb, K, LDH, lymphocytes, MCV, Na, ser alb, Platelet Count, Uric Acid, and WBC (Appendix B).

FORMULAS:

The formulas used in this case study include ideal body weight, percent ideal body weight, percent usual body weight, total lymphocyte count, BEE using the Harris-Benedict equation, stress factors, and total energy and protein needs, all of which can be found in Appendix A, Tables 7, 8, 13, and 17.

MEDICATIONS:

Become familiar with the following medications before reading the case study. Note the diet-drug interactions, dosages and methods of administration, gastrointestinal tract reactions, etc.
1. Fudr (floxuridine); 2. Lomotil (diphenoxylate hydrochloride); 3. Morphine Sulphate
****

PART I: CHEMOTHERAPY

Mrs. S is a 54 YOBF who is a buyer for one of the local department stores. She has lived a healthy life with no major illnesses. She is married and has three children, all of whom are married and well. Mrs. S has a FH of carcinoma. Her mother died of breast cancer at the age of 65 and her sister had a mastectomy for carcinoma when she was 62. Mrs. S has one younger brother who is healthy. She was doing fine until about 6 weeks before her first hospital admission, when she noticed some difficulty swallowing. She paid little attention to the problem at first but, as it seemed to get worse, she began to become concerned. This was a very busy time of the year for her. Christmas was approaching and sales were picking up. Mrs. S stayed in a continuous rush and had to "gulp" her food. She had heard people say that they "had a lump in their throat" when they were upset and decided, because of the stress and the fast eating, that was probably what she had. She tried eating more slowly and taking smaller bites, but it did not work. Her swallowing got worse. As a result, she was eating less and drinking more liquids. Mrs. S noted that she was losing weight but could not find time to go to the doctor.

The week after Christmas, six weeks after she first noticed a problem swallowing, she went to the doctor. She had lost 20 lbs since her last visit. He had some blood work done and did a UGI series on an outpatient basis. The results were as follows:

CBC							
TEST	RESULT	REFERENCE UNITS Conventional	SI	TEST	RESULT	REFERENCE UNITS Conventional	SI
Hgb	11 g/dl	12-16 g/dl	120-160 g/L	WBC	10.2 10^3/µl	4.5-10.5 x 10^3/cells/mm^3	4.5-10.5 x10^9/L
Hct	33 %	36-48%		% Lymph	13%	25 – 40% of total WBC	1500-4000 cells/mm^3
RBC	4.0x10^6/µ	3.6-5.0x10^6/L	3.6-5.0 x10^{12}/L	MCH	28 pg/cell	26-34 pg/cell	0.40-.53 fmol/cell
MCV	82 µm^3	82-98µm^3	82-98 fL	MCHC	33 g/dl	32-36 g/dl	320-360 g/L

BASIC METABOLIC PACKAGE							
TEST	RESULT	REFERENCE UNITS Conventional	SI	TEST	RESULT	REFERENCE UNITS Conventional	SI
Glu	87 mg/dl	70-110 mg/dl	3.8-6.1 mmol/L	Na	138 mEq/L	136-145 mEq/L	136-145 mmol/L
BUN	17 mg/dl	6-20 mg/dl	2.1-7.1 mmol/L	K	3.2 mEq/L	3.5-5.2 mEq/L	3.5-5.2 mmol/L
Cr	0.8 mg/dl	0.6-1.1 mg/dl	53-97 µmol/L	Cl	104 mEq/L	96-106 mEq/L	96-106 mmol/L
Ca	11.2 mg/dl	8.8-10.0 mg/dl	2.20-2.60 mmol/L	Mg	1.8 mEq/L	1.8 - 2.6 mEq/L	136-145 mmol/L
Ser alb	2.8 g/dl	3.5-4.8 g/dl	39-50 g/dl	P	2.7mg/dl	2.7-4.5 mg/dl	4.7-6.0 kPa

LIVER FUNCTION							
TEST	RESULT	REFERENCE UNITS Conventional	SI	TEST	RESULT	REFERENCE UNITS Conventional	SI
AST	12 U/L	10-36 U/L	0.17-0.60 µkat/L	TBIL	0.6 mg/dl	0.3-1.0 mg/dl	5.0-17.0 µmol/L
ALT	8 U/L	7-35 U/L	7-56 U/L	DBIL	0.1 mg/dl	0-0.2 mg/dl	0-3.4 µmol/L
ALP	48 U/L	25-100 U/L	17-142 U/L	CPK	40 IU/L	26–140 U/L	0.42-2.38 µkat/L

The UGI revealed an esophageal lesion. Mrs. S had to go back in two days for a CxR and an esophagogastroscopy. The endoscopy showed the lesion and a narrowing of the distal esophagus just above the LES. A biopsy was taken that proved to be positive for squamous cell carcinoma. The CxR was negative. Mrs. S was admitted to the hospital for more tests and surgery.

Mrs. S's Dx was:
1. Esophageal squamous cell CA
2. Dysphagia and odynophagia 2° to 1.
3. Microcytic, hypochromic anemia
4. Malnutrition

Her height was 5' 6" and she weighed 155 lbs. Her UBW was 175 lbs.
****

CS#30 Esophageal Cancer and Chemotherapy

1. Determine Mrs. S's IBW, percent IBW, and percent UBW. Please show all calculations.

2. Calculate Mrs. S's TLC.

3. Which of the abnormal lab values could be indicative of cancer?

4. Which of the abnormal lab values would be indicative of malnutrition in general?

5. Which of the abnormal lab values would be indicative of anemia?

6. Which of the abnormal lab values would be indicative of microcytic anemia?

7. Briefly define the following:
   Mastectomy:

   Carcinoma:

   Esophageal lesion:

   Endoscopy:

   Esophagogastroscopy:

Squamous cell carcinoma:

Dysphagia:

Odynophagia:

****

Additional radiographic studies suggested that the cancer was not as extensive as the MD originally thought, but Mrs. S was distraught just the same. She was extremely fearful of cancer because of her family history. She had had no idea that she was in such poor shape nutritionally. Mrs. S was so upset that she was not ready for surgery. She asked if she could have a few days to think about it. Considering her poor condition, her physician agreed and allowed the RD to work with her to improve her nutritional status. Meanwhile, he also decided to initiate chemotherapy in an attempt to shrink the tumor prior to surgery. His orders included:

1. High protein, soft diet as tolerated.
2. At least three cans of high protein liquid supplement between meals every day.
3. floxuridine (Fudr) 0.5 mg/kg intraarterial every day.

The hospital was short staffed and was forced to use entry level RDs who did not have the usual orientation and training that the hospital provides before assigning someone to a unit. The RD assigned to Mrs. S had just graduated and had had very little experience with cancer patients. Try to picture the situation the RD is going into, something you should do before entering every hospital room. She is going to talk to a woman who has seen cancer kill several in her family and who went from being very healthy to very sickly in a short period of time. The patient is very upset.

The RD knocked on the patient's door and gained entry appropriately. She properly introduced herself and made sure that she was talking to the right patient. During the introduction, Mrs. S made it clear that she was very upset because she had just been told by her physician that she required surgery for cancer. The RD began her interview:

RD: Mrs. S, I understand you are upset right now, but I need some information about your diet so that we can send you the foods you like to eat.

Mrs. S: Honey, I don't care about eating anything right now, I'm so upset. Everything just sits in my stomach. It's so hard to swallow. It seems like it is getting harder every day, and it burns so.

RD: Well, have you noticed any particular foods that bother you more than others?

Mrs. S: They all bother me. I can only swallow liquids. I just can't. . .

RD: How about blenderized or pureed foods? Have you tried any of them?

Mrs. S: No, but I have tried some mashed potatoes and I still was not . . .

RD: Have you tried diluting the potatoes with milk?

Mrs. S: No, but I don't think that will work.

RD: Well you really don't know if it will work until you have tried it. How about if we send you some very dilute creamed potatoes and some pureed foods? We have very nice pureed food here.

Mrs. S: Honey, nobody has nice pureed food. I hate that stuff!

RD: Well, I want you to try ours before you pass judgment.

Mrs. S: I can't tolerate anything with acid. It burns so much. And I can't take anything that is highly seasoned.

RD: What about for breakfast? Do you eat eggs?

Mrs. S: No. Too high in cholesterol.

RD: Yes, but they are high in protein and very digestible. While you are sick we are not going to worry about cholesterol . . .

Mrs. S: The doctor tells me not to eat it; you tell me to eat it.

RD: What about juice?

Mrs. S: It burns, darling, it burns.

RD: Even grape juice?

Mrs. S: Even grape juice. They all burn. Honey, I don't want to be rude, but I don't feel like talking about food right now. I'm too upset. Just thinking about food makes me nauseous. Please come back tomorrow. Maybe I'll feel better.

RD: Well, OK. I'll let you off this time, but I'll be back. In the meantime, I'm going to send you some pureed food and some liquid supplements between meals. What is your favorite flavor?

Mrs. S: Strawberry.

RD: All right. I'm going to send you some strawberry supplements. You try to drink all of it and be sure to try to eat all the meat, and drink your milk. OK?

Mrs. S: Yea. OK.
****

QUESTIONS CONTINUED:

8. Define intra-arterial. What dangers could accompany this method of administration?

9. List the mistakes the RD made during her conversation with Mrs. S.

10. List the segments of the interview you thought were well done.

11. What would you do differently and how?

12. What energy and protein supplement would you use in this case?

13. Using the Harris-Benedict equation, determine Mrs. S's BEE. Using the appropriate stress factor, calculate her total energy needs (Appendix A, Table 17).

14. Determine her protein needs.

15. Look up the drug floxuridine and list all of the complications that pertain to nutritional status.

16. On a separate sheet of paper, outline a day's menu for Mrs. S.

****

In the week that followed, Mrs. S developed just about every adverse reaction listed for floxuridine, including nausea and diarrhea. She ate very poorly but was able to drink the liquid supplements fairly well. After 10 days of treatment, everything either had a metallic taste or tasted too sweet. The smell of food made her nauseous. She was afraid to drink any more of the supplement because of the diarrhea.

****

QUESTIONS CONTINUED:

17. Is there a different supplement that could be used in these circumstances? If so, identify the supplement and give the scientific basis for using it.

18. There are a few things that can be done to help cancer patients overcome the metallic taste and nausea that occurs with smelling food. Be creative and see if you can think of anything that may be helpful in this respect.

19. Sketch the location of Mrs. S's lesion.

****

Mrs. S was still losing weight and her lab values were getting worse. She was becoming more depressed. The physician decided to make her NPO and initiated TPN. This was continued for one week before surgery and will be discussed in **PART II** of this case study.

****

20. Write a SOAP note for Mrs. S.

S:

O:

A:

P:

****

PART II: TPN, SURGERY AND TF

Ten days after Mrs. S's admission, her weight was 148 lbs (down 7 lbs). Diarrhea was a problem and she was not eating well. The adverse effects of floxuridine combined with her poor intake caused an additional decrease in hgb, hct, MCV, TLC, ser alb, and platelets. Her MD wrote the following orders:

1. D/C floxuridine
2. D/C diet and make pt NPO
3. 2 units of packed cells now
4. Have RD calculate TPN formula and flow rate
5. Schedule surgery in 7 days
6. Diphenoxylate hydrochloride (Lomotil)
7. D_5NS at 50 cc/h

****

QUESTIONS CONTINUED:
21. How many kcals are provided daily by the D_5NS at 50 cc/h?

22. Calculate a TPN formula for Mrs. S. In your calculations include the following:
    a. Calculate the grams of CHO and protein you would give per liter per day.
    b. List any additives you would use.
    c. Explain your flow rate progression from initial flow rate to final flow rate.
    d. Would you use IV lipids? Tell why or why not.
    e. If you used lipids, what percent would you use, how much would you use, and how would you administer (what method of administration and flow rate)?
    f. How many total kcals and how many grams of protein is this per day?
    g. What lab values would you monitor and how often should they be checked?
    h. Discuss the use of prealbumin or retinol binding protein in this case.

23. What is the mechanism of action of diphenoxylate hydrochloride (Lomotil)?

24. What nutritional complications could it have?

****

Mrs. S tolerated the TPN well. The side effects of floxuridine disappeared and Mrs. S felt a lot better. By the time she went to the OR she felt stronger and was in much better spirits. Her surgery was uneventful and she recovered without complications. A resection of the lower esophagus was done. The surrounding lymph nodes checked were negative for metastasis and the surgeons felt confident that they had removed all the cancer. A gastrostomy was also completed in surgery. The TPN was held during the surgery and $D_{10}W$ was hung in its place. TPN was restarted when Mrs. S was in the recovery room.

Post-op orders included:

1. N/G to low intermittent suction
2. Continue NPO
3. Restart TPN at rate RD recommends
4. Have RD evaluate pt for proper TF and administration when BS return
5. MS for pain prn
****

QUESTIONS CONTINUED:

25. At what flow rate and strength would you restart the TPN and how would you progress the flow rate?

26. Discuss the function of the N/G tube to low intermittent suction.

27. Discuss the relationship between surgery, BS, and refeeding. Include in your discussion the effects of hypoalbuminemia and the appropriate tube feeding for this condition.

28. Research the mechanism of action of morphine sulfate. Can you find any interaction this drug could have with the above relationship of BS and refeeding you just discussed?

29. Discuss why you would want to start the tube feeding as soon as possible.

30. Why was TPN discontinued and $D_{10}W$ hung in its place during surgery?

31. Discuss the alternative of using a tube feeding here instead of initiating TPN. In your discussion include the advantages and disadvantages of a tube feeding, what tube feeding you would use and why, and how you would recommend the feeding tube be placed.

32. Describe the gradual increase of TF with the accompanying decrease of TPN and tell how long you would expect to take before meeting Mrs. S's requirements with TF alone.

33. How long would it be before Mrs. S would start to eat again and what progression from TF to po feedings would you recommend?

34. What final diet would you recommend for Mrs. S to go home with?

35. Briefly define the following terms:

Resection:

Metastasis:

Gastrostomy:

ADDITIONAL OPTIONAL QUESTION:
Tube Feeding Drill:

36. Using the table below, compare several of the enteral nutritional supplements that would be appropriate for Mrs. S. (**L** *Hint: remember that everything tastes metallic or sweet and that she wants to swallow as little as possible.*)

Product	Producer	Form	Cal/ml	Non-pro cal/g N	Pro	CHO	Fat	Na mg	K mg	mOsm /kg water	Vol to meet RDA in ml	g of fiber /L	Free H$_2$O /L in ml

37. Complete another SOAP note on Mrs. S, following up on your last SOAP note.

S:

O:

A:

P:

RELATED REFERENCES

1. Chainani-Wu, N. (2002). Diet and oral, pharyngeal, and esophageal cancer. *Nutr Cancer.* 2002;44(2):104-26.

2. Fischbach, F.T. (2003). *A Manual of Laboratory & Diagnostic Tests.* 7th Ed. Philadelphia. J.B. Lippincott Company.

3. Girvin, G.W., Matsumoto, G.H., Bates, D.M., Garcia, J.M., Clyde, J.C., & Lin, P.H. (1995).Treating esophageal cancer with a combination of chemotherapy, radiation, and excision. *Am. J. Surg.* 169(5):557-9.

4. Gurski, R.R., Schirmer, C.C., Rosa, A.R., & Brentano, L. (2003). Nutritional assessment in patients with squamous cell carcinoma of the esophagus. *Hepatogastroenterology.* Nov-Dec;50(54):1943-7.

5. Hung, H.C., Huang, M.C., Lee, J.M., Wu, D.C., Hsu, H.K., & Wu, M.T. (2004). Association between diet and esophageal cancer in Taiwan. *J Gastroenterol Hepatol.* Jun;19(6):632-7.

6. Korn, W.M. (2004). Prevention and management of early esophageal cancer. *Curr Treat Options Oncol.* Oct;5(5):405-16.

7. Lee, J.H., Machtay, M., Unger, L.D., Weinstein, G.S., Weber, R.S., Chalian, A.A., & Rosenthal, D.I. (1998). Prophylactic gastrostomy tubes in patients undergoing intensive irradiation for cancer of the head and neck. *Arch. Otolaryngol. Head Neck Surg.* 124(8): 871-5.

8. Machin, J., & Shaw, C., (1998). A multidisciplinary approach to head and neck cancer. *Eur. J. Cancer Care.* 7(2):93-6.

9. Margolis, M., Alexander, P., Trachiotis, G.D., Gharagozloo, F., & Lipman, T. (2003). Percutaneous endoscopic gastrostomy before multimodality therapy in patients with esophageal cancer. *Ann Thorac Surg.* 2003 Nov;76(5):1694-7; discussion 1697-8.

10. Nelson, G.M. (1998). Biology of taste buds and the clinical problem of taste loss. *Anat. Rec.* 253(3):70-8.

11. Prasad, A.S, Beck., F.W., Doerr, T.D., Shamsa, F.H., Penny, H.S., Marks, S.C., Kaplan, J., Kucuk, O., & Matog, R.H. (1998). Nutritional and zinc status of head and neck cancer patients: an interpretive review. *J. Am. Coll. Nutr.* 17(5);409-18.

12. Prendergast, A. & Fulton, F.L. (1997) *Medical terminology: A Text/Workbook.* 4th Ed. Redwood City, California. Addison-Wesley Nursing.

13. Pronsky, Z.M., Redfern, C.M., Crowe, J. & Epstein, S. (2003) *Food Medication Interactions*, 13th Ed Phoenix, Arizona. Food-Medications Interactions, Publishers and Distributors.

14. Righi, P.D., Reddy, D.K., Weisberger, E.C., Johnson, M.S., Trerotola, S.O., Radpour, S., Johnson, P.E., & Stevens, C.E. (1998). Radiologic percutaneous gastrostomy: results in 56 patients with head and neck cancer. *Laryngoscope.* 108(7):1020-4.

15. Rolfes, S.R., Pinna, K. & Whitney, E. (2006). *Understanding Normal and Clinical Nutrition*, 7th Ed. West/Wadsworth.

16. Sikora, S.S., Ribeiro., U., Kane, J.M. 3rd, Landreneau, R.J., Lembersky, B., & Posner, M.C. (1998). Role of nutrition support during induction chemoradiation therapy in esophageal cancer. *J. Parenter. Enteral Nutr.* 22(1):18-21.

17. Spratto, G.R. & Woods, A.L. (2005). *PDR Nurse's Drug Handbook.* Thompson Delmar Learning, NY.

18. Taylor, P.R., Qiao, Y.L., Abnet, C.C., Dawsey, S.M., Yang, C.S., Gunter, E.W., Wang, W., Blot, W.J., Dong, Z.W., & Mark, S.D. (2003). Prospective study of serum vitamin E levels and esophageal and gastric cancers. *J Natl Cancer Inst.* Sep 17;95(18):1414-6.

19. Weisburger, J.H. (1998). Can cancer risks be altered by changing nutritional traditions? *Cancer.* 83(7):1278-81.

20. Wilkes, J.D. (1998). Prevention and treatment of oral mucositis following cancer chemotherapy. *Semin. Oncol.* 25(5):538-51.

CASE STUDY #31
COLON CANCER AND MALNUTRITION

INTRODUCTION
This is a study of colon cancer that leads to protein-calorie malnutrition and a home health care dilemma. The latest chemotherapy drugs are used. Basic nutrition and advanced nutritional assessment are necessary
****

SKILLS NEEDED

ABBREVIATIONS:
OTC and SC are the only new abbreviations used in the study (Appendix C).

LABORATORY VALUES:
You will need to be able to interpret the nutritional significance of the following laboratory values for this case study: BUN, Cl, Cr, glucose, hct, hgb, K, lymphocytes, MCH, MCHC, MCV, Mg, Na, P, RBC, ser alb, and WBC (Appendix B).

FORMULAS:
The formulas used in this case study include ideal body weight, percent ideal body weight, percent usual body weight, BEE using the Harris-Benedict equation, stress factors, and total energy and protein needs, all of which can be found in Appendix A, Tables 7, 8, 13, and 17.

MEDICATIONS:
Become familiar with the following medications before reading this case study. Note the diet-drug interactions, dosages and method of administration, gastrointestinal tract reactions, etc.
1. Synthroid (levothyroxine); 2. Cordarone (amiodarone hydrochloride); 3. Digoxin (Lanoxin); 4. Advil (ibuprofen); 5. Megace (megestrol acetate); 6. Lomotil (diphenoxylate hydrochloride with atropine sulfate); 7. Donnatal Tablets; 8. Kopectate; 9. Lovenox (enoxaparin); 10. Xeloda (capecitabine).
****

GW is a 75 YOWM who has worked hard as a dairy farmer in the south and, even though his son does most of the work now, he still works hard for his age. The long hours and hard work have kept him active and, unlike his four siblings, he has never had a weight problem. In fact, his weight has been on the low side of normal all of his life, weighing between 138 and 142 consistently. He is 5'7" tall. He has a Hx of hypothyroidism for which he takes Synthroid (levothyroxine). He also has a Hx of arrhythmias for which he takes 200 mg of Cordarone (amiodarone hydrochloride) and 0.25 mg of Digoxin (Lanoxin) daily. Recently, he started having diarrhea and noticed blood in his stool on occasion. He did not have a change in the way he felt other than being tired, but he thought that came with age. Being a stubborn man and not liking doctors, he refused to go see his physician. When the diarrhea and bleeding persisted and got worse, his wife stepped in and convinced him to make an appointment.

His family practitioner sent him to a gastroenterologist who scheduled him for a colonoscopy. A mass was found in the sigmoid colon and a biopsy was taken. The physician felt sure it was malignant and his suspicions were correct. GW was sent to a surgeon and surgery was planned immediately.
****

QUESTIONS:
1. Describe the action and any nutritional side effects of the following drugs:

Digoxin:

Synthroid:

Cordarone:

****

Upon admission GW weighed 135 lbs and his admission labs were as follows.

CBC							
TEST	**RESULT**	**REFERENCE UNITS** **Conventional SI**		**TEST**	**RESULT**	**REFERENCE UNITS** **Conventional SI**	
Hgb	12.8 g/dl	14 - 17.4 g/dl	140-174 g/L	WBC	5.2 10^3/µl	4.5-10.5 x 10^3/cells/ mm^3	4.5-10.5 x 10^9/L
Hct	36%	42 – 52%		% Lymph	23%	25 – 40% of total WBC	1500-4000 cells/mm^3
RBC	4.7x10^6/µ	3.6-5.0x10^6/L	3.6-5.0x10^{12}/L	MCH	27 pg/cell	26-34 pg/cell	0.40-.53 fmol/cell
MCV	76 µm^3	82-98µm^3	82-98 fL	MCHC	36 g/dl	32-36 g/dl	320-360 g/L

BASIC METABOLIC PACKAGE							
TEST	**RESULT**	**REFERENCE UNITS** **Conventional SI**		**TEST**	**RESULT**	**REFERENCE UNITS** **Conventional SI**	
Glu	80 mg/dl	70-110 mg/dl	3.8-6.1 mmol/L	Na	138 mEq/L	136-145 mEq/L	136-145 mmol/L
BUN	5 mg/dl	6-20 mg/dl	2.1-7.1 mmol/L	K	3.8 mEq/L	3.5-5.2 mEq/L	3.5-5.2 mmol/L
Cr	0.9 mg/dl	0.9-1.3 mg/dl	80-115 µmol/L	Cl	103 mEq/L	96-106 mEq/L	96-106 mmol/L
Ca	8.9 mg/dl	8.8-10.0 mg/dl	2.20-2.60 mmol/L	Mg	1.8 mEq/L	1.8 - 2.6 mEq/L	136-145 mmol/L
Ser alb	3.1 g/dl	3.5-4.8 g/dl	39-50 g/dl	P	2.5mg/dl	2.7-4.5 mg/dl	4.7-6.0 kPa

****

QUESTIONS CONTINUED:

2. Compare GW's UBW to his IBW. If his UBW has been slightly lower than his IBW all his life, is that of any major concern? Is the fact that he is now, upon admission to a hospital for colon cancer, a little below his UBW of concern? Explain.

3. Does the additional information obtained from the labs add any concern?

4.   If you were the oncology RD responsible for GW, what, if anything, should you do at this point?

****

The RD reviewed GW's chart and visited him and his wife to perform an admission screening prior to surgery. After an appropriate entry into his room and properly identifying GW, the conversation went something like this:

RD: Well, Mr. W, I want you to take me through a *typical* day when you are at home and feeling well. Tell me what time you get up and what is the first thing you have to eat or drink?

GW: I get up about 3 AM and get a cup of coffee.

RD: Three AM? Do you just get up to get coffee or what?

GW: You don't live on a farm do you? I'm a dairyman. I have to get my cows in for milking.

RD: At 3 AM? Every morning?

GW: Every morning, seven days a week.

RD: Oh, uh… well, uh... what do you put in your coffee?

GW: Nothing, I drink it black.

RD: Do you have anything else with your coffee?

GW: Nothing, I set the automatic coffee maker the night before and when I'm going out the door it's ready to go.

RD: I see. When are you finished with your cows?

GW: I come back in between 6 and 7 AM and my wife has breakfast.

RD: And what does breakfast consist of?

GW: I have cream of wheat every morning, a few strips of bacon, some toast and a cup of hot chocolate.

RD: Hot chocolate huh. Well, do you put anything on your toast?

GW: A little margarine.

RD: When is the next time you eat or drink?

GW: Welllll.... after I read the paper, about 8:30 or so, I usually go down to Corn Crib and sit around with some of my friends and have some more coffee.

RD: The corn crib? Is that in your barn?

GW: Noooo, that's the name of a country store down the road. We have a little corner in there where we get together in the morning and solve the world's problems.

RD: Oh. Do you have anything with your coffee?

GW: Not usually. I still drink it black.

RD: When is the next time you have something to eat or drink?

GW: Lunch time. I go back to the house about 10:30 or 11 and have lunch.

RD: Isn't that early for lunch?

GW: Not when you get up at 3 o'clock it's not.

RD: No, I guess not. What do have to eat then?

GW: Well, we always have a vegetable, like green beans or squash.... always some kind of beans or peas, like butter beans or pink-eye purple-hull Crowder peas.... some kind of meat.... like some ribs or pork chops.... and cornbread, always have to have cornbread.

RD: Wow!... What do you have to drink?

GW: Sweet tea.

RD: When is the next time you have something to eat or drink?

GW: Suppertime, about 5:30. We usually eat light at supper, some soup or cereal, toast, something like that.

RD: How about before you go to bed, do you have anything then?

GW: Usually not.

GW actually did not get up every morning at 3 AM like he used to; his son does most of the early morning milking, but he does get up with him some of the time. Old habits are hard to break. He seldom goes out in the afternoon any more for the afternoon milking like he used to. Lately, he has not been getting up early at all because he has been so tired.

The surgical procedure went as well as could be expected. After surgery, GW received two units of whole blood because of his previous bleeding and the blood lost during surgery. The tumor was in the distal sigmoid. A double barrel colostomy was performed with the proximal descending colon being brought to the outside for defecation. The distal end of the sigmoid was also brought to the outside. The colon in-between was removed. The surgeons planned on giving GW chemotherapy and allowing his colon to heal before performing another surgical procedure in three months to reconnect the two ends of the colon. After resection, GW would be able to have normal bowel movements. After spending a few days in ICU, GW returned to a private room. He was started on clear liquids and advanced to full liquids but everything he drank gave him diarrhea. He was given a nutritional supplement to drink with meals and between meals but he did not like it. He liked chocolate but he said chocolate and vanilla soured on his

stomach. GW now weighed 125 lbs, his serum albumin was 2.7 g/dl, and prealbumin was 7 mg/dl. Iatrogenic malnutrition could now be added to his list of problems. A feeding tube was placed and the physician wrote an order for the dietitian to suggest a tube feeding and a feeding plan.
****
5. Calculate GW's caloric and protein needs.

6. What comments do you have about the dietitian's interview? Point out the good and bad points and tell what you would do differently.

7. What tube feeding would you recommend and why? Would you use a tube feeding with special additives that would be of benefit to GW? What flow rate would you start with and how would you progress?

8. Compare several of the possible appropriate tube feedings for GW.

Product	Producer	Form	Cal/ml	Non-pro cal/g N	g/L			Na mg	K mg	mOsm /kg water	Vol to meet RDA in ml	g of fiber /L	Free H$_2$O /L in ml
					Pro	CHO	Fat						

9. Research prealbumin and describe exactly what it consists of and its relationship to albumin and total protein.

****

Because of the pain GW was having, and because of the weakness he was experiencing from the loss of blood and not eating, he was difficult to get out of bed and walk as was ordered. His inactivity caused stasis in his legs and he started having pain in his left calf and soreness to touch. He had developed thrombophlebitis and had to be put on heparin. The heparin caused his blood to be too thin and he started spontaneous bleeding. This was finally corrected and GW eventually began tolerating his tube feeding better, but still had some problems with diarrhea. He gained three pounds back and the feeding tube was removed. GW was taking some food by mouth and probiotics were initiated but he continued to have diarrhea, severe at times. He did not like the colostomy and complained of abdominal cramps almost continuously. GW's main problem now was eating and gaining his strength back. There was nothing else they could do for him in the hospital and the physician thought that his home environment would be more conducive to GW eating so he discharged him with the following orders:

▶ Advil (ibuprofen) OTC for pain
▶ Megace (megestrol acetate) 4 teas/d 40mg/ml for appetite
▶ Lomotil (diphenoxylate hydrochloride with atropine sulfate) 2.5 mg bid for diarrhea
▶ Donnatal Tablets 1 or 2 qid for diarrhea
▶ Kopectate, OTC for diarrhea
▶ Lovenox (enoxaparin) 0.8 ml (80 mg/0.8 ml) SC every day for blood clots

****

10. Research the following drugs and describe their function, side effects, and nutritional implications.

Megace:

Lomitil:

Donnatal Tablets:

Kopectate:

Advil:

11. What are probiotics and how could they help with diarrhea?

12. Prepare a SOAP note for GW's discharge.

S:
O:
A:
P:

13. Suppose GW was a much younger man that still had to work to support his family, and suppose that he did not have quite as much weight loss and his diarrhea was mild. As an oncology dietitian you are asked to give GW a discharge diet instruction. After a few weeks, GW intends to be back at work at 3 AM in the morning. Knowing GW's likes and dislikes from your interview, how would you instruct GW on the foods and supplements he should take? What would you do about the early morning schedule?

14. On a separate sheet of paper, prepare a menu for GW based on the information listed in question 12.
****

GW went home but continued with diarrhea for several days. Even with the Megace, his appetite was poor. GW was not going to have to get up at 3 AM to attend to his cows because of his age and his condition; his son would do that. His schedule changed to that of a more normal person, getting up around 7 AM, having breakfast, etc. He tried taking supplements between meals but could not tolerate them. He continued to slowly lose weight, constantly being bothered with diarrhea. In less than the planned three months, he went back into the hospital to have his colon reattached. The physicians were thinking that this would help his diarrhea and he would eat more. His hospital stay was uneventful as far as the surgery was concerned, but further tests revealed a suspicious spot on his liver and two on his left lung. Even with this news, GW returned home optimistic that he would be able to eat again. His weight dropped because of the surgery and was now down to 125 lbs. He went home with the same meds as before and a new medication he was to take when he got over the diarrhea..

Once home the second time, his new routine included a light breakfast, a small amount of nutrition at mid-morning and at lunch, a larger evening meal, and a banana and more supplement at night. He alternated between Ensure and Boost because he got tired of the same supplements over and over. He has not been able to take in enough supplements to gain weight or strength. He still has diarrhea though it is not as bad. GW now has protein-calorie malnutrition and is depressed.

The physician's plan was to increase GW's weight and strength and then start Xeloda, an oral chemotherapy medication. Xeloda was ordered to be taken as six 500 mg tablets, three twice a day 12 hours apart, for three weeks. A rest period of one week would be followed by another three-week treatment. This was to be repeated four times. Xeloda could not be started until GW was stronger because the side effects are harsh, including severe diarrhea. GW asked around and found two people that took this drug and had a variety of severe side effects. GW became more depressed and decided he did not want to take the drug.
****

15. Research the medication Xeloda and record its action and side effects.

16. Assume you are a home health dietitian and are assigned to GW. You have access to his chart and all of the information above. You visit him at home and do a complete assessment. Answer the questions below on a separate sheet of paper.

    a. Outline the components of your home health assessment.
    b. Considering protein-calorie malnutrition, what are you going to recommend as a goal for GW's calorie and protein intake?
    c. What route of administration, or combination of routes, are you going to recommend?
    d. Your above assessment may be completely correct and your recommendations may be the best anybody could make, but you have a problem. GW thinks he still has cancer and he thinks the cure is worse than the cause so he thinks he is going to die and does not want to eat. How are you going to handle this problem?

RELATED REFERENCES

1. Breier-Mackie S, & Newell CJ. Home parenteral nutrition: an ethical decision making dilemma. (2002). *Aust J Adv Nurs.* Jun-Sep;19(4):27-32.

2. Chao, A., Connell, C.J., Jacobs, E.J., McCullough, M.L., Patel, A.V., Calle, E.E., Cokkinides, V.E., & Thun, M.J. (2004). Amount, type, and timing of recreational physical activity in relation to colon and rectal cancer in older adults: the Cancer Prevention Study II Nutrition Cohort. *Cancer Epidemiol Biomarkers Prev.* Dec;13(12):2187-95.

3. Fischbach, F.T. (2003). *A Manual of Laboratory & Diagnostic Tests.* 7th Ed. Philadelphia. J.B. Lippincott Company.

4. Junien, C., & Gallou, C. (2004). Cancer nutrigenomics. *World Rev Nutr Diet.* ;93:210-69.

5. Marse, H., Van Cutsem, E., Grothey, A., & Valverde, S. (2004). Management of adverse events and other practical considerations in patients receiving capecitabine (Xeloda). *Eur J Oncol Nurs.* 8 Suppl 1:S16-30.

6. Martinez, M.E. (2005). Primary prevention of colorectal cancer: lifestyle, nutrition, exercise. *Recent Results Cancer Res.* ;166:177-211.

7. Nelson, G.M. (1998). Biology of taste buds and the clinical problem of taste loss. *Anat. Rec.* 253(3):70-8.

8. O'Connell, M.J. (2004). Current status of adjuvant therapy for colorectal cancer. *Oncology* (Huntingt). (6):751-5; discussion 755-8.

9. Okamoto, K., Fukatsu, K., Ueno, C., Shinto, E., Hashiguchi, Y., Nagayoshi, H., Hiraide, H., & Mochizuki, H. (2005). T lymphocyte numbers in human gut associated lymphoid tissue are reduced without enteral nutrition. *JPEN J Parenter Enteral Nutr.* Jan-Feb;29(1):56-8.

10. Ooi, S.E., Chen, G.W., & Chou, C.T. (2004). Adequate nourishment through total parenteral nutrition treatment may augment immune function in patients with colon cancer. *Arch Med Res.* Jul-Aug;35(4):289-93.

11. Prendergast, A. & Fulton, F.L. (1997) *Medical terminology: A Text/Workbook.* 4th Ed. Redwood City, California. Addison-Wesley Nursing.

12. Pronsky, Z.M., Redfern, C.M., Crowe, J. & Epstein, S. (2003) *Food Medication Interactions*, 13th Ed Phoenix, Arizona. Food-Medications Interactions, Publishers and Distributors.

13. Rolfes, S.R., Pinna, K. & Whitney, E. (2006). *Understanding Normal and Clinical Nutrition*, 7th Ed. West/Wadsworth.

14. Scheithauer, W., McKendrick, J., Begbie, S., Borner, M., Burns, W.I., Burris, H.A., Cassidy, J., Jodrell, D., Koralewski, P., Levine, E.L., Marschner, N., Maroun, J., Garcia-Alfonso, P.,Tujakowski, J., Van Hazel, G., Wong, A., Zaluski, J., Twelves, C.; X-ACT Study Group. (2003). Oral capecitabine as an alternative to i.v. 5-fluorouracil-based adjuvant therapy for colon cancer: safety results of a randomized, phase III trial. *Ann Oncol.* Dec;14(12):1735-43.

15. Spratto, G.R. & Woods, A.L. (2005). *PDR Nurse's Drug Handbook.* Thompson Delmar Learning, NY.

16. Willett, W.C. (2005). Diet and cancer: an evolving picture. *JAMA.* Jan 12;293(2):233-4.

17. Weisburger, J.H. (1998). Can cancer risks be altered by changing nutritional traditions? *Cancer.* 83(7):1278-81.

18. Wong, N.S., Chang, B.M., Toh, H.C., & Koo, W.H. (2004). Inflammatory metastatic carcinoma of the colon: a case report and review of the literature. *Tumori.* Mar-Apr;90(2):253-5.

CASE STUDY #32
AIDS

INTRODUCTION

A patient with AIDS could have pneumonia, a liver complication, renal involvement, endocarditis, or any combination of the above. Usually with these problems, diarrhea, GI cramps, and infections of the mouth and esophagus are common. This complicates nutritional therapy and frequently a TF or TPN is necessary. Each case is different and has to be evaluated with the general nutritional goals plus the additional goals for each complication.

****

SKILLS NEEDED

ABBREVIATIONS:

Knowledge of the following abbreviations is required in order to understand this case. You should learn these abbreviations before you begin the study. AIDS, ARC, D_5W, HIV, TF, and TPN (Appendix C).

FORMULAS:

The formulas used in this case study include: ideal body weight, caloric needs using the Harris-Benedict equation, total caloric and protein requirements, simple percentages for tube feeding and I.V. calculations, and flow rates (Appendix A, Tables 7, 8, and 17).

MEDICATIONS:

Become familiar with the following medications before reading the case study. Note the diet-drug interactions, dosages and methods of administration, gastrointestinal tract reactions, etc.
1. Retrovir (zidovudine, or formally AZT); 2. Vincasar PFS (vincristine sulfate);
3. Mycostatin (nystatin).

****

LT is a 35 YOWM who is employed in a major department store. He is a buyer for the men's clothing department and has been successful in his job for the past 10 years. He brags about how hard he works during the week and how hard he parties on weekends. He calls himself a fast-lane single and does not hesitate to admit that he has tried various drugs. As with many drug users, the pills and marijuana led to I.V. drug abuse. About 2 years ago, he started to notice that he was becoming weaker and easily fatigued. His appetite was poor and he was losing weight. He woke up during the night soaking wet with severe sweats. Before the symptoms started, LT weighed 190 lbs and was 6'1". When he was approaching 170 lbs, he went to a physician. Some blood work was done and indicated that he had elevated WBC, elevated sedimentation rate, and a normocytic normochromic anemia. He was admitted to the hospital. Further tests indicated that he had infective endocarditis. He underwent antibiotic therapy and was sick for several weeks. He continued to lose weight to 165 lbs. While in the hospital, he was also tested for AIDS since endocarditis is not an uncommon complication of I.V. drug abuse. LT tested HIV+. LT did not show any symptoms of AIDS in this hospitalization, but his physician told him that he should be evaluated frequently. Any change in his health status should be reported to the physician immediately.

Since LT had been using I.V. drugs for some time, it was not known how long it was since LT had been exposed to the AIDS virus. Not long after LT's discharge from the hospital, he began to have generalized lymphadenopathy. He returned to his physician and was diagnosed as having ARC. During this time his temperature was elevated and he was still losing weight. He was beginning to experience some abdominal cramps and diarrhea. His physician suggested that he start on zidovudine (Retrovir). Not long after this, LT noticed an unusual bump on his chest. When he went back to his physician, it was diagnosed as Kaposi's sarcoma. He was given vincristine sulfate (Vincasar PFS) to treat the Kaposi's sarcoma.

****

QUESTIONS:

1. List the symptoms of AIDS that were manifested in LT.

2. What are the general nutritional goals for a patient with AIDS?

3. Calculate LT's total energy needs using the Harris-Benedict equation and appropriate stress factor (Appendix A, Table 17).

4. Calculate his protein needs.

5. Are there any vitamins or minerals LT should be taking in therapeutic doses? Explain your answer.

6. Give the mechanism of action of the following drugs:

   Vincristine sulfate (Vincasar PFS):

   Zidovudine (Retrovir):

7. List any nutritional complications of each of these drugs:

   Vincristine sulfate (Vincasar PFS):

   Zidovudine (Retrovir):

****

Not long after he had taken these medications, LT's symptoms increased with an elevated temperature (which was now 100.6° F), N/V, headaches, diarrhea, malaise, and extreme fatigue. He had to take a leave of absence from work. He developed a bad cough and chest congestion. His physician admitted him to the hospital for tests and found LT to have a Pneumocystis pneumonia caused by Pneumocystis carinii. During LT's hospital stay, he continued to have complications. He experienced infections such as candidiasis. This made it very difficult for him to eat and required another medication, nystatin (Mycostatin). LT also experienced severe diarrhea and he became very depressed. His ser alb was 2.2 g/dl. His desire to eat was affected, so the RD recommended that LT be given a tube feeding. The physician agreed. A feeding tube was placed into the small bowel and two I.V.s were infusing, one with 3NS @ 25 cc/hr for medications and one with D_5W @ 50 cc/hr.

****

QUESTIONS CONTINUED:

8. What diet therapy would you recommend for LT considering the above conditions? Would his stress factor and energy needs change? Explain your answer.

9. Why would candidiasis make it difficult to eat?

10. What is nystatin (Mycostatin)? List its possible adverse reactions.

11. What is the significance of the ser alb being 2.2 g/dl? Discuss the pathophysiological effects this could have on LT's GI tract.

12. From LT's history, summarize all of the possible causes of diarrhea and explain how they might cause diarrhea.

13. Discuss what could be done, if anything, to check LT's diarrhea.

14. What tube feeding would you recommend for LT? Explain your choice.

15. How many grams of CHO and kcals is LT receiving from the D_5W @ 50 cc/hr? Show your work.

16. How would you manage the TF, i.e., what strength and flow rate would you start with and how would you progress to the final rate? Include the final rate that you hope to achieve.

17. Assuming you reach the final rate in your goals, how many kcals and how much protein will this provide? Show your work.

18. Add to this the kcals from the D_5W and compare the total to the energy requirement you previously calculated. Discuss your results.

19. What criteria would you use to suggest a change from enteral to parenteral nutrition?

20. Define the following terms:

Lymphadenopathy:

Normocytic Normochromic Anemia:

Kaposi's sarcoma:

Endocarditis:

HIV Virus:

Pneumocystis pneumonia:

Pneumocystis carinii:

Malaise:

Candidiasis:

ARC:

ADDITIONAL OPTIONAL QUESTION:
Tube Feeding Drill:

21. Some research indicates that the addition of glutamine, arginine, and/or fish oils may be of some benefit to immunocompromised patients, patients with atrophic GI tracts, and/or edematous guts. Using the table below, compare several of the enteral nutritional supplements that would be appropriate for one or more of these conditions.

Product	Producer	F o r m	Cal/ ml	Non-pro cal/g N	g/L			Na mg	K mg	mOsm /kg water	Vol to meet RDA in ml	g of fiber /L	Free H$_2$O /L in ml
					Pro	CHO	Fat						

22. Using the space below, prepare a SOAP note on LT.

S:
O:
A:
P:

RELATED REFERENCES

1. Anabwani, G. & Navario, P. (2005). Nutrition and HIV/AIDS in sub-Saharan Africa: An overview. *Nutrition.* Jan;21(1):96-9.

2. Barker, D., Younger, N., MooSang, M., & McKenzie, C.A. (2004). HIV serostatus and recovery from severe childhood malnutrition. A retrospective matched case-control study. *West Indian Med. J.* Mar;53(2):89-94.

3. Beaugerie, L., Carbonnel, F., Carrat, F., Rached, A.A., Masio, C., Genre, J.P., Rozenbaum, W., & Cosnes, J. (1998). Factors of weight loss in patients with HIV and chronic diarrhea. *J. Acquir Immune Defic. Syndr. Hum. Retrovirol.* 1;19(1);34-9.

4. Charlin, V., Carrasco, F., Sepulveda, C., Torres, M., & Kehr, J. (2002). Nutritional supplementation according to energy and protein requirements in malnourished HIV-infected patients. *Arch Latinoam Nutr.* Sep;52(3):267-73.

5. Crotty, B., McDonald, J., Mijch, A.M., & Smallwood, R.A. (1998). Percutaneous endoscopic gastrostomy feeding in AIDS. *J. Gastroenterol. Hepatol.* 13(4):371-5.

6. Davidhizar, R. & Dunn, C. (1998). Nutrition and the client with AIDS. *J. Pract. Nurs.* 48(1):16-28.

7. Fields-Gardner, C., Fergusson, P.; & American Dietetic Association; Dietitians of Canada. (2004). Position of the American Dietetic Association and Dietitians of Canada: nutrition intervention in the care of persons with human immunodeficiency virus infection. *J Am Diet Assoc* Sep;104(9):1425-41.

8. Fischbach, F.T. (2003). *A Manual of Laboratory & Diagnostic Tests.* 7th Ed. Philadelphia. J.B. Lippincott Company.

9. Gerrior, J.L., Bell, S.J., & Wanke, C.A. (1997). Oral nutrition for the patient with HIV infection. *Nurs. Clin. North Am.* 32(4):813-30.

10. Griffiths, R.D. (2003). Specialized nutrition support in critically ill patients. *Curr Opin Crit Care.* Aug;9(4):249-59.

11. Grinspoon, S., Mulligan, K.; & Department of Health and Human Services Working Group on the Prevention and Treatment of Wasting and Weight Loss. (2003). Weight loss and wasting in patients infected with human immunodeficiency virus. *Clin Infect Dis.* Apr 1;36(Suppl 2):S69-78.

12. Henry, F.J. (2003). Nutrition in AIDS management. An opportunity being lost. *West Indian Med J.* Jun;52(2):89-90.

13. Kotler, D.P. (1998). Human immunodeficiency virus-related wasting: malabsorption syndromes. *Semin. Oncol.* 25(2 Suppl 6): 70-5.

14. Lee, R.D., Nieman, D.C., & Nieman, D. (2002). *Nutritional Assessment.* 3rd Ed. McGraw-Hill.

15. Matarese, L.E. (1998). Enteral feeding solutions. *Gastrointest. Endosc. Clin. N. Am.* 8(3):593-609.

16. Moscardini, C., Touger-Decker, R., & Ostrowski, M.B. (1997). Nutritional needs in the AIDS patient. Recognizing and treating wasting syndrome. *Adv. Nurse Pract.* 5(6):34-7, 41-2.

17. Pichard, C., Sudre, P., Karsegard, V., Yerly, S., Slosman, D.O., Delley, V., Perrin, L. & Hirschel, B. (1998). A randomized double-blind controlled study of 6 months or oral nutritional supplementation with arginine and omega-3 fatty acids in HIV-infected patients. Swiss HIV Cohort Study. *AIDS.* 1;12(1):53-63.

18. Position of the American Dietetic Association and Dietitians of Canada: Nutrition intervention in the care of persons with human immunodeficiency virus infection http://www.eatright.org/Member/PolicyInitiatives/index_21020.cfm

19. Prendergast, A. & Fulton, F.L. (1997) *Medical terminology: A Text/Workbook.* 4th Ed. Redwood City, California. Addison-Wesley Nursing.

20. Pronsky, Z.M., Redfern, C.M., Crowe, J. & Epstein, S. (2003) *Food Medication Interactions*, 13th Ed Phoenix, Arizona. Food-Medications Interactions, Publishers and Distributors.

21. Rabeneck, L., Palmer, A., Knowles, J.B., Seidehamel, R.J., Harris, C.L., Merkel, K.L., Risser, J.M., & Akrabawi, S.S. (1998). A randomized controlled trial evaluating nutrition counseling with or without oral supplementation in malnourished HIV-infected patients. *J. Am. Diet. Assoc.* 98(4):434-8.

22. Rolfes, S.R., Pinna, K. & Whitney, E. (2006). *Understanding Normal and Clinical Nutrition*, 7th Ed. West/Wadsworth.

23. Salomon, S.B., Jung, J., Voss, T., Suguitan, A., Rowe, W.B., & Madsen, D.C. (1998). An elemental diet containing medium-chain triglycerides and enzymatically hydrolyzed protein can improve gastrointestinal tolerance in people infected with HIV. *J Am Diet* Assoc. *98(4):460-2.*

24. Sherlekar, S., & Udipi, S.A. (2002). Role of nutrition in the management of HIV infection/AIDS *J Indian Med Assoc.* Jun;100(6):385-90.

25. Spratto, G.R. & Woods, A.L. (2005). *PDR Nurse's Drug Handbook.* Thompson Delmar Learning, NY.

26. U.S. National Library of Medicine. (1997). Important Therapeutic Information on Prevention of Recurrent Pneumocystis Carinii Pneumonia in Persons with AIDS. http://www.nlm.nih.gov/

27. Ware, L.J., Wootton, S.A., Morlese, J.M., Gazzard, B.G., & Jackson, A.A. (2002). The paradox of improved antiretroviral therapy in HIV: potential for nutritional modulation? *Proc Nutr Soc* Feb;61(1):131-6.

CASE STUDY #33
PERITONEAL DIALYSIS

INTRODUCTION

This study examines the nutritional treatment of a patient with end stage renal disease who is receiving peritoneal dialysis. The student should review the medical nutrition therapy for the various types of dialysis treatments prior to studying this case.
****

SKILLS NEEDED

ABBREVIATIONS:
Knowledge of the following abbreviations is required in order to understand this case. You should learn these abbreviations before you begin to read the study. CAPD, ESRD, HD, and PD (Appendix C).

LABORATORY VALUES:
You will need to be able to interpret the nutritional significance of the following laboratory values for this case study: BUN, Ca, Cl, Cr, glucose, K, Mg, Na, P, and ser alb (Appendix B).

FORMULAS:
The formulas used in this case study include metric conversions, ideal body weight (Appendix A, Tables 1, 2, 7, and 8 and Information Box 33-1) and energy expenditure for renal patients.

MEDICATIONS:
Become familiar with the following medications before reading the case study. Note the diet-drug interactions, dosages and methods of administration, gastrointestinal tract reactions, etc.
1. Fosrenol (lanthanum carbonate); 2. Aranesp (darbepoetin alfa); 3. Hectorol (doxercalciferol);
4. Aldomet Hydrochloride (methyldopa).
****

BT is a 45 YOWM who is a successful executive and has a history of malignant hypertension. Because of his lifestyle, it was not convenient for him to comply with his diet and medication regimens. As a result, BT was diagnosed with ESRD and required dialysis. Hemodialysis was not an option for him because it required that he sit still for at least three hours three times a week. He is a very busy man and did not have time for hemodialysis. When continuous ambulatory peritoneal dialysis (CAPD) was described to him, it seemed like his best option. A catheter was surgically placed into his peritoneal space and he was instructed on how to complete the procedure of CAPD. BT has been on CAPD for three years. Periodically, BT meets with the dietitian for an evaluation. In his last evaluation the following information was obtained from his medical record:

BT's ht is 177.8 cm and he weighs 75 kg. His usual body weight prior to renal failure was 70 kg. His daily CAPD dialysate prescription is as follows: 2 exchanges of 4.25% dextrose alternating with 2 exchanges of 1.5% dextrose, each exchange to dwell in his peritoneum for 4 hrs during waking hours; 1 exchange of 2.5% dextrose to dwell in his peritoneum for 6 hrs during sleeping hours. An exchange consist of 2 L.

His nutritional prescription included the following: 35 kcals/kg of IBW, 1.2 g of protein per kg of IBW, 3 g of Na, K unrestricted, 2000 ml of fluid + urinary output, Ca supplemented by medication, and 15 mg of Phos per kg of IBW. The dietitian discussed BT's diet with him and obtained a 24-hour recall. She was convinced that BT was complying with his diet and medication plans reasonably well. Upon her evaluation, she recommended reducing his kcals to 25/kg of IBW, increasing his protein to 1.4 g/kg of IBW, increasing Na to 4g, increasing his calcium medication (calcium acetate), and letting K, Phos, and fluid remain the same.

His lab values were as follows:

BASIC METABOLIC PACKAGE							
TEST	**RESULT**	**REFERENCE UNITS** Conventional	**SI**	**TEST**	**RESULT**	**REFERENCE UNITS** Conventional	**SI**
Glu	105 mg/dl	70-110 mg/dl	3.8-6.1 mmol/L	Na	133 mEq/L	136-145 mEq/L	136-145 mmol/L
BUN	60 mg/dl	6-20 mg/dl	2.1-7.1 mmol/L	K	4.8 mEq/L	3.5-5.2 mEq/L	3.5-5.2 mmol/L
Cr	7.0 mg/dl	0.9-1.3 mg/dl	80-115 µmol/L	Cl	100 mEq/L	96-106 mEq/L	96-106 mmol/L
Ca	8.8 mg/dl	8.8-10.0 mg/dl	2.20-2.60 mmol/L	Mg	2.0 mEq/L	1.8 - 2.6 mEq/L	136-145 mmol/L
Ser alb	3.7 g/dl	3.5-4.8 g/dl	39-50 g/dl	P	6.2mg/dl	2.7-4.5 mg/dl	4.7-6.0 kPa

****

QUESTIONS:

1. Define the following terms:

    Malignant hypertension:

    Dialysate:

    Continuous Peritoneal Ambulatory Dialysis:

2. Convert BT's height and weight from metric to English and determine his IBW (Appendix A, Tables 1, 2, 7 and 8).

3. Calculate the kcals and grams of protein, Na, and phos BT should be consuming in the original diet plan and the new plan recommended by the dietitian.

	Original Plan	New Plan
Kcals		
Protein		
Na		
Phos		

****

BT's medications included:

1   Fosrenol (lanthanum carbonate)
2   Aranesp (darbepoetin alfa)
3   Hectorol (doxercalciferol)
4   Aldomet Hydrochloride (methyldopa).
****

Information Box 33 – 1

Peritoneal dialysis effectively removes waste products from the blood by making use of the semi-permeable membrane of the peritoneum. After the surgical implantation of a catheter into the peritoneal cavity, a concentrated dialysate containing dextrose is infused into the peritoneum. Waste products diffuse from the blood across the peritoneum into the dialysate. This method is effective but not perfect. Substances other than waste products also diffuse into the dialysate, such as amino acids. Also, since the concentration of glucose in the dialysate is higher than the concentration of glucose in the blood, glucose diffuses across the peritoneum into the blood. This can be a significant amount of glucose and has to be accounted for. The volume of the dialysate and concentration of glucose in the dialysate varies from treatment to treatment. This makes it difficult to place a constant value on the amount of glucose that may infuse into the blood per treatment. The following formula is used to estimate the calories obtained from peritoneal dialysis:

$Y = [(11.3X) - 10.9] \times L$ of dialysate x 3.7 kcal/g of glucose where:
Y = grams of glucose absorbed per liter of dialysate
X = the concentration of glucose in g/L
L = a liter and 1g of glucose = 3.7 kcals

The possible concentrations of glucose in dialysate include:
1.5% dextrose dialysate = 1.3 g of glucose/dL absorbed
2.5% dextrose dialysate = 2.2 g glucose/dL absorbed
4.25% dextrose dialysate = 3.8 g glucose/dL absorbed

Example: If the dialysate prescription consisted of 3 exchanges of 1.5%, 2 exchanges of 2.5%, and 3 exchanges of 4.25% glucose, how many kcals would diffuse from the dialysate? Each exchange is 2 L.

1.   Determine the grams of glucose absorbed from the various exchanges by multiplying the number of exchanges by the liters per exchange times the glucose concentration.
      3 exchanges x 2L x 1.3 g/dl = 7.8 g
      2 exchanges x 2L x 2.2 g/dl = 8.8 g
      3 exchanges x 2L x 3.8 g/dl = 22.8 g

2.   Add the total grams of glucose diffused.   Total = 7.8 + 8.8 + 22.8 = 34.4 g

3.   Determine the grams of glucose per liter (X) by dividing the total grams by the total liters.
      34.4/16 = 2.15 g glucose/L

4.   Plug X into the formula
      Y   = [11.3 x 2.15 - 10.9] x 16 L x 3.7 kcal/g glucose =
             = 13.4 x 59.2
             = 793 kcals absorbed

For further explanation, see reference #27. There are other methods for making this calculation. An excellent summary and explanation can be found in reference #9.

4. Calculate the kcals BT is receiving from the dialysate described in his prescription.

5. Why is the caloric value for glucose in the above formula 3.7 kcals per gram instead of the usual 4 kcals per gram?

6. Usually the amounts of dietary protein, Na, K, and fluids allowed on CAPD are more than what are allowed for HD and PD. The kcal allotment for CAPD is usually lower than HD and PD. Explain why this is so.

7. If BT was following his diet and medication plans as prescribed, the dietitian was making her determinations based on his anthropometric measurements and lab values. Using these two parameters, give possible explanations for the changes the dietitian recommended in BT's nutrition care plan.

Kcals:

Protein:

Na:

Ca:

8. Why would she recommend K, phos, and fluid remain the same?

9. Compare the differences between hemodialysis, peritoneal dialysis, and continuous ambulatory peritoneal dialysis as related to kcals, protein, Na, K, Phos, and fluid intake.

	HD	PD	CAPD
Kcals			
Protein			
Na			
K			
Phos			
Fluid			

10. List the advantages/disadvantages of hemodialysis, peritoneal dialysis, and continuous ambulatory peritoneal dialysis.

	Advantages	Disadvantages
HD		
PD		
CAPD		

11. It is recommended that at least 50% of the protein fed to PD patients be of HBV. What does that mean and why is it important?

12. Today some are using a new glucose polymer, icodextrin, in peritoneal dialysis in place of glucose. Research icodextrin and describe the results reported thus far for this new polymer. In which patients might this be especially useful?

13. What is the pharmacological classification of BT's drugs?

    Fosrenol:

    Aranesp:

    Hectorol:

    Aldomet:

14. Describe the relationships of Fosrenol, Aranesp, and Hectorol to ESRD.

    Fosrenol

    Aranesp:

    Hectorol:

15. Another medical problem that patients with ESRD have to contend with is renalosteodystrophy. Relate why this is a concern.

16. Calcium acetate is the most effective phosphate binder for ESRD patients. Aluminum hydroxide gels used to be the treatment of choice years ago. Explain why these gels are no longer recommended for ESRD.

RELATED REFERENCES

1. Adamson, J.W. & Eschbach, J.W. (1998). Erythropoietin for end-stage renal disease. *N.Engl. J. Med.* 27;339(9):625-7.

2. Bannister, D.K., Acchiardo, S.R., Moore, L.W., & Kraus, A.P. Jr. (1987). Nutritional effects of peritonitis in continuous ambulatory peritoneal dialysis (CAPD) patient. *J. Am. Diet. Assoc.* 87(1):53-6.

3. Bergstrom, J., Wang, T., & Lindholm, B. (1998). Factors contributing to catabolism in end-stage renal disease patients. *Miner. Electrolyte Metab.* 24(1):92-101.

4. Bennett, C.L., Luminar,i S., Nissenson, A.R., Tallman, M.S., Klinge, S.A., McWilliams, N., McKoy, J.M., Kim, B., Lyons, E.A., Trifilio, S.M., Raisch, D.W., Evens, A.M., Kuzel, T.M., Schumock, G.T.,Belknap, S.M., Locatelli, F., Rossert, J., & Casadevall, N. (2004). Pure red-cell aplasia and epoetin therapy. *N Engl J Med.* Sep 30;351(14):1403-8.

5. Besarab, A., Bolton, W.K., Browne, J.K., Egrie, J.C., Nissenson, A.R., Okamoto, D.M., Schwab, S.J., & Goodkin, D.A. (1998). The effects of normal as compared with low hematocrit values in patients with cardiac disease who are receiving hemodialysis and epoetin. *N. Engl. J. Med.* 27;339(9):584-90.

6. Bodnar, D.M., Busch, S., Fuchs, J., Piedmonte, M., & Schreiber, M. (1993). Estimating glucose absorption in peritoneal dialysis using peritoneal equilibration tests. *Adv Perit Dial.* 9:114-8.

7. Chertow, G.M., Bullard, A., & Lazarus, J.M. (1996). Nutrition and the dialysis patient. *Am. J. Nephrol.* 16(1):79-89.

8. Eknoyan, G. (2003). Meeting the challenges of the new K/DOQI guidelines. *Am J Kidney Dis.* Jun;41(5 Suppl):3-10.

9. Fischbach, F.T. (2003). *A Manual of Laboratory & Diagnostic Tests.* 7th Ed. Philadelphia. J.B. Lippincott Company.

10. Forbes, L. (2004). Glucose Absorption PD. *PD Serve Global Quarterly Newsletter*, Vol 8, No. 1. http://www.pdserve.com/pdserve/pdserve.nsf/AttachmentsByTitle/PDF_PDServe:Vol+8,+No+1/$FILE/PDServe+composite+final+pdf.pdf.

11. Fouque, D. (1997). Causes and interventions for malnutrition in patients undergoing maintenance dialysis. *Blood Purif.* 15(2):112-20.

12. Gradden, C.W., Ahmad, R., & Bell, G.M. (2001). Peritoneal dialysis: new developments and new problems. *Diabetic Medicine*, 18:5; 360-363.

13. Grzegorzewska, A.E., & Mariak, I. (2003). Differences in clinical and laboratory data of peritoneal dialysis patients selected according to body mass index. *Adv Perit Dial.* 19:222-6.

14. Hogg, R.J., Furth, S., Lemley, K.V., Portman, R., Schwartz, G.J., Coresh, J., Balk, E., Lau, J., Levin, A., Kausz, A.T., Eknoyan, G., & Levey, A.S. (2003): National Kidney Foundation's Kidney Disease Outcomes Quality Initiative clinical practice guidelines for chronic kidney disease in children and adolescents: evaluation, classification, and stratification. *Pediatrics.* Jun;111(6 Pt 1):1416-21.

15. Ishizaki, M., Yamashita, A.C., Kawanishi, H., Nakamoto, M., & Hamada, H. (2004). Dialysis dose and nutrition in Japanese peritoneal dialysis patients. *Adv Perit Dial.* 20:141-3.

16. Islam, M.S., Briat, C., Soutif, C., Barnouin, F., & Pollini, J. (1997). More than 17 years of peritoneal dialysis: a case report. *Adv. Perit. Dial.* 13:98-103.

17. Kawabe, T., Zakaria, E.R., Hunt, C.M., Harris, P.D., & Garrison, R.N. (2004). Peritoneal dialysis solutions contract arteries through endothelium-independent prostanoid pathways. *Advances in Peritoneal Dialysis.* 20:177-83.

18. Kopple, J.D. (1997). Nutritional status as a predictor of morbidity and mortality in maintenance dialysis patients. *ASAIO J.* 43(3):246-50.

19. Lazarus, J.M. (1993). Nutrition in hemodialysis patients. *Am J. Kidney Dis.* 21(1):99-05.

20. le Poole, C.Y., van Ittersum, F.J., Weijmer, M.C., Valentijn, R.M., & ter Wee, P.M. (2004). Clinical effects of a peritoneal dialysis regimen low in glucose in new peritoneal dialysis patients: A randomized crossover study. *Advances in Peritoneal Dialysis*, 20:170-76.

21. Levey, A.S., Coresh, J., Balk, E., Kausz, A.T., Levin, A., Steffes, M.W., Hogg, R.J., Perrone, R.D., Lau, J., & Eknoyan, G. (2003). National Kidney Foundation practice guidelines for chronic kidney disease: evaluation, classification, and stratification. *Ann Intern Med.* Jul 15;139(2):137-47.

22. Lindholm, B. & Bergstrom, J. (1992). Nutritional aspects of peritoneal dialysis. *Kidney Int. Suppl.* 38:S165-71.

23. Mahajan, S., Boulton, H., Gokal, R. (2004). A trial of subcutaneous administration of darbepoetin alfa once every other week for the treatment of anemia in peritoneal dialysis patients. *J Nephrol.* Sep-Oct;17(5):687-92.

24. *Manual of Clinical Dietetics.* (2000). 6th Ed. Chicago, IL. The American Dietetic Association.

25. Mehrotra, R., & Kopple, J.D. (2003). Protein and energy nutrition among adult patients treated with chronic peritoneal dialysis. *Adv Ren Replace Ther.* 10(3):194-212.

26. McCusker, F.X. & Teehan, B.P. (1997). Peritoneal dialysis: an evolving understanding. *Semin. Nephrol.* 17(3):226-38.

27. Patel, S.S., Kimmel, P.L., & Singh. A. (2002). New clinical practice guidelines for chronic kidney disease: a framework for K/DOQI. *Semin Nephrol.* Nov;22(6):449-58.

28. Podel, J., Hodelin-Wetzel, R., Saha, D.C., & Burns, G. (2000). Glucose absorption in acute peritoneal dialysis. *J Ren Nutr.* Apr;10(2):93-7.

29. Prendergast, A. & Fulton, F.L. (1997) *Medical terminology: A Text/Workbook.* 4th Ed. Redwood City, California. Addison-Wesley Nursing.

30. Pronsky, Z.M., Redfern, C.M., Crowe, J. & Epstein, S. (2003) *Food Medication Interactions*, 13th Ed Phoenix, Arizona. Food-Medications Interactions, Publishers and Distributors.

31. Quellhorst, E. (2002). Insulin Therapy During Peritoneal Dialysis: Pros and Cons of Various Forms of Administration. *J Am Soc Nephrol* 13:S92-S96.

32. Rayner, B., Hollander, M., & Willett, C. (2002). Adequacy of peritoneal dialysis and nutritional status in patients on continuous ambulatory peritoneal dialysis (CAPD). *S Afr Med J.* Nov;92(11): 887-9.

33. Rolfes, S.R., Pinna, K. & Whitney, E. (2006). *Understanding Normal and Clinical Nutrition*, 7th Ed. West/Wadsworth.

34. Schiro-Harvey, K. (2002). *National Renal Diet: Professional Guide.* 2Ed. The American Dietetic Association. Chicago, IL,

35. Schmicker, R. (1995). Nutritional treatment of hemodialysis and peritoneal dialysis patients. *Artif. Organs.* 19(8):837-41.

36. Showers, D. (2004). Strategies to improve albumin in patients on peritoneal dialysis. *Nephrol Nurs J.* Sep-Oct;31(5):592-3.

37. Snively, C.S. & Gutierrez, C. (2004). Chronic kidney disease: prevention and treatment of common complications. *Am Fam Physician.* Nov 15;70(10):1921-8.

38. Spratto, G.R. & Woods, A.L. (2005). *PDR Nurse's Drug Handbook.* Thompson Delmar Learning, NY.

39. Ueunten, A., & Shovic, A. (2003). Patient education. Improving albumin levels in peritoneal dialysis patients. *J Ren Nutr.* 13(2):105-8.

40. Van Biesen, W., Boer, W., De Greve, B., Dequidt, C., Vijt, D., Faict, D., & Lameire, N. (2004). A randomized clinical trial with a 0.6% amino acid/ 1.4% glycerol peritoneal dialysis solution. *Perit Dial Int.* May-Jun;24(3):222-30.

41 Wang, A.Y., Woo, J., Lam, C.W., Wang, M., Sea, M.M., Lui, S.F., Li, P.K., & Sanderson, J. (2003). Is a single time point C-reactive protein predictive of outcome in peritoneal dialysis patients? *J Am Soc Nephrol.* 14(7):1871-9.

42. Wolfson, M. & Jones, M. (1999). Nutrition Impact of Peritoneal Dialysis Solutions. *Mineral and Electrolyte Metabolism*; 25:4-6. Proceedings of the 9th International Congress on Renal Nutrition and Metabolism, August 29-September 1, 1998, Vienna, Austria.

CASE STUDY #34
HYPERTENSION RESULTING IN RENAL DISEASE, HEMODIALYSIS AND KIDNEY TRANSPLANT

INTRODUCTION
This is a three-part case study about a man with a family history of hypertension and renal disease. The patient is not compliant with diet or medication orders. PART I is a basic study that concerns dietary sodium restriction and teaching techniques. As you read the RD's interview with the patient, pay attention to any inappropriate questions or mannerisms she uses and omissions she may make. If this patient had been compliant with diet and medications, the problems involved in the next two parts may not have occurred. Review foods high in sodium and potassium. PART II demonstrates the possible effects of a patient's noncompliance to medication and diet. It is a good introduction to renal disease, hemodialysis, and the associated diet, drugs, terms, and lab values. PART III is concerned with a kidney transplant and the differences in diet are noted.
****

SKILLS NEEDED

ABBREVIATIONS:
Knowledge of the following abbreviations is required in order to understand this case. You should learn these abbreviations before you begin to read the study.
A-V, D/C, ESRD, HD, qod, S.C., and SG, (Appendix C).

FORMULAS:
The formulas used in this case study include ideal body weight, percent ideal body weight, percent usual body weight, adjusted body weight, body mass index, caloric needs, and protein requirements (Appendix A, Tables 5 through 9 and 17).

LABORATORY VALUES:
You will need to be able to interpret the nutritional significance of the following laboratory values for this case study: BUN, Ca, Cl, Cr, glu, hct, hgb, K, lymph, MCH, MCHC, MCV, Mg, Na, P, RBC, uric acid, Ser alb, WBC and urine glu, ketones, pH, protein, and SG (Appendix B).

MEDICATIONS:
Become familiar with the following medications before reading the case study. Note the diet-drug interactions, dosages and methods of administration, gastrointestinal tract reactions, etc.
1. Capoten (captopril). 2. Lasix (furosemide); 3. Hectorol (doxercalciferol); 4.Epogen (epoetin); 5. Prednisone (prednisone); 6. Sandimmune (cyclosporine alfa); 7. Aldomet Hydrochloride (methyldopa).
****

PART I: HYPERTENSION AND DIET

Mr. G is a 45 YOBM employed as a plant manager in the automobile industry. He enjoys his job, but it is highly stressful because of the pressure to produce as many cars as possible in a short period of time. Recently, the pressure has increased because of increased gas prices and decreased car sales. Mr. G is a worrier. He has been losing sleep over the slow economy and the effect it may have on his job. He is married and has children, one in high school and two in elementary school. His wife works as a cashier in a food store and sometimes has to work evenings. This increased Mr. G's stress since he did not know how to cook and the children always complained when he tried.

He has a history of HTN but has not been checking his BP as he should. He had a routine physical recently and his BP was 175/100. This added to his concern because if it does not go down, he fears the plant physician will force him to take sick leave. His medication included Capoten 50 mg b.i.d. and Lasix,

30 mg qod or prn for pedal edema. He has been on hypertensive medication for five years but the strength of the medication has been increasing for the last two years because of the gradual increase in his BP. Mr. G has not been a compliant patient. He frequently does not take his medication because he feels fine and believes he is too young to have high BP, even though his father died from a stroke at 57. He has an uncle on his father's side who has renal failure secondary to untreated HTN.

MR. G is 5'10" and weighs 225 pounds, has a medium frame, and is moderately active. He has always been on the heavy side but his weight has increased by 20 lbs in the past year. At his last physical, the MD found more pedal edema than usual. Mr. G admitted to noncompliance in respect to his medication. The MD instructed him on the importance of taking his medication, talked to him about the effects of worrying, and told him to see the plant dietitian. It was the dietitian's job to complete a nutritional assessment and determine his energy and protein needs. She also had an order from the MD to instruct him on a 2 g Na diet with appropriate kcals and protein based on her assessment.
****

QUESTIONS:
1. Determine Mr. G's IBW and percent of IBW (Appendix A, Tables 7 and 8).

2. Determine his percent of UBW (Appendix A, Tables 7 and 8).

3. Determine Mr. G's adjusted body weight (Appendix A, Table 9).

4. Calculate his BMI (Appendix A, Tables 10 and 11).

5. Determine his protein needs.

6. Using the Harris-Benedict equation, calculate his BEE (Appendix A, Table 17).

7. Considering Mr. G as moderately active, calculate his total caloric needs for the day.

8. Mr. G's BP was 175/100. What does blood pressure mean? Is 175/100 something to be concerned about? Explain.

9. What are the functions of Capoten and Lasix?

10. List any nutritional complications of Capoten and Lasix.

11. List the principles of a 2 g Na diet.

****

The RD had Mr. G come to his office for a discussion. He obtained a typical day's recall and a food frequency as follows:

RD: Mr. G, the plant MD tells me that you have been gaining weight recently and that your blood pressure has been elevated. Is that correct?

Mr. G: Yes, it is.

RD: OK. He wants me to talk to you about a meal plan. Have you ever been on any kind of meal plan?

Mr. G: Well, yea. I'm supposed to be watching my salt intake right now.

RD: How have you been doing?

Mr. G: Very good. I don't think I use that much.

RD: I see. What about a meal plan for weight reduction? Have you ever been on a weight reduction diet?

Mr. G: Not really. I've tried to lose a few pounds every now and then, but nothing other than that.

RD: OK. When the doctor weighed you the other day, you were 225 lbs and 5'10". Is that correct?

Mr. G: That is what he said.

RD: OK. I want you to take me through a typical day from the time you get up in the morning, to the time you go to bed at night. Tell me everything you have to eat or drink; amounts, how it was prepared, everything. So, when you get up in the morning, what is the first thing you have to eat or drink?

Mr. G: Well, the first thing I have is a cup of coffee while I'm getting ready to go to work. Then I sit down and have some breakfast with my wife. I usually have a couple of sausage-biscuits with another cup of coffee. That's all I really eat in the morning. That's all I have time for.

RD: What is the next thing you have to eat or drink?

Mr. G: Well, I get to work and I start on my paperwork first. Then I have to make my rounds and check my men. I come back to the office and take a little break. I have a cup of coffee.

RD: OK. What is the next thing?

Mr. G: For lunch my wife fixes me a lunch box. I'll have a sandwich, piece of fruit, some cookies, a piece of cake if she made some the night before, you know, something like that. Some coffee.

RD: What kind of sandwich do you have?

Mr. G: Well, some kind of meat, you know, like luncheon meat, boiled ham, bologna, a piece of cheese on it, you know. The stuff you get in the store in the little packs.

RD: Does she put anything else on the sandwich?

Mr. G: Yea, sometimes she puts a little mustard or mayo.

RD: What kind of cheese?

Mr. G: I don't know, my wife gets that.

RD: What kind of fruit?

Mr. G: Usually an apple.

RD: What is the next thing you have to eat or drink?

Mr. G: Well, in the afternoon I usually get a soda.

RD: OK.

MR. G: Then when I go home I eat a good supper. I usually have some kind of meat. Could be meat loaf, chicken, some kind of meat. And we usually . . .

RD: Let me see if I can get you to accurately estimate how much meat you normally eat. These are plastic food models. Look at this model of roast beef and tell me if what you normally eat is smaller than, equal to, or larger than this piece.

Mr. G: Oh, it would be more than that. It would be about twice that.

RD: OK.

MR. G: Is that plastic food? Let me see that. Boy, that feels funny huh?

RD: What else?

Mr. G: Well, then we have some potatoes, you know . . .

RD: How are those potatoes fixed?

Mr. G: Sometimes she boils them, but we have french fries a lot. The kids like french fries.

RD: OK. What else would you have?

Mr. G: She always has some vegetables, like green beans, greens, or squash. Always some vegetables.

RD: How does she fix the vegetables?

Mr. G: Well . . . I don't know how she cooks them . . . what do you mean?

RD: Does she boil them? Fry them? Does she cook them with butter, margarine, bacon fat, or some other seasoning?

Mr. G: Every now and then we have some fried okra or squash, but other than that we don't have much fried foods. She puts lots of seasoning in the vegetables, like fat meat, bacon, stuff like that.

RD: OK. Mr. G, do you know if your wife adds any salt to your food?

Mr. G: Some, I don't know how much. You will have to ask her that.

RD: Does she ever try cooking with other seasonings and no salt?

Mr. G: I don't know. She does all the cooking.

RD: Mr. G, do you have any salad or bread with your meals?

Mr. G: We usually have some bread, some salad every now and then. Sometimes she fixes a pie or a cake.

RD: What do you put on your bread?

Mr. G: I put a little bit of margarine on it.

RD: What about the salad, do you put anything on your salad?

Mr. G: I use a little bit of salad dressing.

RD: What kind do you use, Mr. G?

Mr. G: Oh I don't know, she gets all kinds; whatever she has.

RD: OK. And what do you have to drink with your meal?

Mr. G: Kool Aid.

RD: Sweetened or unsweetened?

Mr. G: Sweetened.

RD: How much sugar does she add to the Kool Aid?

Mr. G: I don't know that. You will have to ask the wife.

RD: After supper is there anything you have to eat or drink before you go to bed?

Mr. G: Well, after we get the kitchen cleaned up, I like to help the kids with their homework. Then I like to relax, you know. I put my feet up and look at some TV. I might snack on some potato chips or peanuts and drink a beer or two before bed. See I really don't eat that much; I really don't know why I'm gaining all this weight.

RD: OK. Mr. G, you only mentioned fruit at lunch. Do you ever have fruit any other time?

Mr. G: No, that's about it. I don't care for fruit that much.

RD: Mr. G, I noticed that you did not mention milk. Do you drink milk?

Mr. G: No, I'm allergic to milk.

RD: You're allergic to milk? What happens when you drink milk?

Mr. G: Oh I get a lot of cramps and gas, you know.

RD: What about cheese or yogurt, do you eat much cheese?

Mr. G: Yogurt? I don't eat that stuff, but I like cheese. Cheese doesn't bother me. I eat some cheese and crackers sometimes at night with my beer.
****

QUESTIONS CONTINUED:

12. Identify any mistakes the RD may have made in this interview.

13. Is there anything you would do differently? Explain.

14. What are some good points about this interview?

15. What are the goals of nutritional therapy for Mr. G?

16. In one column, list the foods that Mr. G eats that are high in sodium. In a second column, list possible substitutes for the foods in column one.

HIGH Na FOODS   **SUGGESTED SUBSTITUTES**

17. In column one, list the foods Mr. G eats that are high in fat. In a second column, list possible substitutes for the foods in column one.

HIGH FAT FOODS	SUGGESTED SUBSTITUTES

18. Based on the recall, approximate Mr. G's energy and protein intake. Is he taking in too much, too little, or an appropriate amount?

19. Approximate Mr. G's sodium intake (high, low, or appropriate).

20. Explain the relationship between BP and pedal edema.

21. Should the RD be concerned about Mr. G's calcium intake? Explain.

22. Considering Mr. G's medication, diet, and recall, on a separate sheet of paper, outline the teaching program you would use for him. Include in your outline behavioral changes you would recommend, foods to avoid with appropriate substitutes, and foods to include. Explain why you are making changes.

****

PART II: HEMODIALYSIS AND DIET

After talking to the dietitian, Mr. G followed his meal plan for a few months, during which time he lost approximately 18 lbs. He gradually felt better about himself but, as time passed, he went off his meal plan. At first, he took his medications as ordered, but then he started to skip them on occasion. He noticed that he had to go to the bathroom more frequently. He also noted that he had been waking up during the night with leg cramps, something he had never experienced in the past. He was not sure why this was happening but it started after he began taking the new medication. He believed the medication was causing the leg cramps, even though he did not know what the relationship was. He observed that if he took Lasix every other day instead of daily, he did not have as many leg cramps. Gradually he started taking Lasix less and less regularly. The pedal edema went away. He knew Lasix helped prevent edema, so he thought he didn't need to take it any longer. His condition remained stable for several months. When edema returned, he would take Lasix until it went away and then he would quit taking it. Every time he had a doctor's appointment he would take Lasix and his blood pressure medication several days before the appointment. He thought this would prevent obvious signs of edema and his blood pressure checks would be normal. It seemed to work. His blood pressure was borderline or slightly elevated. After the doctor's visit, he would quit taking his medication because he thought he did not need it.

This continued for a couple of years. Then he started to notice that when the edema came back and he took Lasix, it would not go away. He did not have to go to the bathroom as much. He also noticed some pain in the lower left flank. The pain persisted but he thought it was because he was not getting enough exercise. He did not relate the pain to renal disease, so he ignored it. The pain continued and the pedal edema got worse. He was gaining weight, but he really did not feel like he was eating any more than usual. He went off his meal plan by eating more fatty foods but continued to watch his sodium intake for almost a year. By then he was completely back to his old eating habits. One day he felt very fatigued and decided to go get his blood pressure checked by the plant nurse. It was 180/105. The nurse made an appointment for him to see his doctor. When the doctor weighed him, he had gained all of his weight back and then some. He now weighed 235 lbs. The doctor made him an appointment to see a nephrologist.

Mr. G went to see the nephrologist who examined him and had the following lab work done:
Urinalysis:
SG 1.001   Protein +2   Glucose neg.   Ketones neg.   pH 8.1

TABLE 1

RENAL PACKAGE							
TEST	**RESULT**	**REFERENCE UNITS** Conventional	SI	**TEST**	**RESULT**	**REFERENCE UNITS** Conventional	SI
Glu	80 mg/dl	70-110 mg/dl	3.8-6.1 mmol/L	Na	148 mEq/L	136-145 mEq/L	136-145 mmol/L
BUN	33 mg/dl	6-20 mg/dl	2.1-7.1 mmol/L	K	5.5 mEq/L	3.5-5.2 mEq/L	3.5-5.2 mmol/L
Cr	2.2 mg/dl	0.9-1.3 mg/dl	80-115 µmol/L	Cl	103 mEq/L	96-106 mEq/L	96-106 mmol/L
Uric Acid	8.6 mg/dl	3.4-7.0 mg/dl	202-416 µmol/L	Ca	9.2 mg/dl	8.8-10.0 mg/dl	2.20-2.60 mmol/L
Ser alb	3.2 g/dl	3.5-4.8 g/dl	39-50 g/dl	P	5.5mg/dl	2.7-4.5 mg/dl	4.7-6.0 kPa

TABLE 2

CBC							
TEST	**RESULT**	**REFERENCE UNITS** Conventional	SI	**TEST**	**RESULT**	**REFERENCE UNITS** Conventional	SI
Hgb	12. g/dl	14 - 17.4 g/dl	140-174 g/L	WBC	5.2 10^3/µl	4.5-10.5 x 10^3/cells/ mm^3	4.5-10.5 x 10^9/L
Hct	37%	42 – 52%		% Lymph	23%	25 – 40% of total WBC	1500-4000 cells/mm^3
RBC	4.5x10^6/µ	3.6-5.0x10^6/L	3.6-5.0x10^{12}/L	MCH	26 pg/cell	26-34 pg/cell	0.40-.53 fmol/cell
MCV	82 µm^3	82-98µm^3	82-98 fL	MCHC	32 g/dl	32-36 g/dl	320-360 g/L

****

QUESTIONS:

23. Explain why Mr. G had leg cramps and explain what he could do to prevent them.

24. Explain the pathophysiology of renal disease and HTN.

25. Look up the anatomy of the kidney and define the following terms:
    Glomerulus:

    Nephron:

    Loop of Henle:

    Medulla:

    Cortex:

26. Which lab values in Table 1 and which results of the urinalysis indicate that Mr. G has a renal problem?

27. Which lab values indicate protein malnutrition? In your answer, give the possible reasons for protein malnutrition and explain the relationship between protein in the urine and renal disease.

****

The nephrologist told Mr. G that his kidneys were failing and that he would have to go on a very strict meal plan and medication schedule. Orders from the nephrologist were as follows:
➢ D/C Tenormin
➢ Aldomet
➢ Lasix
➢ Hectorol
➢ Multivitamin with minerals
➢ 0.6 g of protein per kg of body weight

> kcals per RD's recommendation
> 2g Na
> No K restriction
> No fluid restriction

	DOCTOR'S ORDERS
10/28/95	Tenormin 50mg po q AM & ↑ to 100 mg q AM p̄ ↑d.
	Lasix 40mg p.o. q AM 20 mg po p̄ VIII hr.
	Phos-K 500mg tid c̄ meals
	epogen 50u/kg s.c. 3X/wk
	1 multivit / min qd
	0.6 g prot / kg
	kcal per RD
	2 g Na
	Ø K restriction
	Ø fluid restriction
	JL

Above is a mock page of doctors orders. See if you can transcribe the orders.
****
28. Give the function and nutritional implications of Hectorol.

29. Explain the rationale for Mr. G's meal plan. Include in your discussion the reasons for the following:
> 0.6 g of protein per kg of body weight
> 2 g sodium
> No K restriction
> No fluid restriction

****

The nephrologist had Mr. G see the renal dietitian before he went home. The RD asked him who did the cooking. He told her that his wife did all the cooking and grocery shopping. The RD said that she wanted to talk to Mr. G and his wife together and made an appointment for them. Mr. G came back with his wife and the dietitian instructed them on a meal plan and cooking techniques. She also impressed upon them the importance of following a meal plan and medication orders. Mr. G finally realized the importance of the meal plan and was frightened. He remembered what happened to his uncle who had had total kidney failure. He went home declaring that he would follow his meal plan to the letter. The nephrologist told Mr. G that if he stayed on his meal plan and took his medications, his renal disease may not get any worse and he may not need dialysis, or he may be able to avoid it for years to come. The nephrologist also told him that if he did not follow his meal plan and did not take his medications, he would very likely end up with ESRD.

Mr. G followed his meal plan much more closely than he did last time and he also took all of his medications. The increased dosage of Lasix caused him to go to the bathroom more and he was losing weight. This went on for several months without a problem and then he noticed that he was not going to the bathroom as much. The edema was coming back and so was the weight. His pain in the left lower flank had subsided but was now returning. Mr. G also noticed that he was feeling very tired and would get weak after doing easy tasks. He began to experience anorexia, headaches, and nausea. Mr. G went back to his nephrologist, who obtained another set of lab values. These lab values were as follows:

TABLE 3

RENAL PACKAGE							
TEST	RESULT	REFERENCE UNITS Conventional	SI	TEST	RESULT	REFERENCE UNITS Conventional	SI
Glu	85 mg/dl	70-110 mg/dl	3.8-6.1 mmol/L	Na	149 mEq/L	136-145 mEq/L	136-145 mmol/L
BUN	49 mg/dl	6-20 mg/dl	2.1-7.1 mmol/L	K	5.8 mEq/L	3.5-5.2 mEq/L	3.5-5.2 mmol/L
Cr	2.5 mg/dl	0.9-1.3 mg/dl	80-115 µmol/L	Cl	103 mEq/L	96-106 mEq/L	96-106 mmol/L
Uric Acid	9.2 mg/dl	3.4-7.0 mg/dl	202-416 µmol/L	Ca	9.3 mg/dl	8.8-10.0 mg/dl	2.20-2.60 mmol/L
Ser alb	3.2 g/dl	3.5-4.8 g/dl	39-50 g/dl	P	6.2mg/dl	2.7-4.5 mg/dl	4.7-6.0 kPa

TABLE 4

CBC							
TEST	RESULT	REFERENCE UNITS Conventional	SI	TEST	RESULT	REFERENCE UNITS Conventional	SI
Hgb	11. g/dl	14 - 17.4 g/dl	140-174 g/L	WBC	5.7 10^3/µl	4.5-10.5 x 10^3/cells/ mm^3	4.5-10.5 x 10^9/L
Hct	34%	42 – 52%		% Lymph	24%	25 – 40% of total WBC	1500-4000 cells/mm^3
RBC	4.5x10^6/µ	3.6-5.0x10^6/L	3.6-5.0x10^{12}/L	MCH	24 pg/cell	26-34 pg/cell	0.40-.53 fmol/cell
MCV	77 µm^3	82-98µm^3	82-98 fL	MCHC	32 g/dl	32-36 g/dl	320-360 g/L

Urinalysis: SG 1.001   Protein +1   Glucose neg.   Ketones neg.   pH 8.2

The nephrologist told Mr. G that the results of his tests were not good. His kidneys were going into ESRD and he would have to go on a hemodialysis machine for about 3 hrs 3x/wk. He told Mr. G that he would require minor surgery to have a primary AV fistula created in his arm to provide access to the dialysis machine. He explained what an AV fistula was. Mr. G's weight was now 215 lbs.
****

QUESTIONS CONTINUED:

30. Which lab values indicate Mr. G is anemic?

31. Describe the AV fistula for hemodialysis.

32. Describe hemodialysis and list the complications.

33. List the dietary principles for a patient on hemodialysis.

****

The MD told Mr. G that his new meal plan would be as follows:
- 1.3 g of protein per kg of body weight
- 2 g Na
- 90 mEq K
- Fluid intake = urine output +500 cc

Mr. G's new orders for medications were as follows:
- Continue Hectorol
- Continue antihypertensive
- Start Epogen
- D/C Lasix
- Continue multivitamin

****

34. Describe the function of Epogen and explain the kidney relationship with anemia.

35. Convert 60 mEq K to mg (Appendix A, Table 5).

36. Why did the protein in the diet order increase with ESRD?

****

Mr. G was admitted to the hospital again to have a wrist (radial-cephalic) primary AV fistula created in his left arm. While in the hospital, Mr. G received hemodialysis for the first time. His weight upon admission to the hospital was 215 lbs. This was listed as his wet weight. After dialysis, Mr. G was weighed again and weighed 210 lbs. This was listed as his dry weight.

The renal dietitian met with Mr. G and his wife again and explained the changes in his new meal plan. She emphasized the importance of increasing the protein and restricting sodium and fluid. She also told Mr. G that it was important for him to take in enough energy. To do this, it will now be necessary for him to eat more sweets and fats. She suggested that whenever he eats bread or toast, he should add margarine, and whenever he eats salad, he can add lots of low-sodium salad dressing. She also suggested that he eat more candy that did not have salted nuts in it. He can add sugar to coffee, tea, Kool-Aid, etc.
****

QUESTIONS CONTINUED:
37. Explain the difference between the wet weight and the dry weight.

38. On the next page, create a SOAP note for Mr. G using all of the information since and including Tables 3 and 4. Use any pertinent information prior to Table 3 as his previous history.

PROGRESS NOTES

S:	
O:	

A:

P:

39. Calculate Mr. G's BEE using the Harris-Benedict equation and the appropriate stress factor (Appendix A, Table 17).

40. Mr. G's energy and protein requirements on hemodialysis are higher than his energy and protein requirements without hemodialysis. Explain why.

41 The RD encouraged Mr. G to increase his caloric intake by eating more fat and sugar. Comment on the advantages vs. disadvantages of doing this with a patient who has renal disease.

****

Mr. G's wife asked the MD how long Mr. G would have to stay on his meal plan. The MD replied that he would have to stay on his meal plan for the rest of his life. The only way that he could change his meal plan would be to have a successful kidney transplant. He discussed the possibility of a kidney transplant with Mr. G and his wife. Mr. G decided that he wanted to be put on the list to receive a donor kidney.

****

42. On a separate sheet of paper, using Mr. G's last plan of MNT (1.3 g of protein per kg, 2 g Na, 90 mEq K, and 500 cc fluid + urinary output), plan a day's menu using renal diet exchanges (your textbook, your local diet manual, or reference #33 would be good places to obtain renal diet exchange information).

****

PART III: KIDNEY TRANSPLANT

Mr. G has been doing well on his meal plan and medications for the past eight months. He has been receiving HD 3 x/wk for 4 hrs at a time. He has not had any complications but continues to lose weight. His dry weight is now 196 lbs. He is very much concerned about his weight loss. Mr. G is now in the hospital being prepared for a kidney transplant. His most recent lab values were as follows:

TABLE 5

RENAL PACKAGE							
TEST	RESULT	REFERENCE UNITS Conventional	SI	TEST	RESULT	REFERENCE UNITS Conventional	SI
Glu	120 mg/dl	70-110 mg/dl	3.8-6.1 mmol/L	Na	141 mEq/L	136-145 mEq/L	136-145 mmol/L
BUN	54 mg/dl	6-20 mg/dl	2.1-7.1 mmol/L	K	5.4 mEq/L	3.5-5.2 mEq/L	3.5-5.2 mmol/L
Cr	3.5 mg/dl	0.9-1.3 mg/dl	80-115 µmol/L	Cl	100 mEq/L	96-106 mEq/L	96-106 mmol/L
Uric Acid	8.0 mg/dl	3.4-7.0 mg/dl	202-416 µmol/L	Ca	9.1 mg/dl	8.8-10.0 mg/dl	2.20-2.60 mmol/L
Ser alb	2.3 g/dl	3.5-4.8 g/dl	39-50 g/dl	P	6.3mg/dl	2.7-4.5 mg/dl	4.7-6.0 kPa

TABLE 6

CBC							
TEST	RESULT	REFERENCE UNITS Conventional	SI	TEST	RESULT	REFERENCE UNITS Conventional	SI
Hgb	11.7 dl	14 - 17.4 g/dl	140-174 g/L	WBC	5.3 x 10^3/µl	4.5-10.5 x 10^3/cells/ mm^3	4.5-10.5 x 10^9/L
Hct	34%	42 – 52%		% Lymph	21%	25 – 40% of total WBC	1500-4000 cells/mm^3
RBC	4.6x10^6/µ	3.6-5.0x10^6/L	3.6-5.0x10^{12}/L	MCH	22 pg/cell	26-34 pg/cell	0.40-.53 fmol/cell
MCV	75 µm^3	82-98µm^3	82-98 fL	MCHC	27 g/dl	32-36 g/dl	320-360 g/L

Mr. G is to receive a kidney transplant that was found through the hospital's computerized system. The new kidney is a cadaver transplant from a 30 YOM that was killed in an automobile accident. Mr. G went to surgery and the transplant was completed successfully. After surgery, Mr. G recovered well without incident. His new orders read as follows:

➢ < 1. prednisone
➢ cyclosporine
➢ D/C Hectorol
➢ high protein, low carbohydrate, 2 g Na diet

➢ no K restriction
➢ no fluid restriction

The renal RD again met with Mr. G and his wife and explained the changes in his meal plan. She told him that he now does not need to limit his protein intake. In fact, she encouraged him to take in a lot of protein. She also cautioned him to avoid sweets such as sugar, candy, soft drinks, and desserts. She recommended that he reduce fat intake in his meal plan and emphasized the importance of following the 2 g Na recommendation. At first, Mr. G was confused because this was so different from the HD diet of limited protein, high carbohydrate, high fat, and restricted K.
****

QUESTIONS:

43. The values indicating protein malnutrition are a little lower than they were the last time. Discuss what factors could be responsible for this.

44. Describe the action of prednisone. Discuss the nutritional implications.

45. Describe the action of cyclosporine and discuss the nutritional implications.

46. What are the nutritional goals for a patient who has just had a kidney transplant?

47. Calculate Mr. G's energy and protein needs and compare these values with his needs before dialysis and during dialysis. Show your work.

48. If you were the RD, how would you explain to Mr. G the reasons for the change in his meal plan? (***Hint: Consider Mr. G's medications.***)

****

Mr. G recovered as expected without complications. His renal function improved dramatically. He was not back to normal and never would be, but as long as he stayed on his meal plan and continued his medications, his dietary restrictions should not get any worse. He went home from the hospital, followed his meal plan, and took his medications. He returned to work and was very thankful to have renewed energy and the ability to adequately complete his job. After about five months, Mr. G's weight increased to 216 lbs. He noticed that the weight gain was fat and not muscle. He weighed as much as he did before he was sick, but he did not have the muscle mass he had prior to his illness. He was concerned about this and returned to see his RD. Upon visual examination, the RD could see that Mr. G had an increase in abdominal fat and a very full round face. He appeared to be much healthier than he was when he was receiving HD, but it was obvious that he had gained a considerable amount of fat. The RD explained to Mr. G why this was taking place.

****

QUESTIONS CONTINUED:

49. Explain what is happening to Mr. G.

50. For a patient on prednisone, an increased amount of fat tissue and a round full face is not uncommon. What is this condition called?

51. Define the following terms:
    Cadaver Transplant:

    Sibling Transplant:

ADDITIONAL OPTIONAL QUESTION:

TUBE FEEDING DRILL:

52. Suppose Mr. G became seriously ill prior to receiving his transplant, had to be hospitalized, and could only be fed by a feeding tube. Using the table below, compare several of the enteral nutritional supplements that would be appropriate under these conditions.

Product	Producer	Form	Cal/ml	Non-pro cal/g N	g/L			Na mg	K mg	mOsm /kg water	Vol to meet RDA in ml	g of fiber /L	Free H$_2$O /L in ml
					Pro	CHO	Fat						

RELATED REFERENCES

1. Abdelfatah, A., Ducloux, D., Toubin, G., Motte, G., Alber, D., Chalopin, J.M. (2002). Treatment of hyperhomocysteinemia with folic acid reduces oxidative stress in renal transplant recipients. *Transplantation.* Feb 27;73(4):663-5.

2. Adamson, J.W. & Eschbach, J.W. (1998). Erythropoietin for end-stage renal disease. *N. Engl. J. Med.* 27;339(9):625-7.

3. Ahmad, S. (2004). Dietary sodium restriction for hypertension in dialysis patients. *Semin Dial.* Jul-Aug;17(4):284-7.

4. Bennett, C.L., Luminar,i S., Nissenson, A.R., Tallman, M.S., Klinge, S.A., McWilliams, N., McKoy, J.M., Kim, B., Lyons, E.A., Trifilio, S.M., Raisch, D.W., Evens, A.M., Kuzel, T.M., Schumock, G.T.,Belknap, S.M., Locatelli, F., Rossert, J., and Casadevall, N. (2004). Pure red-cell aplasia and epoetin therapy. *N Engl J Med.* Sep 30;351(14):1403-8.

5. Bergstrom, J., Wang, T., & Lindholm, B. (1998). Factors contributing to catabolism in end-stage renal disease patients. *Miner. Electrolyte Metab.* 24(1):92-101.

6. Bray, G.A., Vollmer, W.M., Sacks, F.M., Obarzanek, E., Svetkey, L.P., and Appel, L.J.; DASH Collaborative Research Group. (2004). A further subgroup analysis of the effects of the DASH diet and three dietary sodium levels on blood pressure: results of the DASH-Sodium Trial. *Am J Cardiol.* Jul 15;94(2):222-7.

7. Chumlea, W.C. (2004). Anthropometric and body composition assessment in dialysis patients. *Semin Dial.* Nov-Dec;17(6):466-70.

8. Coroas, A., Oliveira, J.G., Sampaio, S., Borges, C., Tavares, I., Pestana, M., De Almeida, M.D. (2004). Nutritional status and body composition evolution in early post-renal transplantation - is there a female advantage? *Asia Pac J Clin Nutr.* Aug;13(Suppl):S150.

9. Burdick, C.O. (1998). Prealbumin and prediction of survival in dialysis patients. *Am. J. Kidney Dis.* 31(1):195.

10. Cherla, G. and Jaimes, E.A. (2004). Role of L-arginine in the pathogenesis and treatment of renal disease. *J Nutr.* Oct;134(10 Suppl):2801S-2806S; discussion 2818S-2819S.

11. Cockram, D.B., Hensley, M.K., Rodreguez, M., Agarwal, G., Wennberg, A., Ruey, P.,Ashbach, D., Hebert, L., & Kunan, R. (1998). Safety and tolerance of medical nutritional products as sole sources of nutrition in people on hemodialysis. *J. Ren. Nutr.* 8(1):25-33.

12. Cook, N.R., Kumanyika, S.K., & Cutler, J.A. (1998). Effect of change in sodium excretion on change in blood pressure corrected for measurement error. The Trails of Hypertension Prevention, Phase I. *Am. J. Epidemiol.* 1;148(5):431-44.

13. de Vries, A.P., Bakker, S.J., and, van Son, W.J. (2000). Dietary intervention after renal transplantation. *Transplantation.* Jul 15;70(1):241-2.

14. El Haggan, W., Vendrely, B., Chauveau, P., Barthe, N., Castaing, F., Berger, F., de Precigout, V., Potaux, L., and Aparicio, M. (2002). Early evolution of nutritional status and body composition after kidney transplantation. *Am J Kidney Dis.* Sep;40(3):629-37.

15. Elijovich, F. (2004). Is sodium restriction important to hypertension? The argument against. *Clin Hypertens* Jun;6(6):337-9.

16. Fischbach, F.T. (2003). *A Manual of Laboratory & Diagnostic Tests.* 7th Ed. Philadelphia. J.B. Lippincott Company.

17. Fouque, D. (2003). Why is the diet intervention so critical during chronic kidney disease? *J Ren Nutr.* Jul;13(3):173.

18. Froissart, M., Rossert, J., Jacquot, C., Paillard, M., and Houillier. P. (2005). Predictive Performance of the Modification of Diet in Renal Disease and Cockcroft-Gault Equations for Estimating Renal Function. *J Am Soc Nephrol.* Jan 19.

19. Horowitz, C.R., Tuzzio, L., Rojas, M., Monteith, S.A., and Sisk, J.E. (2004). How do urban African Americans and Latinos view the influence of diet on hypertension? *J Health Care Poor Underserved.* Nov;15(4):631-44.

20. Hunt, S.C., Cook, N.R., Oberman, A., Cutler, J.A., Hennekens, C.H., Allender, P.S., Walker, W.G., Whelton, P.K., & Williams, R.R. (1998). Angiotensinogen genotype, sodium reduction, weight loss, and prevention of hypertension: trials of hypertension prevention, phase II. *Hypertension.* 32(3):393-401.

21. Jones, M., Ibels, L., Schenkel, B., and Zagari, M. (2004). Impact of epoetin alfa on clinical end points in patients with chronic renal failure: a meta-analysis. *Kidney Int.* Mar;65(3):757-67.

22. Katz, J. (1998). Salt wars. *Science.* 25;28(5385):1963.

23. Kaysen, G.A. (1998). Albumin turnover in renal disease. *Miner. Electrolyte Metab.* 24(1):55-63.

24. Lancaster, K.J. (2004). Dietary treatment of blood pressure in kidney disease. Adv Chronic Kidney Dis. Apr;11(2):217-21.

25. Luft, F.C., Morris, C.D., & Weinberger, M.H. (1997). Compliance to a low-salt diet. *Am.J. Clin Nutr.* 65(2 Suppl):698S-703S.

26. .*Manual of Clinical Dietetics.* (2000). 6th Ed. Chicago, IL. The American Dietetic Association.

27. McCarty, M.F. (2004). Should we restrict chloride rather than sodium? *Med Hypotheses*. 63(1):138-48.

28. Modesti, P.A. (2004). Ethnic differences in hypertension and blood pressure control. Issues for prevention strategies. *Saudi Med J*. Sep;25(9):1160-4.

29. McCarron, D.A. (1998). Diet and blood pressure—the paradigm shift. *Science*. 14;281 (5379):933-4.

30. Prendergast, A. & Fulton, F.L. (1997) *Medical terminology: A Text/Workbook*. 4th Ed. Redwood City, California. Addison-Wesley Nursing.

31. Pronsky, Z.M., Redfern, C.M., Crowe, J. & Epstein, S. (2003) *Food Medication Interactions*, 13th Ed Phoenix, Arizona. Food-Medications Interactions, Publishers and Distributors.

32. Rolfes, S.R., Pinna, K. & Whitney, E. (2006). *Understanding Normal and Clinical Nutrition*, 7th Ed. West/Wadsworth.

33. Schiro-Harvey, K. (2002). *National Renal Diet: Professional Guide*. 2Ed. The American Dietetic Association. Chicago, IL,

34. Snively, C.S. and Gutierrez, C. (2004). Chronic kidney disease: prevention and treatment of common complications. *Am Fam Physician*. Nov 15;70(10):1921-8.

35. Spratto, G.R. & Woods, A.L. (2005). *PDR Nurse's Drug Handbook*. Thompson Delmar Learning, NY.

36. Taal, M.W. (2004). Slowing the progression of adult chronic kidney disease: therapeutic advances. *Drugs*; 64(20):2273-89.

37. Tai, T.W.C., Chan, A.M.W., Cochran, C.C., Harbert, G., Lindley, J., & Cotton., J. (1998). Renal Dietitians' Perspective: identification, prevalence, and intervention for malnutrition in dialysis patients in Texas. *J. Ren. Nutr.* 8(4):188-98.

38. Tang, W.W., Stead, R.A., & Goodkin D.A. (1998). Effects of Epoetin alfa on hemostasis in chronic renal failure. *Am. J. Nephrol.* 18(4):263-73.

39. Taubes, G. (1998). The (political) science of salt. *Science.* 14;281(5379):898-901,903-7.

40. Teplan, V., Schuck, O., Stollova, M., and Vitko, S. (2003). Obesity and hyperhomocysteinaemia after kidney transplantation. Nephrol Dial Transplant. 2003 Jul;18 Suppl 5:v71-3.

41. Weir, M.R., & Dworkin, L.D. (1998). Antihypertensive drugs, dietary salt, and renal protection: how low should you go and with which therapy? *Am J Kidney Dis.* 32(1):1-22.

42. Youssef, R.M., and Moubarak, I.I. (2002). Patterns and determinants of treatment compliance among hypertensive patients. *East Mediterr Health J*. Jul-Sep;8(4-5):579-92.

CASE STUDY #35
CROHN'S DISEASE AND TPN

INTRODUCTION

In PART I of this study of Crohn's disease, treatment required surgery that left the patient with an ileostomy and home TPN. This case provides a good introduction to the disorder. PART II provides a more advanced treatment and requires knowledge of TPN
****

SKILLS NEEDED

ABBREVIATIONS:
Knowledge of the following abbreviations is required in order to understand this case. You should learn these abbreviations before you begin to read the study.

AA, amp, $D_{50}W$, IBD, NS, NST, mOsm/kg, MVI, PVC, SBR, SBS, and TPN (Appendix C).

LABORATORY VALUES:
You will need to be able to interpret the nutritional significance of the following laboratory values for this case study: BUN, Ca (total and ionized), Cl, Cr, glucose, hct, hgb, K, lymphocytes, MCH, MCHC, MCV, Mg, Na, P, RBC, ser alb, and WBC (Appendix B).

FORMULAS:
The formulas used in this case study include ideal body weight and percent ideal body weight, total caloric needs using the Harris-Benedict equation and appropriate stress factors; total protein needs and TPN formulation. The formulas can be found in Appendix A, Table7, 8 and 17. Appendix D would also be helpful.

MEDICATIONS:
Become familiar with the following medications before reading the case study. Note the diet-drug interactions, dosages and methods of administration, gastrointestinal tract reactions, etc.
1. Solu-Medrol (methylprednisone sodium succinate); 2. Panasol (prednisone);
3. Azulfidine (sulfasalazine); 4. Lactated Ringers; 5. MVI 12; and 6. MTE.
****

PART I: ILEOSTOMY AND HOME TPN

Mrs. M is a 54 YOWF of Jewish descent from New York City. Her husband is a successful businessman. Both are well respected in the community. Mrs. M is a very active woman, always taking part in Temple activities, charitable fund raisers, etc. She is also a member of the Hadassah, an organization for Jewish women. She is very kind, but very excitable. Everything she does has to be in perfect order, whether it is at home, the Temple, or in civic organizations. She never takes time to rest. She is always on the go.

Mrs. M was diagnosed with regional enteritis (now called Crohn's disease) 30 years ago. The disease cleared up shortly after it was diagnosed and remained in remission for several years, recurring only during times of extreme stress. Mrs. M had surgery three times, but since the surgeries were performed in three different parts of the country, details of her surgical history are incomplete. It is understood that she had a total colectomy and part of the distal ileum was removed. It is not certain how much of the ileum remains. The last surgery was a little over a year ago.

Mrs. M has been on limited solid food intake for the past year. She has been having a difficult time with diarrhea through the ileostomy. Her electrolytes are usually out of line because of this. She has been to the best physicians in the country for help. The final consensus was to place a Hickman/Broviac catheter to provide her with TPN during the night, thus by-passing the GI tract in an attempt to provide her with

324

nourishment and control electrolytes. Mrs. M recently had another flare-up of the disease. She experienced excessive loss of fluid through the ileostomy, as well as fatigue and weakness, and was having PVCs. She was admitted to a hospital. Her height and weight were 5'2" and 97 lbs. Her diagnoses read as follows:

- Recurrent Crohn's disease
- Dehydration
- Hyponatremia
- Hypokalemia
- Hypophosphatemia
- Hypocalcemia
- Hypomagnesemia
- Anemia

Her orders included:
1. SBR
2. Standard TPN via a Hickman/Broviac catheter, start at 25 cc/hr
3. Have NST determine patient's needs and recommend appropriate TPN mixture, flow rate, and diet for SBS
4. NPO
5. Start I.V. with NS, 50 cc/hr
6. Solu-Medrol (methylprednisone sodium succinate), 30 mg I.V. q4h
7. CBC and Metabolic Package

Before starting anything through the GI tract, the MD wants to give the bowel a chance to rest and possibly start an elemental tube feeding.
****

QUESTIONS:
1. Research Crohn's disease and discuss the incidence of the disease, the cause, the symptoms, and the treatment.

2. What is the function of Solu-Medrol and what nutritional implications does it have?

3. What dietary considerations are necessary with an ileostomy? (*Hint: Remember the colon has been removed. {What is the function of the colon?}*)

4. Are there any foods/nutrients that tend to cause diarrhea after the colon is removed?

5. If a person with an ileostomy has excessive loss of fluids, are there any foods that may help electrolyte balance?

6. What is the purpose of bowel rest and the elemental diet?

7. Define the following terms:

Hyponatremia:

Hypokalemia:

Hypophosphatemia:

Hypocalcemia:

Hypomagnesemia:

8. Should there be concern about any vitamins or minerals that are believed to be absorbed in the ileum?

9. Determine Mrs. M's IBW and percent IBW (Appendix A, Tables 7 and 8).

****

The dietitian interviewed Mrs. M and obtained the following information: Mrs. M was not a true Orthodox Jew but was a Conservative Jew and followed many of the rules of the Kashruth (laws based on biblical and rabbinical regulations). The solid foods she ate were in small amounts and were mostly some of her favorite foods, such as gefilte, borscht, latkes, blintzes, and kugel. Mrs. M enjoyed candy, particularly chocolate. She wanted to eat more but, because of the diarrhea, the food went right through her and she felt like it was a waste. She depended heavily on the TPN she received during the night. She did not know what TPN formula was being used. Mrs. M knew that she lost a lot of water through the ileostomy. She believed that she should drink a lot of fluids to replace those that were lost. The fluids she drank as replacements included: approximately 1.5 qts of fruit juice, close to 1 L of a caffeine-containing soda, and 6 to 7 c of coffee (with sugar) per day. She also tried drinking several different kinds of nutritional supplements (she named several of the more popular supplements used). They were either too sweet or tasted awful. She was never instructed by an RD.

****

QUESTIONS CONTINUED:

10. What are the differences between the dietary practices of an Orthodox Jew, a Conservative Jew, and a Reformed Jew?

11. What does Kosher mean? How would Kosher food affect a diet instruction, particularly Kosher meat?

12. Identify the following foods Mrs. M liked to eat and indicate the nutrients contained in these foods in high levels:

Gefilte:

Borscht:

Latkes:

Blintzes:

Kugel:

****

Mrs. M's labs were:

BASIC METABOLIC PACKAGE							
TEST	**RESULT**	**REFERENCE UNITS** Conventional	SI	**TEST**	**RESULT**	**REFERENCE UNITS** Conventional	SI
Glu	140 mg/dl	70-110 mg/dl	3.8-6.1 mmol/L	Na	132 mEq/L	136-145 mEq/L	136-145 mmol/L
BUN	19 mg/dl	6-20 mg/dl	2.1-7.1 mmol/L	K	3.3 mEq/L	3.5-5.2 mEq/L	3.5-5.2 mmol/L
Cr	0.8mg/dl	0.6-1.1 mg/dl	53-97 μmol/L	Cl	100 mEq/L	96-106 mEq/L	96-106 mmol/L
Ca	8.8 mg/dl	8.8-10.0 mg/dl	2.20-2.60 mmol/L	Mg	1.6 mEq/L	1.8 - 2.6 mEq/L	136-145 mmol/L
Ser alb	3.0 g/dl	3.5-4.8 g/dl	39-50 g/dl	P	3.0mg/dl	2.7-4.5 mg/dl	4.7-6.0 kPa

CBC							
TEST	**RESULT**	**REFERENCE UNITS** Conventional	SI	**TEST**	**RESULT**	**REFERENCE UNITS** Conventional	SI
Hgb	11 g/dl	12-16 g/dl	120-160 g/L	WBC	14.2 x 10^3/ μl	4.5-10.5 x 10^3/cells/mm^3	4.5-10.5 x10^9/L
Hct	33 %	36-48%		% Lymph	20%	25 – 40% of total WBC	1500-4000 cells/mm^3
RBC	3.9x10^6/μ	3.6-5.0x10^6/L	3.6-5.0 x10^{12}/L	MCH	28 pg/cell	26-34 pg/cell	0.40-.53 fmol/cell
MCV	84 μm^3	82-98μm^3	82-98 fL	MCHC	33 g/dl	32-36 g/dl	320-360 g/L

****

QUESTIONS CONTINUED:

13. Below is a list of diagnoses. Next to each diagnosis, write the name of the lab(s) that helps to confirm the diagnosis.

DIAGNOSIS	ASSOCIATED LAB(S)
Dehydration	
Hyponatremia	
Hypokalemia	
Hypophosphatemia	
Hypocalcemia	
Hypomagnesemia	
Anemia	
Crohn's Disease	

14. What is the difference between total Ca and ionized Ca?

15. What relationship does Ca have to serum albumin?

16. Using the Harris-Benedict equation (Appendix A, Table 17) and the appropriate stress factor, calculate Mrs. M's daily energy needs. Show your work.

17. Calculate Mrs. M's protein needs (take into consideration any medications Mrs. M may be taking that could affect protein metabolism).

18. List any substances that are in excess in Mrs. M's diet, even non-nutrients.

19. Outline the medical nutrition therapy you would recommend for Mrs. M.

20. Prepare a SOAP note for Mrs. M.

S:
O:
A:
P:

ADDITIONAL OPTIONAL QUESTIONS:

21. Describe a Hickman\Broviac catheter and compare it to a central line catheter.

22. Research a standard TPN solution in one of your local hospitals and describe the components.

23. List the advantages and disadvantages of TPN via a central line catheter and a Hickman\Broviac catheter.

TPN	Advantages	Disadvantages
Central Line		
Hickman\Broviac		

****

PART II: TPN TO PO FEEDINGS

An order has been written for the dietitian to calculate Mrs. M's energy and protein needs and to recommend a TPN mixture, flow rate, and diet. In the meantime, her nutrition orders were standard TPN at 50 cc/h. Standard TPN consist of: 500 cc of $D_{50}W$, 500 cc of 8.5% AA, standard electrolytes with 1 amp of MVI 12, and 3 cc MTE every day (Appendix E). This is to be given via a Hickman/Broviac catheter.

****

QUESTIONS CONTINUED:

24. Would you give Mrs. M I.V. lipids? Why or why not?

25. Differentiate between lipid administration as a three-in-one admixture or as piggy back. Include the advantages, disadvantages, and precautions of each.

26. What lab value(s) are used to monitor lipids?

27. If you decided to give lipids, how much would you give and what flow rate would you use?

28. For TPN, would you use the standard formula or create a new formula? Give reasons for your answer, and regardless of which formula you use, list the constituents and amounts you would recommend be given on a daily basis (assume you are working at a hospital that allows individual formulation of TPN formulas if necessary).

29. For whichever formula you used in question 27, calculate the amount of TPN Mrs. M will need daily to meet her energy and protein requirements. Consider the lipids you are giving in your calculations.

30. Calculate the flow rate that is necessary to deliver the amount of TPN calculated in question 28 in a day.

31. Double check your answer by calculating the total amount of CHO, protein, and fat Mrs. M will receive with the formula and flow rates you determined. Compare these values with your original calculations in question 27. Show all work.

32. Would you add any minerals above the standard amount? If so, which ones and how much? Explain your answer.

33. List the complications of TPN.

34. List the labs that are used to monitor TPN and the frequency in which they should be checked.

****

Mrs. M's ileostomy output slowed down after a few days of bowel rest. With TPN and close monitoring, her electrolytes were soon in normal range. Mrs. M started to feel stronger, so po feedings were restarted. The NST recommended the following diet prescription:

1. Restrict complex CHO to 150 g/d (excluding CHO in the supplement)
2. No sweets
3. No more than 4 oz of fruit juice per day
4. No caffeine
5. Chew food extremely well
6. Restrict total fluids to 1500 cc
7. 50 g protein (excluding protein in the supplement)
8. Low fat (no more than 38 g excluding fat in the supplement)
9. No salt restriction
10. At least 2 potassium sources per day
11. Stress multivitamin/mineral tab qd
12. In addition to above, 2 servings of a supplemental tube feeding appropriate for SBS. The dietitian can choose the appropriate supplement.

****

QUESTIONS CONTINUED:

35. Research the available supplements and suggest several appropriate supplements for SBS. With the supplements you choose, fill in the table below (see Appendix F):

Product	Producer	Form	Cal/ ml	Non-pro cal/g N	g/L			Na mg	K mg	mOsm /kg water	Vol to meet RDA in ml	g of fiber /L	Free H$_2$O /L in ml
					Pro	CHO	Fat						

36. Research the medications prednisone and sulfasalazine. Tell what they are used for and list any nutritional implications.

37. On a separate sheet of paper, briefly give the rationale for of the recommendations made by the NST.
    1. Restrict complex CHO to 150 g/d (excluding CHO in the supplement)
    2. No sweets
    3. No more than 4 oz of fruit juice per day
    4. No caffeine
    5. Chew food extremely well
    6. Restrict total fluids to 1500 cc (excluding liquid in the supplement)
    7. 50 g protein (excluding protein in the supplement)
    8. Low fat (no more than 38 g, excluding fat in the supplement)
    9. No salt restriction
    10. At least 2 potassium sources per day
    11. Stress multivitamin/mineral tab every day

****

This diet was attempted by starting slowly and gradually building up to the amount prescribed. The TPN was decreased gradually until it was no longer needed. The pt tolerated the diet and was D/C without TPN. Her medications included prednisone po and sulfasalazine po. Her diet was changed slightly to include 200 g of CHO and 1 serving of supplement per day.

****

38. For the diet that Mrs. M is being discharged with, calculate:
    1. total kcals and kcals/kg
    2. total grams of CHO
    3. total protein
    4. total fat
    5. grams of protein/kg of body weight
    6. stress factor used
    7. ccs per kcal (fluid allowed plus supplement)

39. Prepare a SOAP note for Mrs. M, building on your last SOAP note.

S:
O:
A:
P:

RELATED REFERENCES

1. Alterescu, K.B. (1985). The ostomy. What about special procedures? *Am. J. Nurs.* 85(12):1363-7.

2. Black, P. (1985). Stoma care. Drugs and diet. *Nurs. Mirror.* 161(11):26-8.

3. Danese, S., Sans, M., and Fiocchi, C. (2004). Inflammatory bowel disease: the role of environmental factors. *Autoimmun Rev.* Jul;3(5):394-400.

4. Duerksen, D.R., Nehra, V., Bistrian, B.R., & Blackburn, G.L. (1998). Appropriate nutritional support in acute and complicated Crohn's disease. *Nutrition.* 14(5):462-5.

5. Elishoov, H., Or, R., Strauss, N., & Engelhard, D. (1998). Nosocomial colonization, septicemia, and Hickman/Broviac catheter-related infections in bone marrow transplant recipients. A 5-year prospective study. *Medicine (Baltimore).* 77(2):83-101.

6. Evans, J.P., Steinhart, A.H., Cohen, Z., & McLeod, R.S. (2003). Home total parenteral nutrition: an alternative to early surgery for complicated inflammatory bowel disease. *J Gastrointest Surg.* May-Jun;7(4):562-6.

7. Fischbach, F.T. (2003). *A Manual of Laboratory & Diagnostic Tests.* 7th Ed. Philadelphia. J.B. Lippincott Company.

8. Fernandez-Banares, F., Cabre, E., Gonzalez-Huix, F., & Gassull, M.A. (1994). Enteral nutrition as primary therapy in Crohn's disease. *Gut.* 35(1 Suppl):S55-9.

9. Forbes, A. (2004). Parenteral nutrition: new advances and observations. *Curr Opin Gastroenterol.* Mar;20(2):114-8.

10. Gassull, M.A. (2004). Review article: the role of nutrition in the treatment of inflammatory bowel disease. *Aliment Pharmacol Ther.* Oct;20 Suppl 4:79-83.

11. Geerling, B.J., Badart-Smook, A., Stockbrugger, R.W., & Brummer, R.J. (1998). Comprehensive nutritional status in patients with long-standing Crohn's disease currently in remission. *Am. J. Clin. Nutr.* 67(5):919-26.

12. Hamilton, H. & Fermo, K. (1998). Assessment of patients requiring I.V. therapy via a central venous route. *Br. J. Nurs.* 7(8):451-4, 456-60.

13. Husain, A. & Korzenik, J.R. (1998). Nutritional issues and therapy in inflammatory bowel disease. *Semin. Gastrointest. Dis.* 9(1):21-30.

14. Ishida, T., Himeno, K., Torigoe, Y., Inoue, M., Wakisaka, O., Tabuki, T., Ono, H., Honda, K., Mori, T., Seike, M., Yoshimatsu, H., & Sakata, T. (2003). Selenium deficiency in a patient with Crohn's disease receiving long-term total parenteral nutrition. *Intern Med.* Feb;42(2):154-7.

15. Keller, J., Panter, H., & Layer P. (2004), Management of the short bowel syndrome after extensive small bowel resection. *Best Pract Res Clin Gastroenterol.* Oct;18(5):977-92.

16. Krok, K.L., & Lichtenstein, G.R. (2003). Nutrition in Crohn's disease. *Curr Opin Gastroenterol.* Mar;19(2):148-53.

17. Loftus, E.V. Jr. (2004). Clinical epidemiology of inflammatory bowel disease: Incidence, prevalence, and environmental influences. *Gastroenterology.* May;126(6):1504-17.

18. Ludvigsson, J.F., Krantz, M., Bodin, L., Stenhammar, L., and Lindquist, B. (2004). Elemental versus polymeric enteral nutrition in paediatric Crohn's disease: a multicentre randomized controlled trial. *Acta Paediatr.* Mar;93(3):327-35.

19. Mingrone, G., Benedetti, G., Capristo, E., De Gaetano, A., Greco, A.V., Tataranni, P.A., & Gasbarrini, G. (1998). Twenty-four-hour energy balance in Crohn's disease patients: metabolic implications of steroid treatment. *Am. J. Clin. Nutr.* 67(1):118-23.

20. O'Sullivan, M., & O'Morain, C. (2001). Nutritional Treatments in Inflammatory Bowel Disease. *Curr Treat Options Gastroenterol.* Jun;4(3):207-213.

21. Prendergast, A. & Fulton, F.L. (1997) *Medical terminology: A Text/Workbook.* 4th Ed. Redwood City, California. Addison-Wesley Nursing.

22. Pronsky, Z.M., Redfern, C.M., Crowe, J. & Epstein, S. (2003) *Food Medication Interactions*, 13th Ed Phoenix, Arizona. Food-Medications Interactions, Publishers and Distributors.

23. Rolfes, S.R., Pinna, K. & Whitney, E. (2006). *Understanding Normal and Clinical Nutrition*, 7th Ed. West/Wadsworth.

24. Sales, T.R., Torres, H.O., Couto, C.M., & Carvalho, E.B. (1998). Intestinal adaptation in short bowel syndrome without tube feeding or home parenteral nutrition: report of four consecutive cases. *Nutrition.* 14(6):508-12.

25. Siegmund, B., & Zeitz, M. (2004). Standards of medical treatment and nutrition in Crohn's disease. *Langenbecks Arch Surg.* Sep 23; [Epub ahead of print]

26. Spratto, G.R. & Woods, A.L. (2005). *PDR Nurse's Drug Handbook.* Thompson Delmar Learning, NY.

INTRODUCTION TO BRIEF CASE STUDIES

In the following section are five new brief case studies. They are very short and to the point and are intended to be used after several of the standard preceding cases are completed, but can easily be used in conjunction with the preceding cases. The brief cases require more in-depth knowledge of clinical nutrition, situations, and procedures. All of the cases are based on actual cases that occurred. The initials have been changed and some medications and lab values have been added or changed to make them more appropriate to challenge dietetic students.

CASE STUDY #36
RENAL FAILURE FROM NSAID ABUSE

INTRODUCTION
This is a short case to introduce the student to real-life hospital experiences that they will see and for which they may be part of the health care team that provides treatment for the patient. This involves renal failure for a patient that damaged their kidneys from excessive NSAID abuse.
****

GN is a 34 YOWF who has an Hx of chronic headaches. For this she has taken numerous over-the-counter pain killers. She has been bothered by headaches for so long that when one pain killer did not work, she would try another. If the label said not to take more than six per day, she assumed that to mean six of that brand and excluded other brands. She has been taking at least three different NSAID a day for the past three years, usually 5 or 6 of each. She developed back pain, which stimulated her to take even more pain killers. When she started having dark urine with a foamy appearance, she went to her doctor. A urinalysis showed her to have >500 mg/dl of protein in her urine and RBCs too numerous to count. Creatinine clearance was 60 cc/min (normal 80 – 110 cc/min). She was referred to a nephrologist who completed an ultrasound and found bilateral small kidneys. A biopsy was performed and showed interstitial nephritis. She was placed on 2 mg/kg/day of prednisone for six months and was to return for reevaluation.
****

QUESTIONS:
1. Describe creatinine clearance, tell what it measures and what it means.

2. Describe interstitial nephritis. How is this going to affect the patient's health?

3. What is the recommended dietary meal plan for someone with interstitial nephritis?

4. Describe the nutritional implications of prednisone taken daily for six months.

5. Would you adjust the diet because of the prednisone?

6. Suppose you had to work with GN on an outpatient basis, counseling her on her diet. Write a SOAP note with emphasis on what you would do for a nutrition care plan.

S:
O:
A:
P:

RELATED READING

1. Fogo, A.B. (2003). Quiz page. Acute interstitial nephritis and minimal change disease lesion, caused by NSAID injury. *Am J Kidney Dis*. Aug;42(2):A41, E1.

2. Szalat, A., Krasilnikov, I., Bloch, A., Meir, K., Rubinger, D., & Mevorach, D. (2004). Acute renal failure and interstitial nephritis in a patient treated with rofecoxib: case report and review of the literature. *Arthritis Rheum*. Aug 15;51(4):670-3.

3. Ulinski, T., Guigonis, V., Dunan, O., & Bensman, A. (2004). Acute renal failure after treatment with non-steroidal anti-inflammatory drugs. *Eur J Pediatr*. Mar;163(3):148-50. Epub 2004 Jan 24.

CASE STUDY #37
CROHN'S DISEASE IN A YOUNG COLLEGE FEMALE

INTRODUCTION
This is an account of a young female college student that presents with Crohn's that was initially misdiagnosed. The latest medications for treating Crohn's are introduced.
****

BH is a 22 YOWF in her senior year of college. She is 5'3" and weighs 115 lbs. She is a very bright student that is active in several campus organizations and holds down three part-time jobs to support her way through school. BH suddenly began running a fever and experiencing abdominal discomfort but did not do anything about it. The fever and discomfort continued and she began feeling tired. After five days of this she went to the campus infirmary and saw a doctor. He obtained a CBC and urinalysis. She had a WBC of 13,000 and a hgb of 6.4. Her temperature was 102° F. She was given Cipro for a UTI and told to take Tylenol for fever and to start taking Slow Fe for anemia. She went to her room and took the meds but the pain got unbearable. She called her parents and they came and took her to the ER. A rectal and pelvic exam revealed a peri-rectal abscess. A surgeon was called in and ordered a CT scan to determine the exact location and size of the abscess. BH was put on IV Cipro and Flagyl and was given morphine. Within two hours she was in surgery to have the abscess drained. The surgeon reported that it was the largest abscess he had ever seen. She continued on po Cipro, 500 mg q12h and Flagyl 500 mg q8h.

BH healed and went home but started having diarrhea after almost every meal. She was having loose and frequent stools prior to the surgery but it seemed to be with high-fat foods, lettuce, and especially corn. She thought it was food allergies. Three weeks passed before she started with abdominal pain and a fever. She called her surgeon and ended up back in the ER. The abscess had returned in the same place and the same size. She went through the same procedures as before, surgery included. Her meds were the same: Flagyl, Cipro, but with added Toradol, 500 mg q6h and Buprenex for pain. After she healed from surgery, a colonoscopy was completed. They found and removed a benign polyp, an unusual occurrence for someone so young. Extreme inflammation and ulcers were also found, consistent with Crohn's and ulcerative colitis. Biopsies were obtained but the pathology was unable to determine if it was Crohn's or ulcerative colitis. Based on what the surgeon saw, he made an assumption it was Crohn's. He started BH on Remicade and kept her in the hospital until her WBC returned to normal and then sent her to a gastroenterologist.

The gastroenterologist performed a sigmoidoscopy and took another biopsy. This time the biopsy revealed Crohn's disease. She D/Ced the Remicade and started BH on a stronger drug, 6-MP 50 mg a day, 250 mg of Flagyl tid, and Niferex. GH lost 14 pounds since her first visit to the infirmary.
****

QUESTIONS:
1. Review the following drugs and describe their action and side effects with emphasis on nutritional side effects.

    Cipro:

    Slow Fe:

Flagyl:

Toradol:

Buprenex:

Remicade:

6-MP:

Niferex:

2. Calculate BH's % of loss of weight and % of UBW.

3. Considering a temperature of 102°, calculate BH's caloric requirements.

4. What advice would you give BH concerning her nutritional intake while she is having diarrhea? Explain the differences, if any, in her meal plan when the diarrhea stops. Take into consideration that when she has diarrhea, she also has a fever of 102°.

5. If BH were to continue to have diarrhea and lose weight, compare some of the tube feedings you would recommend for her.

Product	Producer	Form	Cal/ ml	Non-pro cal/g N	g/L			Na mg	K mg	mOsm /kg water	Vol to meet RDA in ml	g of fiber /L	Free H$_2$O /L in ml
					Pro	CHO	Fat						

RELATED REFERENCES

1. Duerksen, D.R., Nehra, V., Bistrian, B.R., & Blackburn, G.L. (1998). Appropriate nutritional support in acute and complicated Crohn's disease. *Nutrition.* 14(5):462-5.

2. Fernandez-Banares, F., Cabre, E., Gonzalez-Huix, F., & Gassull, M.A. (1994). Enteral nutrition as primary therapy in Crohn's disease. *Gut.* 35(1 Suppl):S55-9.

3. Gassull, M.A. (2004). Review article: the role of nutrition in the treatment of inflammatory bowel disease. *Aliment Pharmacol Ther.* Oct;20 Suppl 4:79-83.

4. Geerling, B.J., Badart-Smook, A., Stockbrugger, R.W., & Brummer, R.J. (1998). Comprehensive nutritional status in patients with long-standing Crohn's disease currently in remission. *Am. J. Clin. Nutr.* 67(5):919-26.

5. Gonvers, J.J., Juillerat, P., Mottet, C., Felley, C., Burnand, B., Vader, J.P., Michetti, P., & Froehlich, F. (2005). Maintenance of Remission in Crohn's Disease. *Digestion.* Feb 4;71(1):41-48 [Epub ahead of print]

6. Griffiths, A.M. (2005). Use of 6-mercapturine/azathioprine as the immunomodulator of choice for moderately active Crohn's disease: con. *Inflamm Bowel Dis.* Feb;11(2):200-2.

7. Hyams, J.S. (2005). Use of 6-mercaptopurine/azathioprine as the immunomodulator of choice for moderately active Crohn's disease: pro. *Inflamm Bowel Dis.* Feb;11(2):197-9.

8. 1 Jacobstein, D.A., & Baldassano, R.N. (2005). Use of 6-mercaptopurine/azathioprine as the immunomodulator of choice for moderately active Crohn's disease: balance. *Inflamm Bowel Dis.* Feb;11(2):203-5.

9. Krok, K.L., & Lichtenstein, G.R. (2003). Nutrition in Crohn disease. *Curr Opin Gastroenterol.* Mar;19(2):148-53.

10. Mingrone, G., Benedetti, G., Capristo, E., De Gaetano, A., Greco, A.V., Tataranni, P.A., & Gasbarrini, G. (1998). Twenty-four-hour energy balance in Crohn's disease patients: metabolic implications of steroid treatment. *Am. J. Clin. Nutr.* 67(1):118-23.

11. O'Sullivan, M., & O'Morain, C. (2001). Nutritional Treatments in Inflammatory Bowel Disease. *Curr Treat Options Gastroenterol.* Jun;4(3):207-213.

CASE STUDY #38
METABOLIC SYNDROME

INTRODUCTION

This is a short case to introduce the advanced student to metabolic syndrome complicated by a cardiovascular emergency.

****

FA is a 48 YOWM who has a Hx of chronic obesity that he claims is uncontrollable by diet. In spite of being obese, he has been healthy and thus saw no reason to see a physician. One evening he reported to the ER with complaints of sudden retosternal chest pain, nausea, diaphoresis, and weakness. On examination, he was found to have a blood pressure of 180/90. His height was 5' 10" and he weighed 295 lbs. His waist was 43 inches. An electrocardiogram revealed an acute anterior myocardial infarction. A chest X-ray revealed mild pulmonary edema. Random blood was drawn and revealed serum glucose to be 240 mg/dl; triglycerides were 320 mg/dl, cholesterol was 280 mg/dl, and HDL was 30 mg/dl. His urinalysis revealed 260 mg/dl albuminuria.

Dx: Metabolic syndrome with acute myocardial infarction.

Tx Plan: Left heart catherization with stent placement. Begin Capoten (captopril) and Crestor (rosuvastatin calcium). Weight reduction and exercise. Workup for diabetes.

****

QUESTIONS:

1. Define the following terms:

   metabolic syndrome:

   retosternal:

   diaphoresis:

2. Calculate FA's LDL.

3. Describe the action and complications of his medications.

   Capoten:

   Crestor:

4. What is a normal blood pressure?

5. What are the symptoms FA displayed that indicated metabolic syndrome?

6. Calculate FA's caloric requirements, describe the diet you would recommend, and tell why.

RELATED READING

1. Martin-Lazaro, J.F., & Becerra-Fernandez, A. (2005). The metabolic syndrome: Uncertain criteria. *Pharmacol Res*. Apr;51(4):385-6.

2. Moller, D.E., & Kaufman, K.D. (2005). Metabolic syndrome: A Clinical and Molecular Perspective. *Annu Rev Med*. 56:45-62.

3. Robinson, L.E., & Graham, T.E. (2004). Metabolic syndrome, a cardiovascular disease risk factor: role of adipocytokines and impact of diet and physical activity. *J Appl Physiol*. Dec;29(6):808-29.

4. Sudhakar, M.K. (2004). Ghost of metabolic syndrome. *J Assoc Physicians India*. Apr;52:342.

5. Zieve, F.J. (2004). The metabolic syndrome: diagnosis and treatment. *Clin Cornerstone*. 6 Suppl 3:S5-13.

CASE STUDY #39
NON-DIABETIC PERIPHERAL NEUROPATHY

INTRODUCTION

This is a study concerned with the continuous use of proton pump inhibitors in someone prone to B_{12} deficiency. Knowledge of physiology, advanced laboratory interpretation and critical thinking are required.

****

WC is a 58 YOWM who has been C/O gastric reflux for years. The GERD almost always occurs during the night while WC sleeps. He is not overweight, being 5'10" and weighing 175 lbs. He is in good physical shape. He talked to a friend who warned him about eating too much before he went to bed. WC was in the habit of having a late-night snack before retiring. He stopped his late-night snacks but it did not help. Another friend informed him about elevating the head of his bed so he was sleeping slightly downhill. He tried that but it did not work either. WC was also feeling tired and he noticed that he got "out of breath" easily. He finally gave in and went to see his family physician who completed blood analyses and found his hgb, hct, and mcv to be low. A stool sample analysis revealed occult blood. The physician put him on Nexium, 40 mg every day at hs and sent him to a gastroenterologist. A gastroduodenoscopy revealed moderate gastritis and a hiatal hernia. The physician told him he would have to be on Nexium the rest of his life and advised him to take over-the-counter iron supplements for three months.

WC followed the orders and the GERD went away. He took the iron for three months and felt fine. Time passed and, about four and one-half years later, WC noticed the bottom of his toes on his left foot did not "feel right" when he walked. He did not pay it much attention because it did not hurt. Over the next few weeks this slowly became more noticeable and the toes of the right foot began to feel the same way. He went to his physician who drew blood and all tests were normal. He sent WC to a neurologist. The neurologist had a series of lab work done (14 tubes of blood) and a nerve conduction test. All of the blood work was negative, but the nerve conduction test revealed slight destruction of the nerve endings in both feet consistent with peripheral neuropathy (PN). The physician completed a physical on WC that was normal. WC's family history was devoid of PN. He told WC that he had a PN of unknown etiology and that the cause of most PNs were unknown. If the condition worsened, he should come back and see him.

Approximately seven months later, WC was shown a textbook that indicated older people absorb less B_{12}. The book further indicated that many older people have problems with GERD and are placed on histamine blockers and proton pump inhibitors. Either of these can block the absorption of B_{12}. WC checked and vitamin B_{12} was not evaluated by the neurologists. By this time, WC had moved to another state and had not established with a physician. On his own he quit taking the Nexium and began taking 400 µg of folic acid, 250 µg of B_{12}, and 50 mg of B_6 in addition to his usual multivitamin. When he saw a physician several weeks later, the physician analyzed his blood for folic acid, B_{12}, and methylmalonic acid. The results indicated his B_{12} was 750 pg/ml (norms = 179-1132) and methylmalonic acid was 169 nmol/L (norms = 88-243). The folic acid results had a special note that read as follows: Diluted 1:10 = 5.87 x 10 = 58.7 (norms = 3.0-45.). The folic acid was so high it was off their scale. They diluted it 1:10 and measured it again and found it to be 5.87. This times the dilution factor of 10 = 58.7.

****

QUESTIONS:

1. Define the following terms:
   gastric reflux

gastroduodenoscopy:

peripheral neuropathy:

GERD:

2. Illustrate the pathway that converts homocysteine to cysteine or to methionine. Show the need for B_6, B_{12}, and folic acid.

3. What part does methylmalonic acid play in the metabolism of B_{12}? Why would the physician analyze for this compound?

4. The theory developed for WC was that the proton inhibitor decreased the possibly already reduced absorption of B_{12}, causing PN. When blood was analyzed, B_{12} was in the normal range but, considering the large doses that WC had been taking for several weeks without taking Nexium, it was assumed that B_{12} should have been higher. A clue that this was correct was the elevation of folic acid. If B_{12} is low, why would folic acid be higher than normal? (Hint: look up the methyl folate trap).

RELATED REFERENCES

1. Ambrosch, A., Dierkes, J., Lobmann, R., Kuhne, W., Konig, W., Luley, C., & Lehnert, H. (2001). Relation between homocysteinaemia and diabetic neuropathy in patients with Type 2 diabetes mellitus. *Diabet Med.* 2001 Mar;18(3):185-92.

2. Arnaud, J., Fleites-Mestre, P., Chassagne, M., Verdura, T., Garcia, I., Hernandez-Fernandez, T., Gautier, H., Favier, A., Perez-Cristia, R., & Barnouin, J. (2001). Vitamin B intake and status in healthy Havanan men, 2 years after the Cuban neuropathy epidemic. *Br J Nutr.* 2001 Jun;85(6):741-8.

3. Hoffbrand, A.V. & Jackson, B.F. (1993). Correction of the DNA synthesis defect in vitamin B_{12} deficiency by tetrahydrofolate: evidence in favour of the methyl-folate trap hypothesis as the cause of megaloblastic anaemia in vitamin B_{12} deficiency. *Br J Haematol.* Apr;83(4):643-7.

4. Sauer, H. & Wilmanns, W. (1977). Cobalamin dependent methionine synthesis and methyl-folate-trap in human vitamin B_{12} deficiency. *Br J Haematol.* Jun;36(2):189-98.

5. Scott, J.M. & Weir, D.G. (1981). The methyl folate trap. A physiological response in man to prevent methyl group deficiency in kwashiorkor (methionine deficiency) and an explanation for folic-acid induced exacerbation of subacute combined degeneration in pernicious anaemia. *Lancet.* Aug 15;2(8242):337-40.

CASE STUDY #40
HERB-DRUG INTERACTIONS

NTRODUCTION

This study gives an example of the improper use of herbs, some false assumptions, and some almost disastrous consequences.

****

LJ is a 47 YOBM who had a kidney transplant three years ago 2° to ESRD, 2° to HTN. The surgery was successful and LJ has been enjoying a much improved quality of life. However, he still has in the back of his mind that he could experience rejection and this creates a lot stress for LJ. It never completely goes away. He has been attending a support group for kidney transplant patients that helps him most of the time. There are times when one of his friends has a problem with rejection and it causes LJ to worry that something similar may happen to him. A friend told him about an over-the-counter herb, St. John's wort, that helps promote calmness. LJ figured that if it was over-the-counter and did not require a prescription, it must be okay to take.

LJ prescription medications included:
▸ Lasix PRN
▸ Prednisone
▸ Cyclosporine
▸ Rapamune

LJ was also told to take multivitamins with minerals, iron supplements, and calcium supplements. On his own imitative, LJ started taking St. John's wort and took the maximum dose indicted on the label. Several days went by and he did not notice a difference in the way he felt. He assumed that it was not working, not because the herb was incapable of helping him, but because he was not taking enough. He thus began taking a larger dose than recommended. In time, he noticed a somewhat calming effect that he attributed to St. John's wort, so he thought he had found the correct dose for him and continued to take it. As time passed his worse fears started to materialize; he was starting to reject his kidney. He was hospitalized to receive stronger I.V. doses of his immunosuppressants. When he told his physicians what he was taking, they told him that St. John's wort can decreases the effectiveness of cyclosporine. He was taken off the herb and his kidney began functioning again.

****

QUESTIONS:

1. Look up the action of the following medications and list their side effects along with any nutritional complications and herbal interactions:

Lasix:

Prednisone:

Cyclosporine:

Rapamune:

2. Look up St. John's wort and describe its indications for use, side effects, and possible drug/food interactions.

3. Explain the effects prednisone, cyclosporine, and rapamune will have on LJ's diet and how his diet should be adjusted accordingly.

4. If the claims made for St. John's wort are true (i.e., beneficial effects, side effects, time it takes to produce an effect), explain why LJ did not feel an effect after taking it a few days.

5. Discuss LJ's attitude, "if a little works, a lot more will work a lot better."

6. Discuss LJ's assumption, "if it's sold over-the-counter, it must be OK."

7. If LJ wanted to take an over-the-counter supplement, herb, vitamin or mineral, what would be the correct way to go about doing it?

RELATED REFERENCES

1. Chueh, S.C. & Kahan, B.D. (2005). Clinical application of sirolimus in renal transplantation: an update. *Transpl Int*. Mar;18(3):261-77.

2. Izzo, A.A. (2005). Herb-drug interactions: an overview of the clinical evidence. *Fundam Clin Pharmacol*. Feb;19(1):1-16.

3. Izzo, A.A. (2004). Drug interactions with St. John's Wort (Hypericum perforatum): a review of the clinical evidence. *Int J Clin Pharmacol Ther*. Mar;42(3):139-48.

4. Kamar, N., Allard, J., Ribes, D., Durand, D., Ader, J.L., & Rostaing, L. (2005). Assessment of glomerular and tubular functions in renal transplant patients receiving cyclosporine A in combination with either sirolimus or everolimus. *Clin Nephrol*. Feb;63(2):80-6.

5. Knuppel, L. & Linde, K. (2004). Adverse effects of St. John's Wort: a systematic review. *J Clin Psychiatry*. Nov;65(11):1470-9.

6. Zhou, S., Chan, E., Pan, S.Q., Huang, M., & Lee, E.J. (2004). Pharmacokinetic interactions of drugs with St John's wort. *J Psychopharmacol*. Jun;18(2):262-76.

CS#40 Herb-Drug Interactions

APPENDIX A

COMMONLY USED FORMULAS AND CONVERSION FACTORS

Table A - 1 Weight Conversions:

1 kilogram (kg) = 1,000 grams (g)	1 ounce (oz) = 28 grams
1 gram (g) = 1,000 milligrams (mg)	16 ounces = 1 pound (lb)
1 milligram = 1,000 micrograms (μg)	1 pound = 454 grams
1 microgram = 1,000 nanograms (ng)	1 kilogram = 2.2 pounds
1 nanogram = 1,000 picograms (pg)	1 teaspoon (tsp) = ~ 5 grams
	3 teaspoons = ~ 1 tablespoon (tbs)

Table A – 2 Volume Conversions:

1 liter (L) = 1,000 milliliters (mL or ml)	1 cup (c) = 8 fluid ounces
1 liter = 1.06 quarts (qt)	1 cup = ~ 240 milliliters
1 quart = 0.95 liters	4 cups = 1 quart
1 milliliter = 1 cubic centimeter (cc)	1 teaspoon (tsp) = ~ 5 milliliters
30 milliliters = 1 fluid ounce	1 tablespoon (tbs) = ~ 15 milliliters
32 ounces = 1 quart	2 tablespoons = ~ 1 ounce

Table A – 3 Length Conversions

1 inch = 2.54 centimeters (cm)
1 foot (ft) = 30.48 centimeters
1 meter (m) = 100 centimeters
1 meter = 39.37 inches
1 meter = 3.28 feet

Table A – 4 Temperature Conversions

To convert Celsius (Centigrade) to Fahrenheit:
$(9/5 \times t_c) + 32 = t_F$

To convert Fahrenheit to Celsius:
$5/9 (t_F - 32) = t_c$

Table A – 5 Milligrams and Milliequivalents:

To convert milliequivalents (mEq) to milligrams (mg), multiply mEq by the element's atomic weight and divide by the valence:

$$mEq \times atomic\ weight/valence = mg$$

To convert milligrams to milliequivalents, divide milligrams by the element's atomic weight and multiply by the valence:

$$mg/atomic\ weight \times valence = mg$$

Example: To convert 2000 mg of Na to mEq: $2000/23 \times 1 = 86.96$ mEq	**Example:** To convert 80 mEq of K to mg: $80 \times 39/1 = 3120$ mg

Table A – 6 Atomic Weights and Valences

	Atomic Weight	Valence		Atomic Weight	Valence
Na	23	1	Mg	24.3	2
K	39	1	P	31	2
Cl	35.4	1	Ca	40	2

Table A – 7 Ideal Body Weight (IBW)

If the Hamwi[1] method is preferred, it recommends the following procedures:

- For males, it allows 106 pounds for the first 5 feet plus 6 pounds for every additional inch over 5 feet.
- For females, 100 pounds is allowed for the first 5 feet plus 5 pounds for each additional inch.
- Up to 10% can be added for a large frame and up to 10% can be subtracted for a small frame. For a comparison of the IBW and the new dietary guidelines for Americans, see **Table A - 9.**

Example: Calculate the IBW of a 5'11" male with a very large frame.	**Example:** Calculate the IBW of a 5'4" female with an average frame.
1. For the first 5' = 106 lbs	1. For the first 5' = 100 lbs
2. For the 11" over 5' add 11 X 6 = 66	2. For the 4" over 5' add 4 X 5 = 20
3. IBW = 106 + 66 = 172 ± 10%	3. IBW = 100 + 20 = 120 ± 10%
4. For a very large frame: 172 X 10% = 17.2 or 17	
5. IBW = 172 + 17 = 189 lbs	

Table A – 8 Percentages

%IBW and %UBW		% of Weight Loss
$\%IBW = \dfrac{\text{Actual Weight}}{\text{Ideal Body Weight}} \times 100$		Original Weight - Final Weight = Loss of Weight
$\%UBW = \dfrac{\text{Actual Weight}}{\text{Usual Weight}} \times 100$		$\dfrac{\text{Loss of Weight}}{\text{Original Weight}} = \%$ of Weight Loss

Table A – 9 Adjusted Body Weight[2] (ABW)

Adjusted Body Weight = [(actual body weight - IBW or RBW) X 0.25[a]] + IBW or RBW

[a] This is based on data that indicates that only 25% of body adipose tissue is metabolically active. When this formula was developed, it was based on the then popular ideal body weight. It was assumed that this formula allowed for a uniform estimation of the caloric needs of the obese. If the assumption is true for IBW, it should be true for RBW also. However, there are some who do not like this assumption and do not use this formula.

Table A – 10 Body Mass Index[3]

Metric	English[4]
BMI = $\dfrac{\text{weight in kg}}{\text{height in cm}^2}$	BMI = $\dfrac{\text{weight in lbs} \times 705}{\text{height in inches}^2}$

Table A - 11 Body Mass Index Categories[5]

Underweight =	<18.5
Normal weight =	18.5-24.9
Overweight =	25-29.9
Obesity =	30 or greater
Morbid Obesity >	40

Table A – 12 Midarm Muscle Circumference (MAMC)[6-7]

MAMC (cm) = midarm circumference (cm) - [3.14* X triceps skinfolds (mm)]

* This factor converts the fatfold measurement to a circumference measurement and millimeters to centimeters.

Table A – 13 Total Lymphocyte Count (TLC)

TLC (mm^3) = WBC mm^3 x % Lymphocytes

Table A – 14 Rule of Nines[14]

The "Rule of Nines" is used to obtain an estimate of the body surface area burned. With this method, each of the following body areas is assumed to cover the indicated percent of the body surface area.

Each arm	= 9%	The posterior trunk	= 18%
Each leg	= 18%	The head	= 9%
The anterior trunk	= 18%	The perineum	= 1%

Table A – 15 Nitrogen Balance[15]

The determination of nitrogen balance requires knowing the 24-hour nitrogen intake and output. To estimate nitrogen from dietary protein, use either of these formulas:

Nitrogen Intake = $\dfrac{\text{Protein Intake (g)}}{6.25}$ or   Protein Intake X 16% = Nitrogen Intake

Nitrogen output per day equals the measured UUN plus a factor of 4 grams to account for nitrogen losses through the lungs, hair, skin, and nails as well as non-urea nitrogen losses in the urine.

Nitrogen output = UUN + 4g

Nitrogen Balance = $\dfrac{\text{Protein Intake (g)}}{6.25}$ - (UUN + 4g)   or   Protein Intake X 16% = Nitrogen Intake

Table A – 16 Waist-to-Hip Ratio:

Divide the waistline measurement by the hip measurement.

$$\dfrac{\text{Waist Measurement}}{\text{Hip Measurement}} = \text{Waist-to-hip ratio}$$

Table A – 17 BEE (Harris-Benedict Equation[10])

Women	Men
BEE = 655 + [9.6 x wt^a] + [1.7 x ht^b] - [4.7 x age^c]	BEE = 66 + [13.7 x wt^a] + [5 x ht^b] - [6.8 x age^c]
^{a}wt is in kg. ^{b}ht is in cm. ^{c}age is in yrs	

Appendix A

Table A – 18 Determining Energy and Protein Needs for a Fever[11]

BEE increases 13% per degree C or 7% per degree F. To calculate, complete the following steps:
1. Determine BEE 2. Normal temperature = 98.6 F. Elevated temp - normal temp = # of degrees F elevated 3. # of degrees F elevated x 7% = % BEE is to be increased 4. BEE x % calculated in 3. = amount BEE needs to be increased 5. BEE + results in 4. = Total kcals Needed
Example: Assume you calculated a BEE of 1500 kcals for someone who has a fever of 101☐ F.
1. BEE = 1500 kcals 2. 101 - 98.6 = 2.4° elevated 3. 2.4 x 7% = 16.8% 4. 1500 x 16.8% = 252 kcals 5. BEE + Needs increase = 1500 + 252 = 1752 total kcals

Table A – 19 Calculation of LDL Cholesterol by the Friedewald Formula[12]

$$LDL = Cholesterol - HDL - \frac{Triglycerides}{5}$$

Table A – 20 TIBC Calculation [13]

$$Transferrin \times 1.25 = TIBC$$

Table A – 21 Transferrin Saturation [12]

$$Transferrin\ Saturation\ \% = \frac{Serum\ Iron \times 100}{TIBC}$$

360

REFERENCES

1. Miller, M.A. (1985). A calculated method for determination of ideal body weight. *Nutri Support Services.* pp. 31-33.

2. Karkeck, J.M. (1984). Adjustment for Obesity, *Am. Diet. Assoc. Renal Practice Group Newsletter*, Winter Issue.

3. Garrow, J.S. & Webster, J. (1985). Quetelet's index (W/H^2) as a measure of fatness. *Int. J. Obesity.* 9:147-153.

4. Stensland, S.H. & Margolis, S. (1990). Simplifying the calculation of body mass index for quick reference. *J. Am. Diet. Assoc.* 90:856.

5. NIH WEB site: http://www.nhlbisupport.com/bmi/.

6. Rolfes, S.R., Pinna, K. & Whitney, E. (2006). *Understanding Normal and Clinical Nutrition*, 7th Ed. West/Wadsworth.

7. Lee, R.D., Nieman, D.C., & Nieman, D. (2002). *Nutritional Assessment.* 3rd Ed. McGraw-Hill.

8. Rakel, R.E. & Conn, H.F. Eds. (1978) The Rule of Nines. Family Practice, 2nd Ed. Philadelphia, W.B. Saunders Company. pg. 536-537.

9. Lee, R.D., Nieman, D.C., & Nieman, D. (2002). *Nutritional Assessment.* 3rd Ed. McGraw-Hill.

10. Harris, J.A. & Benedict, F.G. (1919) A biometric study of basal metabolism in man. *Carnegie Institute, Publication* 279:40.

11. Dubois, E.F.: The Mechanisms of Heat Loss and Temperature Regulation, Stanford University Press, CA, 1937.

12. Kaplan, L.A., Pesce, A.J., & Kazmierczak, S.C. (2003). Clinical Chemistry. Mosby, St. Louis. Pg 625.

13. Kalantar-Zadeh, K., Kleiner, M., Dunne, E., Ahem, K., Nelson, M., Koslowe, R., and Luft, F.C. (1998)Total iron-binding capacity – estimated transferring correlates with the nutritional subjective global assessment in hemodialysis patients. Am. J. Kidney Dis. 31:2, 263-72.

APPENDIX B

BLOOD, PLASMA, OR SERUM LABORATORY VALUES[1]

Reference Ranges

Determination	Conventional Units	SI Units
Albumin	3.5 - 4.8 g/dl	35 - 48 g/L
Alk Phos (ALP)	25 - 100 U/L	17 - 142 U/L
ALT (SGPT)		
Males	10 - 40 U/L	0.17 – 0.68 µkat/L
Females	7 – 35 U/L	0.12 – 0.60 µkat/L
Ammonia	15 - 56 µg/dl	9 - 33 µmol/L
Amylase	25 – 125 U/L	0.4 – 2.1 µkat/L
AST (SGOT)		
Males	14 – 20 U/L	0.23 – 0.33 µkat/L
Females	10 – 36 U/L	0.17 – 0.60 µkat/L
B_{12}	200 – 835 pg/ml	148 – 616 pmol/L
Bilirubin	Total 0.3 - 1.0 mg/dl	5.0 - 17.0 µmol/L
	Direct 0.0 - 0.2 mg/dl	0 - 3.4 µmol/L
BUN	6 - 20 mg/dl	2.1 – 7.1 mmol/L
Ca	Total 8.8 - 10.4 mg/dl	2.20 - 2.60 mmol/L
	Ionized 4.65 - 5.28 mg/dl	1.16 - 1.32 mmol/L
Cholesterol	140 - 199 mg/dl	3.63 – 5.15 mmol/L
CPK		
Men	38 - 174 IU/L	0.63 – 2.90 µkat/L
Women	26 - 140 IU/L	0.46 – 2.38 µkat/L
	Isoenzymes	
	CPK-BB (CPK$_1$) 0%	
	CPK-MB (CPK$_2$) 0 - 6 %	
	CPK-MM (CPK$_3$) 96 - 100 %	
Cl	96 - 106 mEq/L	96 - 106 mmol/L
Cr		
Males	0.9 – 1.3 mg/dl	80 – 115 µmol/L
Females	0.6 – 1.1 mg/dl	53 – 97 µmol/L
Fe		
Males	65 - 175 µg/dl	11.6 - 31.3 µmol/L
Females	50 – 170 µg/d	9.0 – 30.4 µmol/L
Folic acid	2 – 20 ng/ml	4.5 – 45.3 nmol/L
GGT		
Men	7 - 47 U/L	0.12 – 1.80 µkat/L
Women	5 - 25 U/L	0.08 – 0.42 µkat/L
Glucose	fasting 70 - 110 mg/dl	3.8 - 6.1 mmol/L
HCO_3	24 - 28 mEq/l	24 - 28 mmol
Hct	M 42 - 52%	
	F 36 - 48%	
HDL	M 45 - 65 mg/dl	1.17 - 1.68 mmol/L
	F 40 - 85 mg/dl	1.0 - 2.2 mmol/L

Determination	Conventional Units	SI Units
HbA1c		
Nondiabetic	5.5 - 8.5%	
Hgb	M 14 - 17.4 g/dl	140 – 174 g/L
	F 12 - 16 g/dl	120 - 160 g/L
Homocysteine	4 – 17 μmol/L	0.54 – 2.3 mg/L
K	3.5 - 5.2 mEq/L	3.5 - 5.2 mmol/L
LDH	313 - 618 U/L	313 - 618 U/L
	Isoenzymes	
	LD_1 17 - 27%	
	LD_2 29 - 39%	
	LD_3 19 - 27%	
	LD_4 8 - 16%	
	LD_5 6 - 16%	
LDL	<130 mg/dl	<3.4mmol/L
Lymphocytes	25 - 40% of total leukocytes	Relative value = 1500 - 4000 cells/mm^3
MCH	26 - 34 pg/cell	0.40 - 0.53 fmol/cell
MCHC	32 – 36 g/dl	320 – 360 g/L
MCV	82 - 98 μm^3	82 - 98 fL
Methylmalonic acid	88 – 243 nmol/L	
Mg	1.8 - 2.6 mg/dl	0.74 - 1.0 7 mmol/L
Na	136 - 145 mEq/L	136 - 145 mmol/L
Osmolality	280 - 303 mOsm/kg H_2O	280 - 303 mmol/kg H_2O
P	2.7 - 4.5 mg/dl	0.87 - 1.45 mmol/L
$PaCO_2$	35 - 45 mm Hg	4.7 - 6.0 kPa
PaO_2	> 80 mm Hg	>10.6 kPa
pH	7.35 - 7.45	
Platelet Count	140 - 400 x 10^3/mm^3	190 - 380 mg/L
Prealbumin	19 - 38 mg/dl	
PT	10 - 13 secs.	
RBC	3.6 – 5.0 x 10^6/L	3.6 – 5.0 x 10^{12}/L
Sed Rate	Westergren method	
Males	0 - 15 mm/hr (over age 50: 0-20 mm/hr)	
Females	0 - 20 mm/hr (over age 50: 0-30 mm/hr)	
TLC	>1500/mm^3	
Total protein	6.5 – 8.3 g/dl	65 – 83 g/dl
Triglycerides	<150 mg/dl	<1.7 mmol/L
Transferrin	250 - 425 mg/dl	2.5 – 4.2 g/L
Uric Acid		
Males	3.4 - 7.0 mg/dl	202 - 416 μmol/L
Females	2.4 - 6.0 mg/dl	143 - 357 μmol/L
WBC	4.5 10.5 x 10^3/cells/mm^3	4.5 - 10 x 10^9/L

Pediatrics

Albumin 1 - 3 yrs	2.9 - 5.5 g/dl	29 – 55 g/L
BUN child	5 - 18 mg/dl	1.8 – 6.4 mmol/L
Cl same as adult	96 - 106 mEq/L	96 - 106 mmol/L
Cr 3 – 18 years	0.5 – 1.0 mg/dl	44 – 88 µmol/L
Glucose 0 - 2 yr	60 - 110 mg/dl	3.3 – 6.1 mmol/L
Hemoglobin1 - 6 yrs	9.5 - 14.1 g/dl	95 – 141 g/L
K 1 - 18 yrs	3.4 - 4.7 mEq/l	3.4 – 4.7 mmol/L
Na 1 – 16 yrs	136 – 145 mEq/L	136 – 145 mmol/L

Urinalysis

Bili	Neg
Blood	Neg
Glucose	Neg
Ketones	Neg
pH	4.5 - 8
Protein	Neg
SG	1.015 - 1.025

[1] Laboratory reference values will vary from hospital to hospital depending on the type instrumentation used in analysis, reference standards used to calibrate the instrumentation, and other factors. Each hospital produces their own list of "norms." The items in this list are from F. Fischbach's *Laboratory & Diagnostic Tests,* 7th Ed., 2004, Lippincott-Raven. Furthermore, this list is not conclusive but contains only those values that are necessary for answering the case studies in this book. Most of the labs in this book are reported in conventional units. The corresponding SI Units are listed here for your convenience.

APPENDIX C

ABBREVIATIONS

A1c	Glycosylated hemoglobin
AA	Amino acid
ABGs	Arterial blood gasses
ABW	Adjusted body weight
a.c.	Before meals
ACOG	American College of Obstetricians and Gynecologists
ADD	Attention deficit disorder
ADHD	Attention deficit hyperactive disorder
AIDS	Acquired immune deficiency syndrome
Alk Phos (ALP)	Alkaline phosphatase
ALT (formally SGPT)	Alanine aminotransferase
AM	Morning, A.M. snack
amp	Ampule
AODM	Adult onset diabetes mellitus
ARC	AIDS Related Complex
ASA	Acetylsalicylic acid (aspirin)
ASAP	As soon as possible
AST (formally SGOT)	Aspartate aminotransferase
A-V	Arteriovenous shunt or atrioventricular

BCAA	Branched chain amino acids
BE	Barium enema, below the elbow
BEE	Basal energy expenditure
BIA	Bioelectrical impedance
b.i.d.	Twice a day
bili	Bilirubin
BM	Black male
BMR	Basal metabolic rate
BMI	Body mass index
BP	Blood pressure
BPD	Broncopulmonary displesia
BR	Bed rest
BRB	Bright red blood
BS	Bowel sounds, blood sugar, breath sounds
BUN	Blood urea nitrogen
BUT	Biopsy urease test

C	Centigrade
c	Cup
CA	Carcinoma
Ca	Calcium
CABG	Coronary artery by-pass graft
Cap	Capsule
CAPD	Continuous ambulatory peritoneal dialysis

Appendix C

Cardiac cath	Cardiac catheterization
cath	Catheterization
CBC	Complete blood count
CC	Chief compliant
cc	Cubic centimeter
cc/h	Cubic centimeter per hour
CCU	Coronary care unit
CDE	Certified diabetes educator
CF	Cystic fibrosis
CHD	Coronary heart disease
CHF	Congestive heart failure
CHI	Closed head injury
CHO	Carbohydrate
chol	Cholesterol
CICU	Coronary intensive care unit
Cl	Chlorine
cl liqs	Clear liquids
cm	Centimeter
C/O	Complains of
CO_2	Carbon dioxide
CPK	Creatine phosphokinase
CPK_{1-3}	Creatine phosphokinase isoenzymes
Cr	Creatinine
CRP	C-reactive protein
CT	Computed tomography
CxR	Chest X Ray
CVR	Cerebrovascular accident

d	Day
DBIL	Direct bilirubin
DBW	Desirable body weight
D/C	Discontinue
DEXA	Duel energy x-ray absorptiometry
DKA	Diabetic ketoacidosis
dl	Deciliter
DM	Diabetes mellitus
D_5NS	Dextrose, 5% in normal saline
DT	Delirium tremens
D_5W	Dextrose, 5% in water
$D_{10}W$	Dextrose, 10% in water
$D_{50}W$	Dextrose, 50% in water
DVT	Deep vein thrombosis
Dx	Diagnosis

EGD	Esophagogastroduodenoscopy
EKG	Electrocardiogram
Elisa	Enzyme linked immunosorbent assay
ER	Emergency room
ESRD	End stage renal disease

ETOH	Ethanol or alcohol
Exploratory Lap	Exploratory laparotomy

F	Fahrenheit
f	femto (10^{-15})
FBS	Fasting blood sugar
Fe	Iron
FF	Force fluids
FH	Family history
FiO$_2$	Percent oxygen
fL	femtoliter
Fx	Fracture

g	Gram
GB	Gallbladder
GCT	Glucose challenge test
g/dl	grams per deciliter
GDM	Gestational diabetes mellitus
GERD	Gastroesophageal reflux disease
GGTP	Gama glutamyl transpeptidase
GI	Gastrointestinal
glu	Glucose
G-tube	Same as PEG
GTT	Glucose tolerance test
Gtt	Drop

h	Hour
HA	Head ache
HbA1c	Glycosylated hemoglobin
HBC	High branched chain
HCl	Hydrochloric acid
HCO$_3$	Bicarbonate ion
Hct	Hematocrit
H & H	Hematocrit and hemoglobin
HD	Hemodialysis
HDL	High density lipoprotein
Hg	Mercury
Hgb	Hemoglobin
HPRL	Prolactin
HIV	Human immunodeficiency virus
HN	High nitrogen
h.s.	Hour of sleep or evening
Ht	Height
HTN	Hypertension
Hx	History

IBD	Inflammatory bowel disease
IBW	Ideal body weight
ICP	Intracranial pressure

Appendix C

ICU	Intensive care unit
IDDM	Insulin dependent diabetes mellitus
IgG	Immunoglobin g
IHDP	Infant Health and Development Program
IM	Intramuscular
in	Inch
IU	International units
I.V.	Intravenous
IVGTT	Intravenous glucose tolerance test

JODM	Juvenile onset diabetes

K	Potassium
k	kilo
kcals	Kilocalories
kg	Kilogram
KUB	Kidney, ureter, and bladder (X-ray)

L	Liter
LAP	Laparotomy
LBM	Lean body mass
lbs	Pounds
LD_{1-5}	Isoenzymes of LDH
LDH	Lactic dehydrogenase
LDL	Low density lipoprotein
LES	Lower esophageal sphincter
LLQ	Left lower quadrant
LUQ	Left upper quadrant
lymph	Lymphocytes
lytes	Electrolytes

MAC	Midarm circumference
MAMC	Midarm muscle circumference
mcg	microgram
MCH	Mean corpuscular hemoglobin
MCHC	Mean corpuscular hemoglobin concentration
mci	millicuries
MCV	Mean corpuscular volume
MD	Medical doctor
MDI	Multiple daily injections
mech	Mechanical
mEq	Milliequivalent
Mg	Magnesium
mg	Milligram
mg/dl	Milligram per deciliter
$MgSO_4$	Magnesium sulfate
MH	Medical history
MI	Myocardial infarction
milliIU/L	Milliinternational units per iter

min	Minute
m^3	Cubic meters
mm	Millimeter
mm^3	Cubic millimeter
mmol	Millimole
MNT	Medical nutrition therapy
mol	mole
MOM	Milk of magnesia
mOsm	Milliosmole
MTE	Mixture of trace elements
MVA	Motor vehicle accident
MVI	Multiple vitamin infusion

N	Nitrogen
n	nano- (10^{-9})
Na	Sodium
NDDG	National Diabetes Data Group
neg	Negative
ng	Nanogram
N/G	Nasogastric
NH	Nutritional history
NH_3	Ammonia
NIDDM	Noninsulin dependent diabetes mellitus
NPH	Neutral protamine Hagedorn insulin
NPO	Nothing by mouth
NS	Normal saline
NSICU	Neurosurgical intensive care unit
NST	Nutrition support team
NTG	Nitroglycerin
N/V	Nausea and vomiting

O_2	Oxygen
OGTT	Oral glucose tolerance test
OR	Operating room
OTC	Over the counter
oz	Ounce

P	Phosphorous
Pa	Pressure
$PaCO_2$	Partial pressure of carbon dioxide
PaO_2	Partial pressure of oxygen
PC	Packed cells
p.c.	After meals
PD	Peritoneal dialysis
pDEXA	Peripheral duel energy x-ray absorptiometry
PED	Percutaneous endoscopic duodenostomy
PEG	Percutaneous endoscopic gastrostomy
PEJ	Percutaneous endoscopic jejunumostomy
pg	Picogram

pH	The negative logarithm of the hydrogen ion concentration
PICU	Pediatric intensive care unit
PM	Afternoon, P.M. snack
p.o.	By mouth
Post-op	Post-operative
prn	As needed
prot	Protein
PT	Prothrombin time, Physical therapy
pt	Patient
PUD	Peptic ulcer disease
PVC	Premature ventricular contraction
PVD	Peripheral vascular disease

q AM	Every morning
qid	Four times a day
q4h	Every 4 hours
q6h	Every 6 hours
q8h	Every 8 hours
qod	Every other day
qt	Quart
R	Regular
RBC	Red blood cell
RBW	Reference body weight
RD	Registered dietitian
RDA	Recommended dietary allowances
RLQ	Right lower quadrant
Rm	Room
RN	Registered nurse
R/O	Rule out
RUQ	Right upper quadrant
Rx	Prescription

sat	Saturated
SBO	Small bowel obstruction
SBR	Strict bed rest
SBS	Short bowel syndrome
SC	Subcutaneous
sec	Second
Ser alb	Serum albumin
SG	Specific gravity
SGOT	Serum glutamic-oxaloacetic transaminase
SGPT	Serum glutamic-pyruvic transaminase
SH	Social history
SOB	Short of breath
S/P	Status post

T	Tablespoon, temperature
tab	Tablet
TBIL	Total bilirubin

TF	Tube feeding
TG	Triglycerides
t.i.d.	Three times a day
TLC	Total lymphocyte count, tender loving care
tot	Total
TP	Total protein
TPN	Total parenteral nutrition
trach	Tracheostomy
trig	Triglycerides
TSF	Triceps skin fold
TSH	Thyroid-stimulating hormone
tsp	Teaspoon
T_3	Free triiodothyronine
T_4	Free thyroxine

U	Unit
UBW	Usual body weight
U/kg	Units per kilogram
UGI	Upper gastrointestinal
U/L	Units per liter
UTI	Urinary tract infection
UUN	Urinary urea nitrogen

VLCD	Very low calorie diet
VLBW	Very low birth weight

WBC	White blood cell count
Wk	Week
WNL	Within normal limits
Wt	Weight

x	Times
x1d	Times one day
x3	Times three
x3d	Times three days

YO	Year old
YOF	Year old female
YOBF	Year old black female
YOBM	Year old black male
YOM	Year old male
YOW	Year old white
YOWF	Year old white female
YOWM	Year old white male

Symbols

@	At
º	Degree
1h	One hour
1stº	First degree
2ndº	Second degree
2x	Two times
2xd	Two times a day
3rdº	Third degree
3x	Three times
2º	Secondary
μ	Micro
μg	Microgram
μm^3	Cubic microns
μmol	Micromole
¼NS	One fourth strength normal saline
♂	Male
♀	Female
↑	Increase
↓	Decrease
Ø	None
#	Number

Numbers

i	One
ii	Two
iii	Three
iv	Four
v	Five
vi	Six
vii	Seven
viii	Eight
ix	Nine
x	Ten

APPENDIX D

MULTIVITAMIN AND MINERAL I.V. MIXTURES

M.V.I.®-12
MULTI-VITAMIN INFUSION

Description

M.V.I.-12® consist of two vials labeled vial 1 and vial 2 in 5 ml single-dose vials and 50 ml multiple-dose vials.

Each 5 ml in vial 1 provides:

ascorbic acid (vitamin C) .... 100 mg
vitamin A* (retinol).. 1 mg[a]
ergocalciferol* (vitamin D) .... 5 mcg[b]
thiamin (vitamin B_1)(as the hydrochloride)...................................... 3 mg
riboflavin (vitamin B_2) (as riboflavin-5 phosphate sodium)............ 3.6 mg
pyridoxine HCl (vitamin B_6) .... 4 mg
niacinamide .... 40 mg
dexpanthenol (d-pantothenyl alcohol).. 15 mg
vitamin E* (dl-alpha tocopheryl acetate) .... 10 mg[c]

* Oil-soluble vitamins A, D, and E water-solubilized with polysorbate 80.
   a   1 mg vitamin A equals 3,300 USP units.
   b   5 mcg ergocalciferol equals 200 USP units.
   c   10 mg vitamin E equals 10 USP units.

Each 5 ml in vial 2 provides:

biotin...60 mcg
folic acid ....400 mcg
cyanocobalamin (vitamin B_{12})..5 mcg

The contents of both vials should be added to not less than 500 cc of infusion fluid.

There is a new version available: **MVI® Adult** that contains everything **M.V.I.-12®** contains with the addition of 150 mcg of vitamin K per 10 ml.

M.T.E.®-4
Mixture of Four Trace Elements Additive
For IV Use after Dilution

Ingredients	Single Dose Vial (3 ml fill)	Recommend Daily I.V. (TPN) Dose[3]
Zinc (as Zinc Sulfate heptahydrate)	1.0 mg	2.5 - 4 mg
Copper (as Cupric Sulfate pentahydrate)	0.4 mg	0.5 - 1.5 mg
Manganese (as Manganese Sulfate monohydrate)	0.1 mg	0.15 - 0.8 mg
Chromium (as Chromic Chloride hexahydrate)	4.0 mcg	10 - 15 mcg

M.T.E. – 5
Has everything MTE-4 plus 20 mcg of selenium.

M.T.E. – 6
Has everything MTE-5 has plus 25 mcg of iodide.

M.E.T. – 7
Has everything MTE-6 has plus 25 mcg of molybdenum.

Product	Producer	Type	Form*	Cal/ml	Non-pro Cal/g N	Pro (g/L)	Cho (g/L)	Fat (g/L)	Na/L mEq	Na/L mg	K/L mEq	K/L mg	mOs m/kg water	Vol to meet RDIs in ml	g of fiber /L	Free water /L in ml
Advera	Ross	AIDS	L	1.28	108:1	60	215.8	22.8	45.9	1056	72.5	2827	680	1184	8.9	802
AlitraQ	Ross	Elemental/ Glutamine	P	1.0	94:1	52.5	165	15.5	43	1000	31	1200	575	1500	N/A	846
Boost	Novartis	General	L	1.01	128:1	41.7	170.8	16.7	22.8	541.7	42.5	1667	610-670	1180	N/A	833
Boost High Protein	Novartis	High Protein	L	1.01	80:1	62.5	137.5	25	30.8	708	40.4	1583	540-605	946	N/A	833
Boost Plus	Novartis	High Calorie	L	1.52	139:1	58.3	187.5	58.3	30.8	708	40.4	158	720	946	<1	771
Boost with Fiber	Novartis	Fiber	L	1.01	125:1	41.7	175	16.7	30.8	708	40.4	1583	480	1180	12.5	833
Choice	Mead Johnson	Diabetes/ Glucose Intolerance	L	1.06	125:1	45	119	51	37	850	47	1820	300	1120	14.4	850
Compleat	Novartis	Blenderized/ Fiber	L	1.07	114:1	48	128	40	43	1000	44	1720	340	1313	6.0	854
Compleat Pediatric	Novartis	Blenderized/ Fiber Ages 1-10	L	1.0	142:1	38	130	39	33	770	41	1600	380	900	6.8	820
Comply	Novartis	High Calorie	L	1.5	134:1	60	180	61	52	1200	47	1850	460	830	N/A	770
Criticare HN	Novartis	Elemental	L	1.06	149:1	38	220	5.3	27	630	34	1310	650	1890	N/A	850
Crucial	Nestle Nutrition	Elemental	L	1.5	67:1	94	135	67.6	51	1168	48	1872	490	1000	N/A	771
Deliver 2.0	Novartis	High Calorie	L	2.0	145:1	73.7	195.8	100	35	800	40	1600	640	1000	N/A	700

*L = liquid, P = powder

375

Product	Producer	Type	Form*	Cal/ml	Non-pro Cal/g N	g/L Pro	g/L Cho	g/L Fat	Na/L mEq	Na/L mg	K/L mEq	K/L mg	mOs m/kg water	Vol to meet RDIs in ml	g of fiber /L	Free water /L in ml
Diabeti-Source AC	Novartis	Diabetes	L	1.2	95:1	60	100	59	49	1120	49	1920	350	1250	10	818
Ensure	Ross	General	L	1.06	153:1	36.7	166.6	25.4	36.2	833	39.5	1541	590	948	N/A	833
Ensure Fiber with FOS	Ross	Fiber	L	1.06	153:1	36.7	175	25.4	36.2	833	39.5	1541	500	948	11.6	812
Ensure High Calcium	Ross	High Calcium	L	0.95	92:1	50	128.3	25	54.1	1208	54.1	2083	610	948	N/A	846
Ensure High Protein	Ross	High Nitrogen	L	0.95	92:1	50	128.3	25	52.5	1208	53.4	2083	610	948	N/A	846
Ensure Plus	Ross	High Calorie	L	1.5	146:1	54	208.7	57.5	48	1000	52.5	1833	680	1185	N/A	750
Ensure Plus HN	Ross	High Calorie/High Protein	L	1.5	125:1	62	197	49	50.8	1166	45.8	1792	650	947	N/A	769
Fiber-Source	Novartis	Fiber	L	1.2	149:1	43	170	39	52	1200	51	2000	490	1165	10	814
Fiber-Source HN	Novartis	Fiber/High Protein	L	1.2	115:1	53	160	39	52	1200	51	2000	490	1165	10	814
Glucerna	Ross	Diabetes/Glucose Intolerance	L	1.0	125:1	41.8	95.6	54.4	40.5	930	40.2	1570	355	1422	14.4	853
Glutasorb	Nutrition Medical	Elemental/Glutamine	L	1.0	96:1	52	186	6.8	26.5	610	28	1000	575	1800	N/A	732
Glytrol	Nestle Nutrition	Diabetes/Glucose Intolerance	L	1.0	114:1	45.2	100	47.6	32	740	36	1400	280	1400	15.2	840
Impact	Novartis	Critically ill	L	1.0	71:1	56	130	28	48	1100	45	1760	375	1500	N/A	853

* L = liquid, P = powder

Product	Producer	Type	Form*	Cal/ml	Non-pro Cal/g N	g/L Pro	g/L CHO	g/L Fat	Na/L mEq	Na/L mg	K/L mEq	K/L mg	mOs m/kg water	Vol to meet RDIs in ml	g of fiber /L	Free water /L in ml
Impact 1.5	Novartis	Critically ill High Protein	L	1.5	71:1	84	140	69	64	1480	52	2040	550	1250	N/A	780
Impact with Fiber	Novartis	Critically ill Fiber	L	1.0	71:1	56	140	28	48	1100	47	1820	375	1500	10	868
Isocal	Novartis	Isotonic Low Na	L	1.06	168:1	34	135	44	23	530	34	1320	270	1890	N/A	840
Isocal HN	Novartis	Isotonic High Protein	L	1.06	125:1	44	124	45	40	930	41	1610	270	1180	N/A	850
Iso-Source	Novartis	Isotonic	L	1.2	149:1	43	170	39	48	1100	49	1900	490	1165	N/A	819
Iso-Source HN	Novartis	Isotonic High Protein	L	1.2	115:1	53	160	39	48	1100	49	1900	490	1165	N/A	818
Iso-Source VHN	Novartis	Isotonic High Protein	L	1.0	77:1	62	130	29	60	1380	46	1800	300	1250	10	847
Iso-Source 1.5	Novartis	Isotonic High Calorie	L	1.5	116:1	68	170	65	56	1290	58	2250	650	933	N/A	778
Jevity 1 cal	Ross	Isotonic/Fiber	L	1.06	125:1	44.3	154.7	34.7	40.4	930	40.2	1570	300	1321	14.4	829
Jevity 1.2 cal	Ross	High Protein/Fiber	L	1.2	110:1	55.5	171.5	39.3	58.7	1350	47.4	1850	450	1000	22	805
Magnacal Renal	Novartis	High Calorie Hemo-dialysis	L	2.0	144:1	75	200	101	35	800	32	1270	570	1000	N/A	710
Nepro	Ross	Renal	L	2.0	154:1	70	222.7	95.6	37	845	27.1	1055	665	947	N/A	699

*L = liquid, P = powder

Product	Producer	Type	Form*	Cal/ml	Non-pro Cal/g N	Pro g/L	CHO g/L	Fat g/L	Na/L mEq	Na/L mg	K/L mEq	K/L mg	mOsm/kg water	Vol to meet RDIs in ml	g of fiber /L	Free water /L in ml
Nova Source Pulmonary	Novartis	Respiratory Disease/Fiber	L	1.5	102:1	75	150	68	60	1390	68	2670	650	933	8.0	764
Nova Source Renal	Novartis	Renal	L	2.0	140:1	74	200	100	39	900	21	810	700	1000	N/A	709
NuBasics	Nestle Nutrition	General	L	1.0	154:1	35	132.4	36.8	38	876	32	1248	510	2000	N/A	850
NuBasics Plus	Nestle Nutrition	High Calorie	L	1.5	154:1	52.4	176.4	64.8	50.8	1168	48	1868	620-650	1333	N/A	780
Nutren 1.0	Nestle Nutrition	General	L	1.0	131:1	40	127	38	38	876	32.1	1248	315	1500	N/A	848
Nutren 1.0 with Fiber	Nestle Nutrition	Fiber	L	1.0	131:1	40	127	38	38.1	876	32	1240	330	1500	14	838
Nutren 1.5	Nestle Nutrition	High Cal	L	1.5	131:1	60	169.2	67.6	50.8	1168	48	1872	430	1000	N/A	775
Nutren 2.0	Nestle Nutrition	High Cal	L	2.0	134:1	80	196	104	56.6	1300	49.9	1997	720	750	N/A	700
Nutren Junior	Nestle Nutrition	Pediatric 1 - 10 Years	L	1.0	183:1	30	110	49.6	20	460	33.8	1320	350	1000	N/A	852
Nutren Junior with Fiber	Nestle Nutrition	Pediatric 1 - 10 Years	L	1.0	183:1	30	110	49.6	20	460	33.8	1320	350	1000	6	848
NutriHeal	Nestle Nutrition	Wound Healing	L	1.0	75:1	15.6	28.2	8.3	39.5	911	33	1298	N/A	N/A	N/A	882
NutriFocus	Ross	Pressures Sores	L	1.5	125:1	61.7	212.1	48.8	40	917	42	1667	N/A	N/A	10.4	754
NutriRenal	Nestle Nutrition	Renal Disease	L	2.0	151:1	70	204	104	32	740	32	1256	650	750	N/A	704
NutriHep	Nestle Nutrition	Liver	L	1.5	209:1	40	290	21.2	6.9	160	33.9	1320	N/A	1000	N/A	760

* L = liquid, P = powder

Product	Producer	Type	Form*	Cal/ml	Non-pro Cal/g N	g/L Pro	g/L CHO	g/L Fat	Na/L mEq	Na/L mg	K/L mEq	K/L mg	mOsm/kg water	Vol to meet RDIs in ml	g of fiber/L	Free water/L in ml
NutriVent	Nestle Nutrition	Pulmonary	L	1.5	115:1	67.5	100	94	51	1170	48	1872	330	1000	N/A	775
Optimental	Ross	Elemental/ Malabsorption Elemental/	L	1.0	97:1	51.3	138.5	28.4	46	1060	45	1760	540	1422	N/A	835
Osmolite	Ross	Isotonic	L	1.06	153:1	37.1	151	34.7	28	640	26.1	1020	300	1887	N/A	841
Osmolite 1 cal	Ross	Isotonic/ High Protein	L	1.06	125:1	44.3	143.9	34.7	40	930	40	1570	300	1321	N/A	842
Osmolite 1.2 cals	Ross	High Protein/Cal	L	1.2	110:1	55.5	157.5	39.3	62	1420	50	1940	360	1000	N/A	820
Oxepa	Ross	ARDS	L	1.5	125:1	62.5	105.5	93.7	57	1310	50	1960	493	947	N/A	785
PediaSure	Ross	Pediatric 1 - 10 Years	L	1.0	185:1	30	109.7	49.7	17	380	34	1310	335	1000[1] 1300	N/A	844
PediaSure with Fiber	Ross	Pediatric 1 - 10 years Fiber	L	1.0	185:1	30	113.5	49.7	17	380	34	1310	345	1000[1] 1300	5	844
Peptamen	Nestle Nutrition	Elemental	L	1.0	131:1	40	127	39	24	560	38	1500	270	1500	N/A	848
Peptamen Junior	Nestle Nutrition	Elemental Pediatric 1 - 10 Years	L	1.0	183:1	30	137.6	38.4	20	460	34	1320	260	1000[2]	N/A	848
Peptamen VHP	Nestle Nutrition	High Protein	L	1.0	75:1	62.5	104.5	39	24	560	38	1500	270	1500	N/A	844
Perative	Ross	Critical Care	L	1.3	97:1	66.7	180.3	37.3	45	1040	44	1735	460	1155	N/A	790
Pivot	Ross	Metabolic Stress	L	1.5	75:1	93.8	172.4	50.8	61	1400	51	2000	595	1000	7.5	759
Pro-Balance	Nestle Nutrition	Fiber	L	1.2	114:1	54	156	40.8	33	764	40	1560	350-450	1000	10	810

[1] 1-6 = 1000cc 7-10 = 1300cc   [2] 7-10 years

* L = liquid, P = powder

379

Product	Producer	Type	Form*	Cal/ml	Non-pro Cal/g N	g/L Pro	g/L CHO	g/L Fat	Na/L mEq	Na/L mg	K/L mEq	K/L mg	mOsm /kg water	Vol to meet RDAs in ml	g of fiber /L	Free water/ L in ml
Promote	Ross	High Protein	L	1.0	75:1	62.5	130	26	43	1000	51	1980	340	1000	N/A	837
Promote with Fiber	Ross	Fiber	L	1.0	75:1	62.5	138.3	28.2	57	1300	51	1980	380	1000	14.4	830
Protain XL	Novartis	Wound Healing/Fiber	L	1.0	86:1	57	145	30	40	920	45	1760	340	1250	9.1	830
Pulmocare	Ross	Pulmonary	L	1.5	125:1	62.6	105.7	93.3	57	1310	50	1960	475	947	N/A	785
Renalcal	Nestle Nutrition	Renal	L	2.0	300:1	34.4	290.4	82.4	N/A	N/A	N/A	N/A	600	1000[1]	N/A	700
Replete	Nestle Nutrition	HN/Healing	L	1.0	75:1	62.4	113.2	34	38.1	876	38.5	1500	N/A	1000	N/A	845
Replete with Fiber	Nestle Nutrition	HN/Fiber	L	1.0	75:1	62.4	113.2	34	38.1	876	38.5	1500	N/A	1000	14	835
ReSource Diabetic	Novaris	Diabetes/ Glucose Intolerance	L	1.06	79:1	63	100	47	51	1170	35	1360	300	1180	12.8	847
ReSource Just for Kids	Novartis	Pediatric 1-10 Years	L	1.0	185:1	30	110	50	26	590	29	1140	390	1000[2]	N/A	853
ReSource Just for Kids with Fiber	Novartis	Pediatric 1-10 Years	L	1.0	185:1	30	110	50	26	590	29	1140	390	1000[2]	6.0	853
ReSource Just for Kids 1.5 cal	Novartis	Pediatric 1-10 Years	L	1.5	199:1	42	165	75	30	690	33	1310	390	870[2]	N/A	720
ReSource Just for Kids 1.5 cal with Fiber	Novartis	Pediatric 1-10 Years	L	1.5	199:1	42	165	75	30	690	33	1310	390	870[2]	9	720
ReSource Standard	Novartis	General	L	1.06	149:1	37.4	183	25	49	915	37	1456	600	1180	N/A	828
ReSource Plus	Novartis	High Caorie	L	1.5	148.1	54	216	46	56	1310	49	1940	870	946	N/A	752

* L= liquid, P = powder

[1] For water soluble vitamins only

[2] 1-10 years

Product	Producer	Type	Form*	Cal/ml	Non-pro Cal/g N	g/L Pro	g/L CHO	g/L Fat	Na/L mEq	Na/L mg	K/L mEq	K/L mg	mOs m/kg water	Vol to meet RDIs in ml	g of fiber /L	Free water /L in ml
Suplena	Ross	Renal	L	2.0	393:1	30	255.2	95.6	34	790	29	1120	600	947	N/A	713
Tolerex	Novartis	Elemental	P	1.0	282:1	21	230	1.5	20	470	30	1170	550	1800	N/A	864
TramaCal	Mead Johnson	Critical Care	L	1.5	91:1	82	144	68	51	1180	36	1390	560	2000	<1	780
Two-Cal HN	Ross	High Calorie High Protein	L	2.0	125:1	83.3	212.5	87.5	62.5	1437	61.7	2416	725	948	N/A	692
Ultracal	Novatis	Fiber/High Protein/ Isotonic	L	1.06	124:1	45	142	39	59	1350	47	1850	300	1120	14.4	830
Vital HN	Ross	Elemental	P	1.0	125:1	41.7	185	10.8	25	566	36	1400	500	1500	N/A	867
Vivonex Plus	Novartis	Elemental	P	1.0	115:1	45	190	6.7	27	610	27	1060	650	1800	N/A	864
Vivonex T.E.N.	Novartis	Elemental/ Glutamine	P	1.0	149:1	38	210	2.8	26	600	24	950	630	2000	N/A	853

* L = liquid, P = powder

[1] 1-6 = 1000cc   7-10 = 1300cc

APPENDIX F
ELECTRONIC RESOURCES RELATED TO NUTRITION

Source	Electronic Address
AIDS, ADA Position Paper	http://www.eatright.org/Member/PolicyInitiatives/index_21020.cfm
Alternative Diabetes	http://www.alternativediabetes.com/
Alzheimer's Association	http://www.alz.org/
Alzheimer's Disease Education and Referral Center	http://www.alzheimers.org/
American Academy of Allergy, Asthma & Immunology	http://www.aaaai.org/
American Academy of Pediatrics	http://www.aap.org/
American Association for Cancer Research	http://www.aacr.org/
American Botanical Council	http://www.herbalgram.org/browse.php/defaulthome
American Burn Association	http://www.ameriburn.org/
American Cancer Society	http://www.cancer.org
American College of Gastroenterology	http://www.acg.gi.org/
American College of Obstetricians and Gynecologists	http://www.acog.com
American College of Sports Medicine	http://www.acsm.org/
American Council on Exercise	http://www.acefitness.org/default.aspx
American Dental Association	http://www.ada.org/
American Diabetes Association	http://www.diabetes.org/home.jsp
American Dietetic Association	http://www.eatright.org
American Foundation for Urologic Disease	http://www.afud.org./
American Geriatrics Society	http://www.americangeriatrics.org/
American Heart Association – Diet and Nutrition	http://www.americanheart.org/presenter.jhtml?identifier=1200010
American Journal of Clinical Nutrition	http://www.ajcn.org/
American Journal of Sports Medicine	http://journal.ajsm.org/
American Liver Foundation	http://www.liverfoundation.org/
American Lung Association	http://www.lungusa.org
American Medical Association	http://www.ama-assn.org
American Public Health Association	http://www.apha.org
American Society for Bariatric Surgery	http://www.asbs.org/
American Society for Clinical Nutrition	http://www.ascn.org/
American Society for Nutritional Sciences	http://www.nutrition.org/
American Society for Parenteral and Enteral Nutrition	http://www.nutritioncare.org/
American Thyroid Association	http://www.thyroid.org
Anorexia nervosa, bulimia nervosa, and eating disorder not otherwise specified, ADA Position Paper	http://www.eatright.org/Public/NutritionInformation/92_adap0701.cfm
Archives of Gynecology and Obstetrics	http://link.springer.de/link/service/journals/00404/index.htm
Arthritis Foundation	http://www.arthritis.org/
Binge eating disorders, NIH	http://win.niddk.nih.gov/publications/binge.htm
Canadian Diabetes Association	http://www.diabetes.ca/Section_Main/welcome.asp
Canadian Eating Disorders Sites (National Eating Disorders Center)	http://www.nedic.ca
Canadian Liver Foundation	http://www.liver.ca./

Source	Electronic Address
Canadian Paediatric Society	http://www.cps.ca/
Canadian Parenteral-Enteral Nutrition Association	http://www.cpena.ca/home.html
Celiac Disease Foundation	http://www.celiac.org/
Celiac Sprue Association	http://www.csaceliacs.org/
Center for Disease Control & Prevention	http://wonder.cdc.gov
Center for Drug Evaluation and Research	http://www.fda.gov/cder/
Center for Food Safety and Applied Nutrition: Protecting Yourself against Health Fraud	http://vm.cfsan.fda.gov/~dms/wh-fraud.html
Center for Science in the Public Interest	http://www.cspinet.org
Choosing a Safe and Successful Weight-Loss Program	http://win.niddk.nih.gov/publications/choosing.htm
Clinical Guidelines on the Identification, Evaluation, and Treatment of Overweight and Obesity in Adult. NHLBI, NIH	http://www.nhlbi.nih.gov/guidelines/obesity/ob_gdlns.htm
Cornell University Food Science and Technology	http://www.nysaes.cornell.edu/fst/
Crohn's and Colitis Foundation of America	http://www.ccfa.org/
Crohn's Disease	http://www.med.utah.edu/healthinfo/adult/digest/ibdcro1.htm
Crohn's Disease/Ulcerative Colitis/Inflammatory Bowel Disease Pages	http://qurlyjoe.bu.edu/cduchome.html
Dietary Guidelines, AHA	http://circ.ahajournals.org/cgi/content/full/102/18/2284 http://www.americanheart.org/presenter.jhtml?identifier=4764
Dietary Guidelines for Americans 2005	http://www.healthierus.gov/dietaryguidelines/
Dietary Supplements	http://vm.cfsan.fda.gov/~dms/supplmnt.html
Dietetics Online	http://www.dietetics.com
Duke Diet and Fitness Center	http://www.cfl.duke.edu/dfc/
Duke University: Alcohol and Health Page	http://www.duke.edu/~amwhite/Resources/index.html
Dysphagia Resource Center	http://www.dysphagia.com/
Fat-Free: USDA Nutrient Values	http://cgi.fatfree.com/cgi-bin/fatfree/usda/usda.cgi
Fat-Free: The Low-Fat Vegetarian Recipe Archive	http://www.fatfree.com/
FDA Consumer Magazine	http://www.fda.gov/fdac/796_toc.html
Federal Register	http://www.gpoaccess.gov/fr/index.html
Federal Trade Commission	http://www.ftc.gov
Food Allergy and Anaphylaxis Network	http://www.foodallergy.org/
Food and Agriculture Association of the United Nations	http://www.fao.org/
Food fortification and dietary supplements.	http://www.eatright.org/Public/NutritionInformation/92_8343.cfm
Food and Nutrition Information Center	http://www.nal.usda.gov/fnic/
Food and Drug Administration	http://www.fda.gov/
Food and water safety, ADA Position Paper	http://www.eatright.org/Public/GovernmentAffairs/92_adap0297.cfm
Food Processors of Canada	http://foodnet.fic.ca/
Food Resource	http://food.oregonstate.edu/food.html
Food Safety Information Center	http://www.nalusda.gov/foodsafety/

Appendix F

Source	Electronic Address
GERD Information Resource Center	http://www.gerd.com/
Glucose Absorption in PD	http://www.pdserve.com/pdserve/pdserve.nsf/AttachmentsByTitle/PDF_PDServe:Vol+8,+No+1/$FILE/PDServe+composite+final+pdf.pdf
Health Canada	http://www.hc-sc.gc.ca/
Healthfinder	http://www.healthfinder.gov/
Healthy People 2010	http://www.healthypeople.gov/
Healthy School Meals Resource System	http://schoolmeals.nal.usda.gov/
Helicobacter Foundation	http://www.helico.com/
Hepatitis B Foundation	http://www.hepb.org/
Hershey Foods Corporation	http://www.hersheyfoods.com/
Information for Pregnant Women	http://vm.cfsan.fda.gov/~dms/wh-preg.html
Institute of Food Technologists	http://www.ift.org/cms/
International Food Information Council	http://www.ific.org/
Iron Overload Diseases Association	http://www.ironoverload.org/
Jean Mayer USDA Human Nutrition Research Center on Aging at Tufts University	http://www.hnrc.tufts.edu
Joslin Diabetes Center	http://www.joslin.org/
Kidney Foundation of Canada	http://www.kidney.ca/
Library of Congress	http://www.loc.gov/
Mayo Clinic	http://www.mayoclinic.com/
Medscape	http://www.medscape.com/px/urlinfo
National Cancer Institute	http://www.nci.nih.gov/
National Center for Complementary and Alternative Medicine	http://nccam.nih.gov/
National Center for Education in Maternal and Child Health	http://www.ncemch.org/
National Clearinghouse for Alcohol and Drug Information	http://www.health.org
National Council against Health Fraud	http://www.ncahf.org/
National Council on Alcoholism and Drug Dependence	http://www.ncadd.org/
National Eating Disorders Association	http://www.nationaleatingdisorders.org/p.asp?WebPage_ID=337
National Food Safety Database	http://www.agen.ufl.edu/~foodsaf/foodsaf.html
National Health and Nutrition Examination Survey	http://www.cdc.gov/nchs/nhanes.htm
National Heart, Lung, and Blood Institute	http://www.nhlbi.nih.gov/
National Institute of Arthritis and Musculoskeletal and Skin Diseases	http://www.niams.nih.gov/
National Institute of Dental and Craniofacial Research	http://www.nidcr.nih.gov/
National Institute of Diabetic & Digestive & Kidney Diseases	http://www.niddk.nih.gov
National Institute on Aging	http://www.nia.nih.gov/
National Institutes of Health	http://www.nih.gov/
National Kidney Foundation	http://www.kidney.org/
National Library of Medicine	http://www.nlm.nih.gov/
National Osteoporosis Foundation	http://www.nof.org
National Stroke Association	http://www.stroke.org
New England Journal of Medicine	http://content.nejm.org/
NIH Office of Aids Research	http://www.nih.gov/od/oar/
NIH Office of Dietary Supplements	http://dietary-supplements.info.nih.gov/

Source	Electronic Address
NIH Osteoporosis and Related Bone Diseases National Resource Center	http://www.osteo.org/
North American Association for the Study of Obesity	http://www.naaso.org/
Nutrigenomics	http://nutrigenomics.ucdavis.edu/ and http://nutrigenomics.ucdavis.edu/pressarticles.htm
Nutrition and the Athlete from the University of Nebraska	http://ianrpubs.unl.edu/foods/nf66.htm
Nutrition Screening Initiative	http://www.eatright.org/Public/NutritionInformation/92_nsi.cfm
Oldways: The Food Issues Think Tank	http://www.oldwayspt.org/
OncoLink: Abramson Cancer Center of the University of Pennsylvania	http://oncolink.upenn.edu/
Office of Minority Health Resource Center	http://www.omhrc.gov/OMHRC/index.htm
Oxalosis and Hyperoxaluria Foundation	http://www.ohf.org/
Physician and Sports Medicine Online	http://www.physsportsmed.com/index.html
PUB-MED Literature research	http://pub-med.com
Purdue University's Extension Publications	http://www.ces.purdue.edu/extmedia/menu.htm
Quackwatch: Your Guide to Quackery, Health Fraud, and Intelligent Decisions	http://www.quackwatch.org/
Rx List	http://www.rxlist.com/
Sickle Cell Disease Association of America	http://www.sicklecelldisease.org/
The Body: The Complete HIV/AIDS Resource	http://www.thebody.com/index.shtml
Tobacco Information and Prevention Source	http://www.cdc.gov/tobacco/
Traditional Food, Health and Nutrition	http://www.kstrom.net/isk/food/foodmenu.html
Ulcerative Colitis	http://www.med.utah.edu/healthinfo/adult/digest/ibdulc1.htm
USDA	http://www.usda.gov
USDA Agricultural Research Service	http://www.ars.usda.gov/main/main.htm
USDA Cooperative State Research, Education and Extension Service	http://csrees.usda.gov/
USDA Nutrient Data Library	http://www.nal.usda.gov/fnic/foodcomp/
US Pharmacopeial Convention	http://www.usp.org/
Vegetarian diets, ADA Position Paper	http://www.eatright.org/Public/NutritionInformation/92_17084.cfm
Vegetarian Resource Group	http://www.vrg.org/
Very low calorie diets, NIH	http://win.niddk.nih.gov/publications/low_calorie.htm
Weight-control Information Network, Understanding Adult Obesity	http://win.niddk.nih.gov/publications/understanding.htm
Weight-control Information Network, Weight Cycling	http://win.niddk.nih.gov/publications/cycling.htm
Weight-control Information Network, Health Risks	http://win.niddk.nih.gov/publications/health_risks.htm
Weight-loss and Nutrition Myths, NIDDK	http://win.niddk.nih.gov/publications/myths.htm
Weight Watchers	http://www.weightwatchers.com/index.aspx
What We Eat in America: Food Surveys Research Group	http://www.barc.usda.gov/bhnrc/foodsurvey/
World Health Organization	http://www.who.int/en/